458-4574

Changing American Psychiatry

A Personal Perspective

Changing American Psychiatry

A Personal Perspective

Melvin Sabshin, M.D.

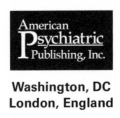

Washington, DC
London, England

Manufactured in the United States of America on acid-free paper
12 11 10 09 08   5 4 3 2 1
First Edition

Typeset in Georgia.

American Psychiatric Publishing, Inc.
1000 Wilson Boulevard
Arlington, VA 22209-3901
www.appi.org

Library of Congress Cataloging-in-Publication Data
Sabshin, Melvin, 1925–
    Changing American psychiatry : a personal perspective / Melvin Sabshin. — 1st ed.
        p. ; cm.
    Includes bibliographical references and index.
    ISBN 978-1-58562-307-5 (alk. paper)
    1. Psychiatry—United States—History—20th century. 2. American Psychiatric Association—History—20th century. 3. Sabshin, Melvin, 1925– 4. Psychiatrists—United States—Biography. I. Title.
    [DNLM: 1. Psychiatry—history—United States—Personal Narratives. 2. History, 20th Century—United States—Personal Narratives. 3. Psychiatry—trends—United States—Personal Narratives. WM 11 AA1 S118c 2008]
    RC443.S23 2008
    616.89—dc22

                                                        2008004460

British Library Cataloguing in Publication Data
A CIP record is available from the British Library.

Contents

List of Plates

About the Author

Mel Sabshin studied medicine at Tulane University after gaining a Bachelor of Science degree at the age of 17 and completing brief service in the U.S. Army. After postgraduate training and a research post at Tulane's Department of Psychiatry, he received an appointment at the Michael Reese Hospital in Chicago, a center of psychiatric research and psychodynamically oriented practice.

While at Michael Reese, where he completed psychoanalytic training, Dr. Sabshin became concerned by the schisms in psychiatry whereby ideologically based assertions took precedence over evidence-based practice and patient care depended more on the psychiatrist's theoretical orientation than on a reliable system of diagnosis and therapeutics. In 1961 he was appointed Professor and Head of the Department of Psychiatry at the University of Illinois College of Medicine. During that time, he became an active leader in the American Psychiatric Association (APA), where he was elected to the Board of Trustees, and chaired several of its major committees.

By 1974, when the post of Medical Director of the American Psychiatric Association became vacant, there was an effort to find a new leader who could help to unify the badly divided field. Psychiatry needed to become a scientifically respected part of medicine. Dr. Sabshin's experience and professional perspectives—his work on the deleterious impact of professional ideologies and his strong emphasis on science and a new image for psychiatry—were seen as fitting him for the job and led to his selection.

On his appointment that same year he inherited a well-run professional support group with highly dedicated staff and officers. But to inform policy makers, and to convince federal and state legislatures of the importance of proper care for the mentally ill, it was necessary to promote psychiatry with efficient advocacy and to stimulate the research and new education that could produce

evidence of effective treatment. Gradually, with great support from senior officers and a most able staff, the APA was transformed into a greatly
respected and effective organization that helped to shape a new American psychiatry.

Important achievements during Dr. Sabshin's tenure at the APA included the publication of new editions of the *Diagnostic and Statistical
Manual of Mental Disorders* and development of practice guidelines;
the creation of American Psychiatric Press, Inc., now the world's premier psychiatric publisher; the significant strengthening of psychiatric
research and education; the much more efficient governance by the
Board of Trustees and the Assembly; powerful professional advocacy;
the development of a closer relationship with the rest of medicine; and
the rapid growth of APA membership.

Dr. Sabshin was particularly interested in links with psychiatry in
the rest of the world. He worked actively with the World Psychiatric Association, taking a central part in the struggle to stop the use of psychiatry to suppress political dissent in many parts of the world, particularly
in the Soviet Union. He also built up a strong Office of International Affairs, which promoted much interchange between the United States and
other countries.

Since his retirement from the APA in 1997, Dr. Sabshin has kept in
close touch with family and old APA friends and attended all Annual
Meetings, while living in London for much of the year with his English
wife. There he enjoys the theatre and exploring the city. Dr. Sabshin is
an Honorary Fellow of the Royal College of Psychiatrists. His American
identity remains strong, with his devotion to presidential politics and its
underlying premises. He also remains faithful, through bad years and
good, to the Chicago Bears.

Foreword

The title of this book, *Changing American Psychiatry: A Personal Perspective,* is most apt. Mel Sabshin was at the helm of the American Psychiatric Association (APA) during a period of perhaps the greatest change in psychiatry since the Freud lectures at Clark University in 1909 introduced psychoanalysis to America. His role in leading the change and his insights into the process and some of the personalities involved, including his own, enliven the history in a personal way.

Dr. Sabshin's incredible intellect was noted early in his academic career. He finished high school at age 14. In college, at the University of Florida, he was elected to Phi Beta Kappa as a junior, placed in advanced classes, and was on his way to medical school when the United States entered World War II. As a 17-year-old college senior, he joined the Army and put off his matriculation to Tulane Medical School.

For those generations of us that experienced Mel Sabshin as the powerful, senior eminence (and transference object) APA medical director, it is intriguing to imagine the brilliant adolescent and young adult making his way through Florida and New Orleans as he started on his career.

This book weaves his personal journey with the history of the intellectual conflicts and changes in the field of psychiatry in the postwar era, describing how they culminated in the remedicalization of psychiatry and the development of DSM-III, and its impact on not only the APA but the world at large.

The story is also about Dr. Sabshin's role in international psychiatry and the Soviet Union and in the growth and development of the APA, including its meetings, journals, and membership. He describes, in these engaging chapters, some of the personalities who were involved with the leadership of our association during his 23 years as medical director.

Psychoanalysis captured the hearts and minds of American psychiatry in the postwar era. Dr. Sabshin discusses the excitement and promises of these times but also emphasizes how the theories that made psychopathology universal had an impact on insurance coverage and the credibility of our diagnoses (since everyone has conflicts, what then is "normal" and what is a disorder?).

In his first few years at the APA, the organization undertook a revision of the *Diagnostic and Statistical Manual of Mental Disorders* (DSM). At that time there had been two editions published, but they had not had much impact. Diagnosis was ideologically based and not deemed very important. But the field was changing, and by the mid-1970s psychiatric research was expanding. There were calls for a more scientifically based system of diagnosis and treatment. Although many histories of DSM-III and its development have been written, the narrative in this book gives the perspective of a consummate insider and adds a special view of what really happened.

Of course, once DSM-III was published, the DSM became very important indeed. Many articles, books, and even doctoral dissertations have been written about the DSM and its impact on not only psychiatry but also law, economics, and popular culture. Many have criticized both the DSM and the APA for what in the end is really the intellectual strength of the DSM and the real gap it filled in enabling clinicians, researchers, and others to do their work. Now, as we undertake the development of the fifth edition of the manual, the focus of attention is even greater than ever, and we have a new challenge to deal with: the influence of the pharmaceutical industry.

Dr. Sabshin describes in his book how the decision to add the industry-supported symposia at the annual meeting was made. These symposia have been very popular for a long time, but in the years since his retirement there has been increasing concern about the influence of industry on medicine. Psychiatry has come under some intense criticism, which has been directed at both the association and its members. During Dr. Sabshin's tenure, the issues were more ideological than economic, and those who believed in different psychological etiologies of mental illness based on a theoretical belief in how the mind worked were the main critics.

Another ideology that concerned the world during the years of Dr. Sabshin's tenure was Soviet communism. The Soviet Union used psychiatry to punish political dissidents. Dr. Sabshin and other leaders of the APA organized meetings with the World Psychiatric Association that began the process of confronting and ultimately ending abuse of these people and indeed the abuse of psychiatry. In the chapter on international affairs (see Chapter 7), Dr. Sabshin explains his interest in psychiatry in the rest of the world and why the APA should not fall back into an isolationist posture in the current era.

Finally, for those interested in the inner workings of organized psychiatry and the APA, Mel Sabshin gives us the consummate insider's view of how things worked at the APA. He describes many of the leaders of our profession, some of the administrative and political challenges, and even a few of the crises he dealt with while he led the association through a doubling of membership, moving the association's headquarters to 1400 K Street, N.W., and bringing psychiatry into a new scientific era.

James H. Scully Jr., M.D.
Medical Director
American Psychiatric Association

Introduction

During the latter half of the twentieth century, psychiatry in the United States experienced two extraordinary periods of change. The first period began during the decade after World War II and lasted until the mid-1970s. Evidence suggests that the change during this period was due primarily to the high rate of rejections for military service based on mental illness and, even more convincingly, to the large number of psychiatric casualties among those who served. With the ending of World War II a remarkable wave of optimism regarding many social and health issues, including psychiatric problems, swept through America. Genuine concern seemed to overcome the bulwark of stigma, apathy, and denial.

There was also an influx of new ideas brought by refugees from Central Europe, including strong interests in psychoanalytic explanations of mental functions. For some of my older colleagues, this period is still perceived as the Golden Age when practice was unfettered, community treatment programs arose, academic departments of psychiatry flourished, and psychoanalytic theory and practice thrived. Others, however, perceive this period as an era of disastrous mistakes that severed psychiatry from its medical roots and overwhelmed the field with questionable formulations.

The majority of American psychiatrists in the 1950s and 1960s accepted the general direction of psychodynamic change and saw it as progress compared with the more conservative perspectives of pre-war psychiatry. The optimism of this majority, however, faded as the practice of psychiatry became increasingly demedicalized. Initially grounded in the medical sciences, psychiatrists became alarmed by the lack of clarity in diagnosing specific mental illnesses, the absence of clear treatment guidelines, and an emerging assumption that almost all of us suffered from some degree of mental disorder. Normal adaptation was a far-fetched ideal if it existed at all!

By the 1970s, the postwar optimism had been replaced by the disturbing realization that actual psychiatric practice was far from the ideal. The tragic conditions in many of our state psychiatric facilities had become a national disgrace. Drastic changes in reimbursement for medical care had begun. Medical insurance, most often provided by one's employers, replaced the relatively free market as the basic reimbursement system. Over time, approval for payment became enormously regulated and constrained by the payers, and we entered an era of "managed care." There is no question that psychiatry was challenged in the last quarter of the twentieth century by these enormous external pressures. Every conceivable way to limit costs of psychiatric care was attempted.

Some historians have regarded these social, economic, and political factors as the basic cause of the subsequent changes in psychiatry. They believe that psychiatrists in a submissive attempt to cope reacted to these dire events by reverting to the old nosological ideas of the "St. Louis Group," which had strongly advocated a medical model for psychiatry. But the decision in the 1970s for a scientifically based nosology was much more active and complex than most historians of psychiatry portray. Somewhat surprisingly, these scholars do not seem to understand that the majority of psychiatrists and their leadership desired a "remedicalization" and a scientific foundation for the profession. This growing majority deplored the frequent public displays of incompatible and competing theories, and they sought a new mental health system in which diagnosis and treatment would be based on objective evidence and would continue to change as new evidence was established. They cringed when they were castigated as a profession of competing ideologues. They also recognized that the lack of a clear and reliable diagnostic classification and empirically derived therapeutics was a fundamental weakness for public understanding, for the evolution of the science, and for purposes of reimbursement. Psychiatry had come close to alienating itself from the rest of medicine. Demedicalization had too many negative consequences; a radical change was necessary, and such change needed to be led by the psychiatric profession. Submitting to the pressures was not enough. This set of conditions cannot easily be appreciated by the current generation of psychiatrists, who are absorbed by a new set of problems. Part of my motivation for writing this book was the wish to emphasize my perspective on why psychiatry elected to remedicalize. For the residual antiscientific ideologues inside and outside of psychiatry, I recognize that my perspective will not be persuasive.

The steps taken by the American Psychiatric Association (APA) were not simply a passive compliance to harsh external forces. As an active participant in the many steps in the establishment of DSM-III (American Psychiatric Association 1980) and DSM-IV (American Psychiatric Association 1994), I joined other psychiatric leaders in advocating a new, evidence-based profession. One of my motives in accepting the post of Medical Director of the APA was to assist in a transition from an ideologically oriented profession to one that developed and maintained a genuine scientific base.

My previous work on ideology among psychiatrists and my concerns about how our ambiguous definitions of normality and health posed major conceptual and practical problems for the profession had led me to advocate changes (Sabshin 1974; Strauss et al. 1964) long before the problems became so evident.

The realities of the current managed care era impose many limitations on practice. Psychiatry has had to "remedicalize" to be granted parity with other medical specialities. Such remedicalization must include commitment to an empirically derived system of diagnosis and therapeutics, clearer definition of the boundaries between health and illness, a plausible epidemiological database, compliance with professional standards and ethics, and a powerful commitment to new research. This is a much more ambitious model than existed in the postwar period of American psychiatry, and the profession is now well on the way to achieving these goals. If psychiatry had not been motivated to make radical changes in its basic concepts and in its practice, the adaptation to the new management systems would have been much more restrictive and the field's prospects of parity with the rest of medicine would have been remote.

Like much of American medicine, however, psychiatry is constrained by our current managed care system. It should be noted, however, that during this period it has been the psychosocial aspects of the field that have suffered most. The loss of public trust emanating from the postwar ideological period has taken its toll and is still having a deleterious impact. It is time for many of those psychiatrists with psychosocial interests to acknowledge that some of the problems had been due to our lack of scientific rigor. One of the main purposes of this book is to suggest how a scientific, psychosocial renaissance might be encouraged and why such a development is important for the field as a whole.

The response to the current problems in American psychiatry and in medicine as a whole requires changes at many levels, including a reformulation of care for our large uninsured population. In addition, psychiatry needs to be a stronger advocate of understanding the relevance of biopsychosocial factors to normal human development and resilience as well as to psychopathology. The twenty-first century will include a strong surge in this direction.

The next period of a changing American psychiatry will include a newly emerging group that wishes to see psychological hypotheses integrated systematically with social and biological variables. Academic psychiatry, in my opinion, will ultimately need to support this new generation of empiricists who must also fully comprehend the fundamental importance of neuroscience. The new psychiatry will require a modification from current practice of what Sharfstein has called a "bio-bio-bio" approach as compared with a genuine "bio-psycho-social" foundation (Sharfstein 2005). As a leader of American psychiatry, he and others will continue to shape a field that will facilitate new hypotheses, new data, and a new rational health system that gives parity to a scientific psychiatry. Changing American psychiatry in this direction will be a worthwhile, and I believe necessary, goal. I hope that during the next decades, search committees seeking to identify new academic leadership for psychiatry will begin to consider candidates with this perspective.

This book is an attempt to describe some major events in American psychiatry during the last half century, and I write as a participant in the process, with all the strengths and weaknesses of such a position. I have tried to demonstrate that the profession has not been merely a passive victim of managed care as has frequently been implied; rather it has been energetic in shaping its own direction. I believe that reiteration of our active role is important at many levels. Many talented and dedicated people, including leaders, members, and staff of the APA, care greatly about our profession and have supported a move to build a future-oriented, evidence-based psychiatry that will be relevant during and after our current national health system.

The timing of this book deserves special comment. I completed it a decade after my retirement, having served as Medical Director of the APA from 1974 to 1997. As occasionally occurs with executive transitions, I found myself estranged from some of the organization's leadership after my retirement and, rightly or wrongly, was not ready to write about events that took place during my time as Medical Director. With the appointment of Jay Scully as Medical Director in 2003 I no longer felt estranged and was delighted with his appointment. I am also delighted that he has agreed to write the foreword to this book. The last decade of my relatively quiet reflection about the APA has been useful in permitting me to formulate the longer-term consequences of some of the actions taken during my tenure as Medical Director. I comment on some of the policies and structures that have been particularly useful, but I also discuss some of my decisions that had negative consequences. I have included discussion of some current issues that the organization is facing and have made suggestions that I hope may affect the deliberations. I recognize that I am much less knowledgeable about the nuances of today's decisions, but I have nevertheless included a few comments about questions that seem to relate to previous changes.

Relatively few histories of American psychiatry have been written covering the latter half of the twentieth century. Several recent publications, however, have appeared, and I have found them to be most stimulating. I disagree, however, with some of their interpretations and have offered my own perspectives. Historians will, of course, make their own evaluation of our respective formulations. They will decide whether the changes in American psychiatry during the last quarter of the twentieth century were driven entirely by external forces or shaped primarily by psychiatric leadership to make the field a full partner in medical science. They will also observe whether psychoanalysis was only a hiatus and assess how important psychosocial issues are for a new psychiatry. I hope the predictions I make in this book, as well as the history I recount, will be useful to those who follow us.

Melvin Sabshin, M.D.

REFERENCES

American Psychiatric Association: Diagnostic and Statistical Manual of Mental Disorders, 3rd Edition. Washington, DC, American Psychiatric Association, 1980

American Psychiatric Association: Diagnostic and Statistical Manual of Mental Disorders, 4th Edition. Washington, DC, American Psychiatric Association, 1994

Sabshin M: Current issues affecting the mental health field. National Association of Private Psychiatric Hospitals Journal 6:12–16, 1974

Sharfstein SS: Response to the presidential address: advocacy for our patients and our profession. Am J Psychiatry 162:2045–2047, 2005

Strauss A, Schatzman L, Bucher R, Ehrlich D, Sabshin M (eds): Psychiatric Ideologies and Institutions. New York, Free Press, 1964

Acknowledgments

This book would never have been attempted or completed without my wife, Marion Bennathan. She has provided inspiration, new ideas, editorial skills, tough criticism, and even typing skills. She grasped what I hoped to accomplish and made it possible.

I am also very grateful to Robert E. Hales, Editor-in-Chief of American Psychiatric Publishing, Inc. (APPI), for his personal and conceptual support and to the other leaders and staff of APPI, John McDuffie, Ron McMillen, Bessie Jones, and Greg Kuny, who dealt with my questions and concerns most promptly and helpfully.

Ellen Mercer was important in encouraging me to write the book and helped a great deal with the chapter on international affairs. Carol Davis filled in many of the gaps in my organizational memories. Gary McMillan was most helpful with identifying and tracking down the relevant references, and Julie Young, M.D., provided invaluable assistance both with editing and with bibliographic work.

It was good to work again with current and past APA staff and APA leaders who shared my enthusiasms. They include John Blamphin; Eugene Cassel; Harold Eist, M.D.; Robert Freedman, M.D.; Edward Goldfarb, M.D.; Carol Lewis; Claudia Hart; Lawrence Hartmann, M.D.; Susan Kuper; Robert Leon, M.D.; JoAnn Macbeth; Michael Murphy; Irvin Muszynski; Nicholas Meyers; Evelyn Myers; Cathy Nash; Judith Nowak, M.D.; Harold Pincus, M.D.; Darrel Regier, M.D.; Jeanne Robb; Carolyn Robinowitz, M.D.; Jay Scully, M.D.; Lydia Sermons-Ward; the late Henry Work, M.D.; and Jason Young.

Of course, none of them is responsible for my occasionally controversial opinions about the history and future prospects for psychiatry. My memory is still good but far from perfect. Old, hazy memories keep recurring, and I realize that I have omitted many important people and events. For this I apologize, but I am proud and pleased that I am able to remember so much of the past and to have strong opinions about the future.

Melvin Sabshin, M.D.

1

Post–World War II Scene in American Psychiatry

*T*here was a glorious period of exultation and optimism in many countries in the immediate aftermath of World War II. Americans and their allies were proud of the preservation of democracy brought about by the defeat of German Nazism, Italian fascism, and Japanese imperialism. Victory in the war seemed to unleash enormous interest in confronting old as well as newly emerging issues. To the extent that "paradigm shifts" in many fields are influenced profoundly by their social contexts (Kuhn 1962), psychiatry was one field that was profoundly influenced by World War II. Some of the new directions in the profession had begun before the war (Meyer 1948). The prevailing bastions of biological psychiatry and of asylums had been challenged, but the upheaval after the war produced major qualitative differences from prewar psychiatry (Meyer 1950).

Psychiatric casualties have been recognized since at least the American Civil War, when the Union army officially documented nearly 8,000 cases of psychiatric disorders in which the individuals required inpatient treatment (Jones 2000). However, the extraordinary types and incidence of traumatic war experiences and neuropsychiatric disorders began to be broadly reconceptualized after World War II (Heaton et al. 1966–1973). Many of the new concepts involved psychodynamic formulations of repressed conflicts as a central feature. Attempts to bring unacceptable thoughts and feelings to consciousness so that they could be mastered with appropriate clinical assistance became an important technique that, in turn, opened up many new theoretical questions. The U.S. Army began screening for psychiatric vulnerability during World War I, with 72,000 (2%) of U.S. recruits being rejected because of neuropsychiatric reasons (Jones et al. 2003).

Ignoring attempts by the American Psychiatric Association (APA) to prepare for massive psychiatric casualties during World War II, American military planners assumed that mental health screening prior to induction would suffice in managing troops' psychiatric problems (Jones 2000). In 1940, psychoanalytic psychiatrist Harry Stack Sullivan was appointed by the Selective Service to develop a psychiatric screening program for military recruits (Pols 2006). Despite screening out those considered to be at highest risk of mental breakdown, the rates of "war neuroses," "battle fatigue," and "combat stress" during World War II far exceeded those during World War I. Recognizing that even "sturdy, well-adjusted" (Pols 2006) soldiers were succumbing to psychiatric *exhaustion,* a group of civilian psychiatrists were commissioned to start providing psychiatric care for American troops on the frontline (Jones 2000).

After the war, there was a strong motivation to develop a new national program that would be therapeutic for those servicemen and servicewomen disabled by their wartime experiences. Gratitude for our troops and pride in what they had accomplished played an important role in the creation of a much stronger national veterans' medical program with intensive treatment and rehabilitation components. Research to understand the basis of the veterans' illnesses was also strongly supported. Psychiatric care was broadly accepted as a central part of this effort, and increased commitment to new approaches for those with mental illness led to a surge of interest in psychiatric treatment. The Veterans Administration's attention to these problems provided an early form of parity for mental health benefits on a par with other health problems—a parity rarely achieved in civilian medical systems. With the creation of the National Center for PTSD in 1989, the Veterans Administration continues to conduct research and to provide education and treatment for the psychiatric casualties of war (U.S. Department of Veterans Affairs 2006).

A significant part of the surge of interest involved explorations of the implications of stress and the psychological aspects of battlefield trauma. American psychiatrists such as Roy R. Grinker and John P. Spiegel, in their book *Men Under Stress* (Grinker and Spiegel 1945), and M. Ralph Kaufman (1947) contributed greatly to the recognition of the importance of psychological factors in the understanding of wartime neuroses.

These leaders had an interest in broadening the application of psycho-analytic concepts to understand the "traumatic" neuroses. Postwar inter-est in these conditions, as well as in the high incidence of mental illness di-agnosed in potential soldiers, began to spread across the United States. Understanding the powerful impact of stressful experiences on the hu-man psyche, as well as determining what could be done for those suffer-ing, became urgent national priorities. Not surprisingly, psychiatry as a career choice increased among physician veterans of the war as they sought to understand the psychological aspects of what they had seen on the battlefield. The number of psychiatric residency positions grew from only 400 before the War World II to more than 1,800 by 1951 (Scully et al. 2000). American psychoanalysts who had been trained before the war and were followers of Adolf Meyer were invigorated by the new surge of interest in psychiatry and recognized a considerable opportu-nity for influence in their field.

Accompanying these exciting trends within American psychiatry it-self was an extremely poignant occurrence, namely, the emigration of many European psychiatrists to the United States. Among this group was a high percentage of Jewish psychoanalysts seeking refuge from Nazi persecution. They had begun to leave Central and Eastern Europe with the rise of Nazism, and their numbers grew dramatically during and af-ter the war. This able group included many bright, ambitious, and tal-ented leaders. Their presence in the United States became a vital part of the subsequent transformation of American psychiatry. Before the war, Adolf Meyer helped prepare the way for at least partial acceptance of de-velopmental and psychological factors as relevant to psychiatric disor-ders. As classical psychoanalytic concepts became widely employed, Meyer paved the way for the acceptance of analytic principles and continued in his advocacy even though his own formulations and methods were soon discarded in a sweep toward the classical model of psychoanalysis.

Many newly arrived psychoanalysts sought appointments in existing psychoanalytic institutes, while others played a key role in creating new ones. The alliance of this group with invigorated native-born colleagues in the United States within the new postwar milieu was a vital compo-nent in the systemic change in postwar American psychiatry. Much has been written on the subject of why and how psychoanalysts became so prominent in American psychiatry; an intriguing explanation appears in Edward Shorter's *A History of Psychiatry: From the Era of the Asylum to the Age of Prozac* (Shorter 1997). He suggests that the acceptance of psychoanalysis, particularly by Jewish women, may have some rele-vance, but this viewpoint overlooks a variety of more significant social and economic variables. Furthermore, to attribute the later decline of psychoanalysis, as Shorter implies, mainly to the assimilation of Jewish women in the American culture seems even less plausible.

The postwar social climate of compassion and commitment to veterans' health and welfare, in conjunction with the excitement about new possibilities for treatment, provided a backdrop for fundamental changes in psychiatry. In addition, the influx of the new group of psychoanalytical leadership helped to create a national movement that shaped new images of psychiatry. The lack of plausible alternative therapeutic models at that time also opened the way for a new approach.

Even during this time of relatively positive acceptance of psychoanalytic concepts, there was great opposition to psychoanalytic theory and practice at many levels, and alternative ideologies became stronger over time. In the book *Psychiatric Ideologies and Institutions* (Strauss et al. 1964), Strauss and I and our co-authors discussed the significance of three dominant ideologies; psychotherapeutic, somatotherapeutic, and sociotherapeutic. We developed a scale to measure the presence of these ideological influences among various groups of psychiatrists. Most often the somatotherapists and the sociotherapists were quite critical of psychoanalytic treatment.

Despite this opposition, psychoanalysis became a dominant force in American psychiatry during the postwar years. Many of the psychoanalysts in the vanguard had achieved this high acceptance despite their own tendency to present themselves primarily as a beleaguered minority. Of course, to describe analysis as fully accepted would be naive. It was frequently attacked (see, e.g., Eysenck 1953; Sabshin 1990; Schoenfeld 1962; Shevrin 1995; Webster 1995), but for at least two decades analysts shaped the predominant direction of postwar psychiatry in the United States.

By and large, psychoanalysts do not accept this formulation of their relative power; they tend to focus upon the ambivalence toward them, whether conscious or unconscious. Therapeutic experiences have made them wary of those who profess positive feelings toward them. Nevertheless, it would be difficult to find such positive attitudes toward psychoanalysis in any other country or at any other time than in postwar America. The strong influence of psychoanalysis pertained despite many contradictions and misunderstandings. Ideological opponents to analysis overestimated the psychoanalysts' power, while many analysts denied or underestimated their own influence. This curious balance persisted during the 1950s and 1960s. Looking back from a new century perspective, however, the period from 1945 to 1970 was the peak of psychoanalytic influence in psychiatry in America or, indeed, in any other nation.

The influence of psychoanalysis was seen most profoundly in psychiatric education. Residency training and medical school teaching programs significantly altered their clinical programs and didactic courses to include psychodynamic principles. Robert Wallerstein, for example, reports that during his residency in the mid-1940s, half of trainees' time was given to "individual psychotherapeutic work with patients" (Wallerstein 1991). Analysts joined many psychiatric department faculties and provided much of the clinical supervision for a newly emphasized psychotherapy. New departments of psychiatry were formed in many medical schools. Approximately half of new psychiatry department Chairs appointed during the 1950s, 1960s, and 1970s were psychoanalysts or deeply committed to psychodynamic education. This tendency was present in many of the most prestigious medical centers. Some critics of psychoanalysis have claimed that almost all departmental Chairs during that time were analysts, but that was not the case. Non-analysts and ideological opponents of analysis were also appointed, albeit less frequently. The tendency by some to claim that the domination by analysts was complete is not accurate and distorts the reality of the complex forces and multiple ideologies then present within American psychiatry.

Psychotherapy, however, became a centerpiece in many residency programs, and much greater attention began to be paid to this form of treatment. The absence of other effective psychological treatments also played a role in making dynamic psychotherapy more popular. The APA and the Association of American Medical Colleges presented a series of special conferences on psychiatric education at Cornell University, reflecting the importance of the dominant psychodynamic milieu on psychiatric education (Earley et al. 1969; Krug and Lourie 1964; Mitchell and Whitehorn 1952, 1953). Psychoanalytic training itself received special attention in the United States and became quite relevant to psychiatric pedagogy. Although trainees were not required to undergo a personal analysis to complete psychiatric training, as had become mandatory in psychoanalytic training, the potential benefit of such an analytical experience for all psychiatrists was broadly supported. "Psychological mindedness," or what might today be called "mentalization capacity" (Fonagy and Target 2006; Twemlow et al. 2005), was an important basic skill for an applicant to have in order to be selected as a psychiatry resident at many of the most highly respected psychiatric programs, where competition to enter psychiatric training had become keen.

Relationships between psychoanalytic institutes and departments of psychiatry became very close in some training programs. Indeed, there were several formal training agreements between academic institutions and analytic institutes. Several psychoanalytic institutes were geographically located in academic psychiatry departments, for example, at Columbia University and the University of Pittsburgh. In Chicago, three institutions—the University of Chicago, the University of Illinois, and Michael Reese Hospital—had a joint program with the Chicago Psychoanalytic Institute; each year the departments of psychiatry selected one resident to spend one year at each of their facilities. Subsequently these residents went on to train as analysts at the institute. The Analytic Institute continues to be located at Columbia but is no longer in Pittsburgh or at Chicago. In all three academic settings, psychiatric residency is no longer a direct pathway to a psychoanalytic career.

That these special relationships evolved at prestigious academic institutions and hospitals was very important. Psychoanalytic leaders gave status to many academic departments; in addition to writing textbooks and many journal articles, they also played a key role in psychiatric education. At that time psychiatric education was the most important function in academic departments of psychiatry; research was a much lower priority in most departments.

Psychiatry grew rapidly in size, complexity, and areas of special concern during the postwar years. The development of subspecialties within psychiatry became important for the field after World War II. Child psychiatry was the first of these subspecialties to differentiate itself from the rest of the field (Berlin 2004). Its postwar history demonstrated some significant parallels with the vicissitudes of adult psychiatry as well as notable differences. Child psychiatry was also very much affected by psychoanalysis, both theoretically and clinically. Treatment for children incorporated central parts of psychodynamic theory. Adolescence was perceived as a period of significant psychological stress and regressive components. Psychoanalytic concepts of adolescence had another major impact that has not been widely perceived; the high incidence of psychological problems during adolescence, as portrayed by Erik Erikson (1968) in *Identity, Youth, and Crisis,* helped to support an implicit belief by analysts during this tumultuous period that psychopathology was extremely common. Even though the analysts often denied that their model was one of illness, the implications of their theory of widespread psychopathology became very influential far beyond adolescence. These implications have been of tremendous influence, leading in part to the assertion by E. Fuller Torrey in *The Death of Psychiatry* (Torrey 1974), by the National Alliance on Mental Illness (NAMI, formerly the National Alliance for the Mentally Ill), and others that analysts deal with the "worried well" while ignoring the seriously mentally ill such as patients with schizophrenia.

Psychoanalysts have rarely discussed the crucial importance of the implications of the high incidence of psychopathology, except to assert that they do indeed employ a model of normal behavior and often tell prospective patients that they do not need treatment since they function well. Nevertheless, in my opinion, psychoanalysts have not responded adequately to criticism that their basic concepts, if taken seriously, had enormous policy implications. Similarly, they have not adequately discussed the epidemiological implications of their basic formulations. Some analysts have defined epidemiology as outside of their interest. Indeed, epidemiology has yet to develop as a serious area of interest for them.

Yet without epidemiology it is not possible to ascertain the distribution of disorders or the size of the normal population. Only in recent years have leaders in psychoanalysis begun to elaborate on their concepts of healthy behavior, but this issue is still not a central subject or one that is clearly enough formulated to be employed in epidemiological studies. While the psychoanalysts themselves did not carry out such epidemiological studies, there was a tendency in the postwar years to use psychoanalytic concepts in such investigations. Consequently, prior to the publication by the APA of the third edition of the *Diagnostic and Statistical Manual of Mental Disorders* (DSM-III; American Psychiatric Association 1980), it was difficult to conduct adequate epidemiological studies.

The *Psychodynamic Diagnostic Manual,* recently published by a group of organizations representing psychoanalytic and psychodynamic therapists, is intended to add psychological depth to the DSM classifications (Alliance of Psychoanalytic Organizations 2006). While it may complement the DSM, it seems unlikely that it can be employed to collect significant epidemiological data in the absence of reliability studies, and it would be difficult to achieve high reliability without clear ways to include and exclude people. Without a proven system utilizing this manual and without good quantitative data, the manual's importance for mental health policy will be limited. It would also be limited in its use for actuarial purposes.

The history of other subspecialties is quite relevant to postwar development. Geriatric psychiatry tended to be perceived in psychobiological terms earlier than most areas of psychiatry; declining biological capacities and bodily functions in older people could not be denied. Nevertheless, the lack of detailed understanding of the biology of aging made it somewhat easier to explain many geriatric problems in psychological terms. The life cycle of psychiatric problems was heavily weighted by analysts toward the significance of early childhood influences; there was a tendency to pay insufficient attention to the problems of geriatric patients. Later, the remarkable increase in life expectancy and the development of a scientifically based gerontology became a central stimulus for a new geriatrics.

The issues of psychogenetic causality affected the field of psychosomatic medicine. Formulations of specific conflicts in childhood and their pathological impact on bodily functions were enunciated by a significant group of psychoanalysts (Alexander 1950). Not all analysts subscribed to the validity of the "specificity" hypotheses, but many agreed that the etiology of illnesses like hypertension, asthma, peptic ulcers, dermatitis, ulcerative colitis, and thyrotoxicosis was significantly affected by psychological conflicts and persistent character problems. The gradual metamorphosis of psychosomatic concepts in American psychiatry and medicine as a whole is relevant to the changing psychiatric scene and is a good indicator of the paradigm shifts. Indeed, the metamorphosis of psychosomatic medicine in the latter part of the twentieth century is a good reflection of overall changes in psychiatry (Levenson 2005). Ideological formulations have been replaced by a practical, evidence-based approach.

Before World War II, most of the severely mentally ill were treated in mental hospitals, and the majority in the United States were housed in large state institutions. This pattern continued until the 1970s, when reforms and economically driven regulations coalesced into a major dehospitalization trend (Lamb 2000). The postwar developments also produced a much increased interest in a less severely ill population. Nevertheless, a new surge of interest in private psychiatric hospitals developed after the war. Long-term use of dynamically oriented psychotherapy for patients with schizophrenia became important in some of these institutions. A cadre of psychoanalysts assumed leadership in advocating psychotherapy as a useful method of dealing with schizophrenia and other severe psychiatric illnesses. The evolution of this movement and its subsequent downfall is another major indicator of changing psychiatry. The rise and fall of long-term psychotherapeutic treatment of patients with schizophrenia and other severe psychiatric illnesses is prototypic of the two major paradigm shifts of the late twentieth century. A surge of psychoanalytic interest in severely ill patients had developed in the first two decades after World War II, but this interest declined significantly after the 1970s. The *Osheroff* case, discussed in Chapter 8 ("Psychoanalysis"), which involved a prestigious psychoanalytic hospital's being sued for inappropriate treatment, was a significant sign of the changing times.

Psychiatric divisions and sections of general hospitals had begun to function before War War II, but they grew quickly in number and popularity after the war. Many of the old state hospitals had originally been constructed away from the centers of big cities. This location was determined in part by stigma against those with mental illness. Keeping mentally ill people locked up and separated from the rest of the population served old myths and beliefs about the dangers of close proximity to the mentally ill. These distant locations also reflected profound pessimism about what could be done to help these patients. General hospitals, in contrast, were mostly located in or near central parts of cities, and the decision to include a psychiatric unit in such a setting indicated some lessening of the fear of mental patients and recognition of the importance of keeping the patient close to his or her family, and led to a considerable decline in stigma. It did not, however, indicate the overcoming of all stigma. Protection of our citizenry from the psychiatric patients in general hospitals has remained a significant concern in many communities to this day, and this is part of a larger public fear about discharged mental patients returning to the community. Even though stigma had declined by the end of the century, the location of psychiatric facilities is still a tender subject.

Physical treatments, such as electroconvulsive therapy and insulin therapy, were frequently employed for individuals cared for in the general hospital psychiatric facilities, even in the post-war years. But a considerable number of general hospital units began to use the combination of psychotherapy and pharmacology, especially after chlorpromazine became available (Riba and Balon 2004; Schatzberg and Nemeroff 2004). (Length of stay in psychiatric sections of general hospitals was at first much shorter than in private psychiatric hospitals, but by the end of the century, length of stay had been severely reduced in both settings [Grob 1994].) The significant decrease in length of stay for hospitalized psychiatric patients is another major indicator of remarkable changes in American psychiatry. Hospitalization has become the last resort after most other efforts have failed, and its goal is behavioral stabilization, not cure.

Psychiatric liaison services in the general hospital became more common in the postwar years. Many of these services emphasized the search for the psychogenic etiology of the anxiety or depression accompanying patients' physical illness. When patients were seen by psychiatric consultants on medical, surgical, and children's wards, the recommendations were often perceived as unhelpful by the other services, who were seeking "practical suggestions." Later, as psychopharmacology and cognitive therapies developed, liaison psychiatrists became more practical and genuinely therapeutic. *Psychosomatics,* previously called *consultation-liaison psychiatry,* became a formal subspecialty in 2003. During the 1940s, 1950s, and 1960s, the impact of psychoanalysis and psychodynamic psychiatry spread broadly across a wide variety of cultural sectors in the United States. Many artists, novelists, and dramatists became devotees of analysis. Films, plays, novels, and other art forms demonstrated powerful psychoanalytic influences (Gabbard and Gabbard 1999). As with psychiatry itself, however, segments of the humanities and arts also became critical of psychoanalysis, and over time more critics appeared. Not all the criticism, however, was based on misconception or stigma; a series of more rational critiques of analysis had begun to appear by the 1970s, although many analysts tended to see all criticism as based on irrational ideological grounds or even as unconsciously based resistance to disturbing analytic ideas. Distinguishing rational questions from ideologies or mythology was not simple, especially if strong ideologies or irrational concerns were involved in response to the questions. Treating all criticism as being symptoms of resistance ultimately was unsuccessful. Resistances can be very subtle, and the objective rationality of science may not be clear enough. Scientific investigation is still the best long-term solution to such dilemmas.

From my perspective, psychiatry in America became heavily dominated by ideologies in the postwar years (Erhlich and Sabshin 1964; Strauss et al. 1964). Ultimately these ideologies became increasingly visible to the public and contributed to a more negative perception of the field. The belief that psychiatry was dominated by ideologies became quite common but was persistently and significantly underestimated and resisted by many psychiatrists for at least three decades after World War II.

As dominance by ideologies became more prominent in American psychiatry, it became harder for the general public, decision makers, and medical colleagues to believe that psychiatry was a legitimate part of medicine or that empirical research was an important part of the field. For a short time after World War II, not much attention was given to the emerging ideologies. By the middle of the 1960s, however, they became hard to ignore, and concern over the ideologies played a role in the efforts to control and regulate the field. For many psychiatrists who believed profoundly in a particular ideology, the criticism of their belief system was perceived as being based primarily on stigma, prejudice, and misunderstanding. Of course, such prejudice existed, but, hard as it may be to accept, it was not the only source of the criticism. The various ideologues in psychiatry were perhaps the strongest critics of other ideologies in the field. The biological ideologues claimed superiority of scientific "validity," but many of them exhibited strong rejection of almost any psychological variables or concepts. By emphasizing that all psychological phenomena could be reduced to their biological base, they denied the implications of social and psychological impact on psychiatric disorder or severely reduced their importance. The social psychiatric ideologues included some who denied the importance of psychological or biological variables, as compared with social or economic forces, in determining human behavior. In this context, Marxists during the peak of the Cold War were particularly critical of psychoanalysis as a capitalist ideology; we saw Chinese patients in the early 1970s who had been given the works of Mao Tse-tung to read while lying in bed for much of the day.

Some psychoanalytic ideologues prominently displayed their beliefs with a certitude that denigrated opposing positions. By and large they did not pose questions that lent themselves to investigation. Some believed that their clinical formulations were undoubtedly correct and, furthermore, that the complexity of these ideas rendered them untestable by current or even future clinical methodology. Some viewed the research side of psychiatry as either trivial or composed of unanalyzable variables. The ideologues were often the public representatives of the field and spoke in passionate tones. Those who used moderate language were often perceived by the ideologues as ambivalent and were not accepted by the "true believers." The public heard the passionate ideologies and assumed that the field was more of a cult than a science.

During the first decade after War World II, however, the ideologies received less attention by the public in the context of the widespread passionate concern for veterans and the need for a system of care for the psychiatric patient. The role of the federal government in supporting the revitalization of the field became increasingly prominent. Creation of the National Institute of Mental Health (NIMH), discussed further in Chapter 10 ("Evidence-Based Diagnosis and Treatment"), was a powerful emerging support for psychiatry and all of mental health. Indeed, over time the NIMH became a driving force for a scientific psychiatry.

The post–World War II boom in academic psychiatry was very much supported by the NIMH, especially in the area of training. For three decades after the war, education was the dominant function of the NIMH. By 1980, however, new leadership had begun to emphasize the research functions of the institute.

The tumultuous developments in psychiatry during the three decades after World War II brought progress on many fronts; the number of psychiatrists increased, and more medical students entered psychiatry than ever before. People began to be treated closer to their home. Psychotherapy began to be used in many cases, subspecialty groups in psychiatry were formed, and public attitudes to psychiatry were, on the whole, positive. As the years went by, greater attention was given to the absence of research, but the decision makers and the general public ultimately became skeptical about permitting psychiatry to grow without stronger regulations.

As public efforts to curb medical expenditures increased, discrimination against psychiatry emerged again as one of the field's most visible problems. Residual mythology about psychiatrists and their patients, plus the antipsychiatry of special groups, such as adherents of Thomas Szasz, Scientologists, and Marxists, and the questions raised about the reliability of psychiatric diagnosis and treatment, combined to weaken the postwar exuberance (Scheff 1966; Szasz 1961). Ideological divisions among psychiatrists played into the growing public criticism of the field. Initial efforts to counter the rising criticism were attempted but were insufficient; the need for a qualitative change became increasingly apparent (Wilson 1993).

My own perspective on these issues was stimulated by many people and institutions. In the next four chapters I describe some of the internal and external influences that led me to psychiatry and ultimately to a post where I could play a part in the recognition of the problems and some potential solutions.

REFERENCES

Alexander F: Psychosomatic Medicine, Its Principles and Applications. New York, WW Norton, 1950

Alliance of Psychoanalytic Organizations, PDM Task Force: Psychodynamic Diagnostic Manual. Silver Spring, MD, Alliance of Psychoanalytic Organizations, 2006

American Psychiatric Association: Diagnostic and Statistical Manual of Mental Disorders (DSM-III), 3rd Edition. Washington, DC, American Psychiatric Association, 1980

Berlin IN: Development of the subspecialty of child and adolescent psychiatry in the United States, in Textbook of Child and Adolescent Psychiatry, 3rd Edition. Edited by Wiener JM, Dulcan MK. Washington, DC, American Psychiatric Press, 2004, pp 3–12

Earley LW, et al: Psychiatry and medical education. Report of a conference held in Atlanta, Georgia, under the auspices of the American Psychiatric Association and the Association of American Medical Colleges.Washington, DC, American Psychiatric Association, 1969

Ehrlich D, Sabshin M: A study of sociotherapeutically oriented psychiatrists. Am J Orthopsychiatry 34:469–480, 1964

Erikson EH: Identity, Youth, and Crisis. New York, WW Norton, 1968

Eysenck HJ: Uses and Abuses of Psychology. London, Penguin, 1953

Fonagy P, Target M: The mentalization-focused approach to self pathology. J Pers Disord 20:544–576, 2006

Gabbard GO, Gabbard K: Psychiatry and the Cinema, 2nd Edition. Washington, DC, American Psychiatric Press, 1999

Grinker RR, Spiegel JP: Men Under Stress. Philadelphia, PA, Blakiston, 1945

Grob G: The Mad Among Us: A History of the Care of America's Mentally Ill. New York, Free Press, 1994, p 287

Hale NG: The Rise and Crisis of Psychoanalysis in the United States. New York, Oxford University Press, 1995

Hammersley DW (ed): Training the psychiatrist to meet changing needs. Report of the Conference on Graduate Psychiatric Education, Washington, DC, December 2–6, 1962, with the co-sponsorship of the Canadian Psychiatric Association, Washington, DC, American Psychiatric Association, 1963

Heaton LD, Anderson RS, Glass AJ, et al: Neuropsychiatry in World War II. Washington, DC, Office of the Surgeon General, Department of the Army, 1966–1973

Jones E, Hyams KC, Wessely S: Screening for vulnerability to psychological disorders in the military: an historical survey. J Med Screen 10:40–46, 2003

Jones FD: Military Psychiatry since World War II, in American Psychiatry After World War II: 1944–1994. Edited by Menninger RW, Nemiah JC. Washington, DC, American Psychiatric Press, 2000, pp 3–36

Kaufman MR: Ill health as an expression of anxiety in a combat unit. Psychosom Med 9:92–97, 1947

Krug O, Lourie RS (eds): Career Training in Child Psychiatry. Report of the Conference on Training in Child Psychiatry, Washington, DC, January 10–15, under the auspices of the American Academy of Child Psychiatry and the American Psychiatric Association. Washington, DC, American Psychiatric Association, 1964

Kuhn TS: The Structure of Scientific Revolutions. Chicago, IL, University of Chicago Press, 1962

Lamb HR: Deinstitutionalization and public policy, in American Psychiatry After World War II: 1944–1994. Edited by Menninger RW, Nemiah JC. Washington, DC, American Psychiatric Press, 2000, pp 259–276

Levenson JL: Introduction, in The American Psychiatric Publishing Textbook of Psychosomatic Medicine. Edited by Levenson JL. Washington, DC, American Psychiatric Publishing, 2005, pp xix–xxi

Meyer A: The Commonsense Psychiatry of Dr. Adolf Meyer. New York, McGraw-Hill, 1948

Meyer A: The Collected Papers of Adolf Meyer. Edited by Winters EE. Baltimore, MD, Johns Hopkins Press, 1950

Mitchell J McK, Whitehorn JC (eds): Psychiatry and medical education. Report of a conference held at Cornell University in 1951 under the auspices of the American Psychiatric Association and the Association of American Medical Colleges. Washington, DC, American Psychiatric Association, 1952

Mitchell J McK, Whitehorn JC (eds): The psychiatrist: his training and development. Report of a conference held at Cornell University in 1952 under the auspices of the American Psychiatric Association and the Association of American Medical Colleges. Washington, DC, American Psychiatric Association, 1953

Pols H: Waking up to shell shock: psychiatry in the US military during World War II. Endeavor 30(4):144–149, 2006

Riba MB, Balon R: Competency in Combining Pharmacotherapy and Psychotherapy: Integrated and Split Treatment. Washington, DC, American Psychiatric Publishing, 2005

Sabshin M: Turning points in twentieth-century American psychiatry. Am J Psychiatry 147:1267–1274, 1990

Schatzberg AF, Nemeroff CB: The American Psychiatric Publishing Textbook of Psychopharmacology, 3rd Edition. Washington, DC, American Psychiatric Publishing, 2004

Scheff T: Being Mentally Ill: A Sociological Theory. Chicago, IL, Aldine de Gruyter, 1966

Schoenfeld CG: Three fallacious attacks upon psychoanalysis as science. Psychoanal Rev 49:35–47, 1962

Scully JH, Robinowitz CB, Shore JH: Psychiatric education after World War II, in American Psychiatry After World War II: 1944–1994. Edited by Menninger RW, Nemiah JC. Washington, DC, American Psychiatric Press, 2000, pp 124–151

Sharfstein SS: Utilization management: managed or mangled psychiatric care? Am J Psychiatry 147:965–966, 1990

Shevrin H: Is psychoanalysis one science, two sciences, or no science at all? A discourse among friendly antagonists. J Am Psychoanal Assoc 43:963–1049, 1995

Shorter E: A History of Psychiatry: From the Era of the Asylum to the Age of Prozac. New York, Wiley, 1997

Strauss A, Schatzman L, Bucher R, et al: Psychiatric Ideologies and Institutions. New York, Free Press, 1964

Sussex JN, et al.: The Working Papers of the 1975 Conference on Education of Psychiatrists: as prepared by members of the Preparatory Commissions for the Conference (Lake of the Ozarks, MO). Washington, DC, American Psychiatric Association, 1976

Szasz T: The Myth of Mental Illness: Foundation of a Theory of Personal Conduct. New York, Harper & Row, 1961

Torrey EF: The Death of Psychiatry. Radnor, PA, Chilton, 1974

Twemlow SW, Fonagy P, Sacco FC: A developmental approach to mentalizing communities, I: a model for social change. Bull Menninger Clin 69:265–281, 2005

U.S. Department of Veterans Affairs, Office of Public Affairs Media Relations: Veterans With Posttraumatic Stress Disorder Fact Sheet. Washington, DC, U.S. Department of Veterans Affairs, March 2006

Wallerstein RS: The future of psychotherapy. Bull Menninger Clin 55:421–443, 1991

Webster R: Why Freud Was Wrong. New York, Basic Books, 1995

Wilson M: DSM-III and the transformation of American psychiatry: a history. Am J Psychiatry 150:399–410, 1993

2

A Pathway to Psychiatry

I was ordained to become a physician even before I was born. My parents, Zalman and Sonia Sabshin, wanted their son to become a distinguished medical specialist rising, in their judgment, above the general practitioner level achieved by my father. His own career pathway evolved from a poor immigrant family who somehow managed to support him through a scientific education that culminated in 1917 with an M.D. degree. He worked in the public health service during the influenza epidemic in 1919 and subsequently entered general practice in the Bronx borough of New York City. My mother was even more ambitious for me, perhaps because, given the limitations for women's education in those days, she had not entered a profession herself. She poured the full measure of her hopes into me. She lived for 103 years and rarely swerved from her idealization of her son. It was extremely important for her and also for me. My sister, Billie, born two years before me, was also highly regarded but without the unambivalent fervor bestowed upon me. Billie was intensively involved in public education as a teacher and, later, as a school board member. Her husband was a general medical practitioner, very much like my father, and their son, Earl, became a lawyer and married another very able attorney.

My mother assisted my father in the management of his medical practice. He rewarded his patients by charging them only two dollars a visit if they came to the office; if he saw them at their home, the fee was increased to three dollars. We lived in a three-story house; my father's office took up most of the space on the middle floor, with the children's bedrooms above and the living room, dining room, and kitchen below. In the office there was a small surgical area, a large consultation desk, a room with bulky X-ray machines, and a dark developing chamber where my father would develop and read the X rays. As a small child I was fascinated by that dark, mysterious chamber. From an early age, I frequently accompanied my father on his house calls, and I enjoyed these opportunities to visit what seemed like far off places in the big city. It was a very special time to be with my father. I also enjoyed being with my family on the relatively rare holiday times we had together. I have fond memories of a few cruise boat trips and visits to lovely parks. I enjoyed playing chess with both my parents; my father was beatable, but I still believe that my mother let me win.

Both of my parents had come to the United States from Russia. To a significant degree, their families had experienced anti-Semitism and fled the country in the early 1900s. My father's family came through Ellis Island in 1910, and my mother's family had the same experience in 1912. My parents met in New York City around 1920. My father came from a very small town, Beshinkovitch, in what is now Belarus. In the 1980s, I was at a psychiatric meeting in Smolensk, where I told my Rusian colleagues about my father. They suggested that we immediately drive to his home town. Arriving in Beshenkovich we realized that it had lain in the path of the German advance to Moscow and that very little of the old city was left. A local surgeon took us to the old cemetery, but there was no trace of any Jewish graves. My mother was born in Slonim, a moderate-sized city in what is now Ukraine. She was the second oldest child of a modestly comfortable family that, before coming to the United States, included three brothers and one sister. My mother's father went to the United States alone and stayed for two years before the rest of his family was able to come. The sixth and last child was born in the United States. My mother's brothers were college educated; one became an engineer, the second became a lawyer, and the third became a businessman. The sister who had accompanied my mother from Russia did not have a professional career but was a particularly loving aunt for me. Lillian, my mother's youngest sister, went to Hunter College and was extraordinarily sophisticated; however, in the eyes of my mother, she always remained the very bright youngest child of the family and was treated as such, even when she was in her 80s.

My father's family had fewer financial resources than my mother's and was really quite poor when they arrived in the United States. They all pooled their money to support my father's education, including his medical school training. As my father's father had died in Russia, and the family had very little income, this was a daunting challenge. My father had one older brother, who was a storekeeper, and two younger sisters, both of whom married early. He was supported for medical school because he seemed more intellectually adept at taking on this challenge. My father's mother lived in our house where I was born, but there was tension between her and my mother. So, in time, she moved to an apartment of her own, provided by my father, who was very grateful for the sacrifices and help that she had provided, in return for which he supported his family for the rest of his life.

My parents' social life was dominated by being part of a group of local Jewish physicians and their spouses in the Bronx. They organized a special "study group" that met once a month in various homes. In effect, it was a small literary society. My mother was the permanent "secretary" of the group, and I had the privilege of seeing notes of the meetings that she kept until her death at 103. The group was highly inclined toward leftist politics. My mother and father had strongly positive feelings toward the Soviet Union, especially since it replaced the Tsarist regime. I never had any evidence that they were members of the Communist Party, but I grew up in a home that was visibly pro-Communist, at least in regard to the party in the U.S.S.R. My mother retained her pro-Soviet position even after the reforms of the early 1990s. I was deeply influenced by these political persuasions, at least until the end of my adolescence. Occasionally during my teenage years I rebelled by taking on a few conservative positions.

I attended public school in the Bronx, as did my sister. One of my special childhood memories is that when it rained, my father would drive me to school. I would hide in the back seat of the car because I was embarrassed to have these special privileges witnessed by my schoolmates, who tended to be less affluent than the physician's son. My father retired from medical practice because of malignant hypertension prior to his 50th birthday. His prognosis upon retirement was seen as poor, but he surprised his physicians and lived for another 16 years. My parents stayed in New York for two more years following his retirement in order to allow me to finish high school, after which they moved to Miami Beach. My mother and father, though proud of their Jewish identity, were uninterested in religion; but my father was deeply committed to Yiddish poetry and published a book of poems written during his retirement.

I had been fortunate in passing the admissions examination for Townsend Harris High School, named after the first U.S. Ambassador to Japan, at the age of 10. This school was located in the "downtown" facility of City College of New York before its closure in 1943. In this school system, it was possible to skip grades, and I was promoted this way five times, thereby allowing me to graduate high school in 1940, shortly after turning 14. Before going to Townsend Harris, I was interviewed for a scholarship to Horace Mann High School. My mother later was aghast to find out that one of her women "friends" in the group of physicians who was on the Board of Horace Mann had vetoed my appointment. While a shock to my mother, this event turned out to be an advantage in that I received a superb education at Townsend Harris High School, perhaps even superior to what I might have experienced at Horace Mann.

The decision to move to Florida was made after a trip to Los Angeles, where my father had close relatives; we almost moved there but decided in the context of the late 1930s that it was too far away from New York. How different that perception would be today. We had spent several months in Los Angeles in 1939, and I had been enthralled by it for many reasons, including the fact that a World Fair had taken place there. Nevertheless, to leave New York City at the beginning of adolescence was somewhat traumatic for me; I did not want to leave my friends or to miss the possibilities of exploring the city even more as I grew older. I think that for much of my life, I have sought to live in the biggest cities to make up for not having stayed in New York. Living in London, as I do today, makes me feel that I have almost come back to New York.

With strong input from my parents, I gained admission to the University of Florida in Gainesville, about 350 miles from Miami, so that, at age 14, I would not be too far from home. I was accepted as a member of Pi Lambda Phi fraternity (the more "integrated" of the two Jewish fraternities at the University of Florida). On the surface my age was not a strong deterrent, as I looked and acted somewhat older than I was, but the adjustment to college was more difficult than I admitted. At that time, the University of Florida had adopted the comprehensive educational system pioneered at the University of Chicago, so in my first two years I took comprehensive courses ("C1–C6") and did very well academically. Because of my age and my mother's "careful supervision," I was given very special attention by several members of the faculty. The Department of Psychology was very interested in me; its chair, Professor Harold Hinckley, and Professor Stanley Wimberly were very kind to me and increased my interest in behavioral science. The remarkably able president of the University, John Tigert, paid particular attention to me, stimulated by a couple of letters from my energetic mother. Later, when I applied to medical school, he wrote a special letter to the Admission Committee at Tulane University, which I am certain facilitated my admission. Because of my good grades at Florida in my freshman year, I was permitted to enroll in a class on international relations that was ordinarily limited to upper classmen. It was a fascinating class taught by William Carlton, called affectionately by the students "Wild Bill." I remember scoring 100% on a very long objective examination, which impressed the professor, and he gave me a number of opportunities to talk with him that provided me a more sophisticated appreciation of international affairs. Of course, I was ultimately enrolled in an overall premedical curriculum; the ordination by my parents in those early years held very strongly, even though I experienced a strong wish to consider a career in political science and international work.

The University of Florida, as a land-grant college, had been authorized to provide military training to all healthy students. At that time, Florida was an all-male school, and for my Reserve Officer Training Corps (ROTC) training, I was enrolled in horse-drawn field artillery. I think that our military authorities were preparing once again to fight the Spanish-American War of 1898. One of the special problems for me in this type of field artillery was that I had hardly ever seen a horse before, let alone ridden one. Naturally, I was determined to do as well as my classmates, as I believed that the grade in that "course" counted on my grade-point average. The practical part of the final exam found about 50 of us on horseback in a large quadrangle, required to walk, trot, canter, and gallop around the four sides. When it was my turn, my horse took off at a full gallop going diagonally. I was very embarrassed, especially so when Lieutenant Lazonby said to me, "Get off that horse, son. Let me show you how to ride him." The Lieutenant was dressed marvelously in his khaki uniform and his *kepi*, a French military cap with a flat circular top and a visor, and looked splendid with his fine mustache and bravado. However, the horse again took off diagonally and threw him. My classmates applauded, but not wanting the Lieutenant to feel badly, I was quiet. I got a good grade in horse drawn artillery, and perhaps this was a symbol of adapting to the less urban atmosphere of the University of Florida in those days.

When I was elected to Phi Beta Kappa in my junior year, I understood that I had a better chance of getting into medical school with that kind of academic performance. This was a period, however, when Jewish students with good grades could not be secure about being accepted into medical school. I had been fortunate throughout my life in very rarely meeting anti-Semitism directly. My difficulty in getting into medical school (several turned me down) was one of the few examples of what I deemed to be anti-Semitism, even though that, too, was indirect. My last year at the University of Florida, when I was 17, was, of course, affected by the United States having entered World War II. I decided to postpone my medical education temporarily and volunteered for the Army, where I started at Camp Blanding, Florida, and was soon transferred to Fort McPherson, outside of Atlanta. At Fort McPherson, I had several experiences that made me wonder if I should have volunteered.

The most memorable involved a large assembly of soldiers standing at attention and the sergeant saying, "Would all college graduates step forward." I was one of the four of the several hundred soldiers who stepped forward. We were taken to a truck and transported to a forest to do heavy digging and carrying of trees.

After a day of brooding, I walked into the Fort's post office and asked if they needed an experienced postman. Lo and behold, I was accepted right away. While it may be an exaggeration to say that my capacity to read and write well was unusual at Fort McPherson, I was certainly better than average in forwarding mail. I stayed there for about a month, during which time I forwarded my medical school application to Tulane University, including the letter from President Tigert. I was transferred from Georgia to New York City, where in early 1944 there was a military compound at the Uptown Campus of City College. There was a good deal of processing activity, and I was ultimately sent to LaGarde General Hospital in New Orleans almost simultaneously with my being accepted at Tulane Medical School for the class entering later that year. I could have gone on to enter the Army Special Training Programs (ASTP) in medical school, a program established and funded by the government to increase the number of doctors. This was, however, near the end of the war, and the Army changed its policy about letting those with admissions to medical school enter as members of the military. I was honorably discharged from the service to go to Tulane Medical School late in 1944, having spent only one year in the Army. The GI Bill of Rights paid for about the first two years of my medical school.

At LaGarde General Hospital, I became friendly with William Sorum and James Rogers, both of whom had also been accepted at Tulane Medical School. Rogers came from Morrow, Georgia, just outside of Atlanta, and was modest and relatively quiet but exceedingly intelligent. Sorum was very large, rambunctious, and an omnivorous reader. He became the lifeguard at the hospital's swimming pool and was also on the hospital football team. Rogers, also, made the team. Before coming to LaGarde Hospital, Sorum had flunked out of Officers Training but remained a corporal. Nothing made him happier than to wake me in the barracks in the morning with the loud cry of "*Rausschmitt!*" (Get up!); if I didn't comply immediately, he would turn the bed over. Among my accomplishments during that time, I dated a sergeant of the Motor Pool, Technical Sergeant Laura McQueen, which helped to ensure good local transportation.

At LaGarde I was assigned to a dermatology division that was primarily involved in diagnosing and treating patients with venereal disease. Any soldier found to have a positive blood test for syphilis was investigated for central nervous system syphilis by having his spinal fluid, as well as blood, tested. As an 18-year-old member of the medical team, I learned how to do the spinal taps myself and assisted Major Stoller, who headed the Dermatology unit. Occasionally, I was also given the additional duty of working on an internal medicine ward at the hospital. While I was on duty there, one soldier was diagnosed with fatal coccidiomycosis. When he died, I was very upset and remember one of the internists taking me aside and telling me that if I went into medicine, I would have to get used to such things happening. Several years after this event, when I was a junior medical student at Charity Hospital in New Orleans, I made a diagnosis of the rarely occurring coccidiomycosis that turned out to be correct. This astounded the staff and was probably one of the reasons that I finished first in my class.

The period at LaGarde General Hospital occurred during the time of much uncertainty about the war in Europe, and we all followed the progress of the battles in the Soviet Union as well as North Africa. It was a time of generally warm feelings toward the Soviet Union. Sorum, Rogers, and I were influenced by several soldiers who had strong pro-Communist leanings. For the next seven or eight years, I remained interested in these activities in New Orleans, only to change my political opinions radically by events of the mid-1950s.

My medical school education at Tulane was on a somewhat accelerated wartime basis, so the length of the training was about 3½ rather than 4 years. For the initial two years of basic medical sciences, I was at the uptown campus of Tulane, and I completed the last two years in a facility next to Charity Hospital in downtown New Orleans. The first-year course in gross anatomy was regarded as the most difficult freshman course, and there was a good deal of anxiety on my part about not being able to pass the course. I also had some anxiety about working on the cadavers. My roommate, Jim Rogers, and I were dissection partners; he was much better at the work than I was, but I probably remembered the details better than he did. The chief instructor in gross anatomy, Wilbur "Bull" Smith, was an absolute tyrant who loved to walk around the class and tell students how badly they were doing. He seemed to enjoy grabbing me by the shirt collar and taking me to another part of the room to view a superior dissection, saying, "Sabshin, this is the way you do it." I, of course, was terrified. For the final practical exam, once again, as with my horse-drawn artillery, I had a traumatic but successful experience. There was a cadaver in Smith's office, bedecked with hundreds of pins placed in different areas, and he would question four students at a time about what they observed. When we arrived in his office, he said, "Sabshin, I think it would do you good to have to repeat this whole year, so I'm not going to ask you any questions." I sat through the entire exam without being asked a single question and with great anxiety about failing medical school. I had done well, however, in all of the other exams, and had I been more empathic, I would have understood that he was teasing me and that I should not have been so afraid. I ended up passing with a very high grade.

I continued to do well in medical school, achieving my highest status at the end of the junior year when it was reported on the school bulletin board that I finished first in the class of 130. I did not do quite so well in my senior year, but I did have the honor at the beginning of that year of being selected as the first student to present a case at Professor Ochsner's surgical Grand Rounds. Alton Ochsner, of course, was the famous founder of the Ochsner Clinic and chairman of the Department of Surgery at Tulane Medical School. Each Saturday morning, a medical student was assigned the task of examining a surgical patient and appearing in an amphitheater with the patient in front of the entire junior and senior classes, to be interrogated by Professor Ochsner. I still remember the 55-year-old male patient who had circulatory problems in one of his legs along with a diagnosis of diabetes. I had hoped to steer the conversation toward the diabetes, about which I thought I knew something, and away from the gross anatomy of the leg, but Ochsner was, of course, way ahead of me. I remember him drawing pictures of the blood vessels of the leg on the blackboard and quizzing me about them and their pathology. At the end, he congratulated me for my courage. He was one of the charismatic people who, quite early in anti-cigarette policies, would become exceptionally angry when seeing someone smoke. In addition, if you walked into one of his lectures late, he might throw a blackboard eraser at you. He was an unforgettable teacher.

My work on the coccidiomycosis patient made me popular in the Department of Internal Medicine. During my time at Tulane, there was a change in the chairmanship of the department when John Musser, the prolific writer of a great textbook of internal medicine (Musser 1934), stepped down and was replaced by the young George Burch, a pioneer of electrocardiography (Burch 1953).

I was most influenced, however, by the appointment of Robert Heath as chairman of the Department of Psychiatry and Neurology. I was fortunate to have the opportunity for significant contact with Heath. By the beginning of my senior year, I had decided that I would go into psychiatry. While I had complied with my parents' wishes to be in medical school, I found psychiatry to be much more absorbing and intellectually stimulating than other specialties. Whereas the previous leadership in the Department of Psychiatry had been part-time and less charismatic,

Heath was involved in developing a broadly based department of psychiatry, including psychoanalysis and neuroscience. When I decided upon going into psychiatry, I chose first to seek an internship at Bellevue Hospital in New York, and then to take a psychiatric residency there, as well. That was one of the first indicators of my desire to return to my home city of New York for nostalgic reasons as well as professional opportunities. Heath, however, convinced me to apply to his new program at Tulane, and I made a fateful decision to stay in New Orleans. I took my internship at Charity Hospital during 1948–49 and enjoyed it thoroughly, including the two 6-week experiences in the emergency room that included the old-fashioned experience of interns riding on the ambulances. I did some home obstetric deliveries and carried out a great deal of suturing work after ordinary Saturday nights in the many bars of that exciting city.

I was elected as one of the officers of the residents' group and participated in one "major" victory. The entire Charity Hospital had been segregated between the W (white) and C (colored) sides. The only place where segregation did not occur was in the Blood Bank, but an effort had begun to segregate that area as well. I led the fight against that segregation and was successful. Charity Hospital had been a special project of Governor Huey Long, and it was a great teaching facility, but its segregation policy was a terrible flaw.

I began my three-year residency in psychiatry at Tulane. The kind of work that I did reflected the composite hodgepodge of approaches that existed in the psychiatry of that time. We used insulin treatment for quite psychotic patients with schizophrenia. We treated depressed people with electric shock and used the induction of malaria to produce fever in patients with psychosis due to central nervous system syphilis. At the same time, the new faculty that Heath brought down from Columbia included several psychoanalysts and neurophysiologists. I entered into psychoanalysis myself with one of the staff analysts who was exceptionally interested in both psychoanalysis and anthropology. Norman Rucker had come from Tennessee to train at Columbia University in New York and moved down to Tulane along with Bob Heath, Harold Leif, and Russell Monroe. Rucker was very deeply interested in the work of Abram Kardiner, whose books *The Individual and His Society* and *The Psychological Frontiers of Society* (Kardiner 1939, 1945) attempted to formulate basic personality styles in different cultures. I was very much impressed with the implications of Kardiner's work. Cultural factors had an important impact on human development!

Heath's own investigation of neural functions and schizophrenia was significantly innovative and daring. He led a group of investigators studying subcortical stimulation of patients with severe schizophrenia. His books on this subject, such as *Studies in Schizophrenia: A Multidisciplinary Approach to Mind-Brain Relationships* (Heath et al. 1954), which, of course, preceded the late-century neuropsychiatric revolution, were interesting at several levels. He encouraged all of the residents in psychiatry to become involved in the work, and the research aura that surrounded his department was particularly influential upon my own career. The eclecticism and the openness to new ideas shaped many of my professional choices.

During my internship at Charity Hospital, before I entered the psychiatric residency and while serving on a pediatric ward, I met Bettye Smith, who was working on a pediatric rotation to Charity Hospital from Laurel General Hospital in Laurel, Mississippi. She had beautiful red hair, a deep southern drawl, and a very strong interest in the young children hospitalized at that time. The complexities of pediatrics included being able to insert a needle into a baby's very small cranial veins, and during this procedure Bettye often assisted me (or vice versa). We developed strong feelings for each other while working with these children, and we eloped on impulse, going to Mississippi for a quick wedding. My parents, as well as hers, were somewhat shocked at the time. Both set of relatives ultimately adapted, but Bettye and I gradually drifted apart; the difference in interests was larger than either of us had previously realized. Our son, Jim, named after James Rogers, was born in November 1950, and Bettye was a marvelous mother. But we both knew that we were part of an incompatible marriage that was not going to last. We finally separated in 1952, and Bettye moved to California, where she married a previous suitor. Jim had gone with her. I was able to visit California often and remained friendly with Bettye and her family, which soon included two more sons. Subsequent to the death of her second husband, she had a lot of difficulties and sadly died at a relatively young age in California.

After the separation, my friends in New Orleans were very helpful to me. Bill Sorum had entered the psychiatric residency at Tulane one year after I did. He and his wife, Monica, were dear friends. Jim Rogers had difficulties in finding a medical career and undertook several periods of *locum tenens* (temporary practice). He named his first son Melvin and moved back to Georgia ultimately, where he died prematurely. Also particularly helpful to me were my colleague Arthur Epstein and his future wife, Leona Cruz. Arthur, after completing neurology training, entered psychiatric residency one year after me. He was very able in teaching both psychiatry and neurology. In addition he wrote novels. Leona was a very dear friend and was particularly helpful to me after my separation from Bettye and from my son Jim.

I was fortunate to be able to see Jim frequently during his childhood in California, and we also spent time together on marvelous vacations, most notably in Jackson Hole, Wyoming. Despite my repeated comments about his freedom to choose whatever career he wished, I was delighted by his choice of medicine and of neurosurgery. He is now a leading practitioner and educator in New Haven. Three of his four daughters have entered the mental health field, two as psychiatrists and one as a psychotherapist.

Many of the events that I have described as occurring in my residency took place during the height of the McCarthy era in the United States. I had had several contacts with agents of the FBI and staff members of the House Un-American Activities Committee. It turned out that I was never important enough to be called before the committee for national testimony, but I will never forget some of the committee staff members' particular perspective. I have vivid memories of one telling me about the extramarital sexual affairs of black leaders in the United States, hoping that I would agree how bad they were.

During the latter part of my psychiatric residency, there were unique opportunities but also special problems. One opportunity was my traveling weekly to Lafayette, Louisiana, to examine psychiatric referrals to that facility. I would fly from New Orleans to Baton Rouge and on to Lafayette every Thursday morning and then back at night after having seen patients all day long. The patients were selected by a clinical psychologist, Richard Miles, in that clinic. There were no other psychiatrists in Lafayette at that time. The patients I saw were quite similar to those previously untreated people seen in Charcot's hospital, in Paris at the turn of the twentieth century. They included people with hysterical syndromes and severe anxiety disorders. A few of the patients only spoke French, and there were two that I remember vividly who did not comprehend that English was spoken as the dominant language in Louisiana. They lived in remarkable rural isolation. The Cajun influence was pervasive. Lafayette, of course, has long since become a thriving city with a strong psychiatric contingent.

During the McCarthy era pressure was placed upon the medical school and the Department of Psychiatry to take some action against a professor of neurophysiology in the department named Robert Hodes. Hodes had been with Heath at Columbia University before coming to Tulane and was a key figure in implementing the subcortical studies in schizophrenia. Allegations had been made about Hodes's Communist activities and trumped-up charges were made about his professional competency. Efforts were begun to take away his faculty position. Several of us rallied to defend him, and I was one of the leaders of that effort. We called for an investigation by the American Association of University Professors (AAUP), and, indeed, to the embarrassment of the medical school and the Department of Psychiatry, a "formal" hearing was held. Somewhere in the long course of that hearing, Professor Hodes and his wife disappeared. It was months before I found out that they had defected to Communist China. I was shocked and had strong feelings of betrayal by the Hodes. The combination of those feelings and my divorce from Bettye Smith convinced me that I needed to leave New Orleans and to seek some new starts.

I chose two superb facilities to investigate for a possible position: the Western Psychiatric Institute at the University of Pittsburgh and the Psychiatric and Psychosomatic Institute of Michael Reese Hospital of Chicago. I had read a good deal about the faculty at Pittsburgh, which included major psychoanalytic programs and biological research. But Roy Grinker, who headed the Institute in Chicago, was a brilliant neurologist as well as psychoanalyst with a very deep interest in major philosophical and psychiatric questions (Grinker and Spiegel 1945). He accepted me as a salaried staff member of his Institute even though he had been warned by the FBI of my political involvement. That he still chose me played a decisive role in my subsequent life.

REFERENCES

Burch GE: A Primer of Cardiology, 2nd Edition. Philadelphia, PA, Lea & Febiger, 1953

Grinker RR, Spiegel J: Men Under Stress. Philadelphia, PA, Blakiston, 1945

Heath RG: Studies in Schizophrenia: A Multidisciplinary Approach to Mind-Brain Relationships. Cambridge, MA, Harvard University Press, 1954

Kardiner A: The Individual and His Society: The Psychodynamics of Primitive Social Organization. New York, Columbia University Press, 1939

Kardiner A: The Psychological Frontiers of Society. New York, Columbia University Press, 1945

Musser JH (ed): Internal Medicine: Its Theory and Practice in Contributions by American Authors, 2nd Edition. Philadelphia, PA, Lea & Febiger, 1934

3

Implicit Preparations for a Leadership Role in Psychiatry

*I*n the middle 1950s I was not fully aware of how fortunate I was in working for Roy Grinker. In later years, I have often thought of his extraordinary talents and how much I learned from him. Roy was the Director of the Institute for Psychosomatic Research and Training (known as the PPI) at Michael Reese Hospital. His career had been distinguished in its breadth and in his remarkable ability to conceptualize and measure the integration of multiple systems. After training in neurology he became interested in psychiatry and psychoanalysis. He had a period of analysis with Sigmund Freud in Vienna and simultaneously became absorbed in general systems theory, which eventually resulted in *Towards a Unified Theory of Human Behavior* (Grinker 1967). As noted earlier, Grinker became a major psychiatric leader in World War II and, along with John Spiegel, authored the book *Men Under Stress,* which played a key role in helping to understand the psychiatric casualties of the war (Grinker and Spiegel 1945). The studies reported in that book were central for many of the major modifications in postwar psychiatry. Grinker's dream of creating a facility in Chicago, where psychosomatic processes could be studied at multiple levels, was actually achieved with the opening of the Psychosomatic and Psychiatric Institute, or PPI, in 1951. Stimulated by his wartime experiences, he had become particularly interested in research on anxiety, which he formulated in "transactional" terms, or as the simultaneous and sequential interplay of multiple variables. He emphasized that there were many biochemical, physiological, psychological, and sociological variables involved in the etiology and treatment of anxiety. This transactional model called for evaluating how a complex interaction of multiple variables produced psychiatric and somatic symptoms. Engel's "biopsychosocial" model (Engel 1980) has become a popular way of specifying a multivariable system that has produced a sequential series of changes.

In the early 1950s, Grinker and several members of his staff published the results of a study of paratroopers training at Fort Benning, Georgia. Grinker and his colleagues investigated the soldiers' adaptation and maladaptation to the stressful conditions of training for parachute jumping (see Basowitz 1955 for summary). Incorporating his interest in general systems theory, Grinker formulated a novel conceptual and systematic method of studying anxiety. He studied subjects who frequently experienced very high anxiety, and measured a wide variety of accompanying physiological, chemical, and psychological changes over time. The measurements were repeated when the subjects' anxiety had been reduced. He also attempted to induce anxiety in research volunteers after learning what psychological stimuli might produce the concerns in each individual. Along with colleagues, I stood behind a two-way mirror and rated levels of anxiety, anger, and depression before and after stressful experiences, using empirically derived rating systems. We were very interested in the reliability of such scales and published our findings (Hamburg et al. 1958).

For this research project, Grinker brought together a superb group of psychologists, chemists, physiologists, and psychiatrists. When I came to Michael Reese Hospital as a research psychiatrist, David Hamburg had just been appointed associate director of the Institute, and he became a close colleague, as did Donald Oken, Daniel Offer, Sheldon Korchin, Harold Basowitz, Harold Persky, James Toman, and John Spiegel (Basowitz et al. 1956; Grinker et al. 1956).

One special attribute that Grinker brought to bear in his study of psychosomatic processes was his intense interest in the application of general systems theory. He was the leader of a small national group of theoreticians who met regularly to discuss a general systems theory in a wide variety of contexts, and published extensively in the field of the philosophy of science (Grinker 1967). The research at Michael Reese Hospital reflected Grinker's strong belief that scientific theory was an integral part of modern psychiatry. Grinker's major formulations were about psychosomatic processes; his broad scope and his innovative research methodologies were extraordinary and far ahead of his time. His attempt to find an integrated understanding of complex behavior contrasted markedly with the work of those who studied simpler, two-dimensional inter-actions. Grinker's theoretical model and his transactional research seem applicable in contemporary psychiatric research, yet his research meth-odology is seldom mentioned in the literature today. Perhaps his theo-retical constructs for the empirical research are a barrier.

In addition to its many contributions to research, the PPI had a large clinical program. It took care of about 75 psychiatric inpatients at a time, administered a fine outpatient clinic, and maintained several high-level advanced educational programs. The psychiatric residency was particu-larly relevant in reflecting the psychiatry of the 1950s. Grinker had ar-ranged for an affiliation of the Michael Reese Residency Program with the residency programs in the Departments of Psychiatry at the University of Chicago and the University of Illinois. The overall program had been ini-tiated and originated by the Chicago Institute for Psychoanalysis headed by Franz Alexander. The three residents selected for this program annu-ally spent a year at each of the three institutions and were accepted for concurrent psychoanalytic training at the Institute. This close relation-ship between analytic and psychiatric training was an excellent example of the close ties between the analytic and psychiatric training programs that existed at that time. The other psychiatric trainees at PPI also spent much of their time in psychodynamic work (Wallerstein 1991). A psychi-atric institute headed by a brilliant critic of analysis had established a residency program that was dominated by psychoanalytic principles. Joan Fleming, Director of Training at the Psychoanalytic Institute, held a weekly case seminar at PPI that was very popular and stimulating. For me the Fleming clinical seminar represented a peak experience of the res-idency program. Fleming was a charismatic clinician who been trained as a teacher before going to medical school. She taught with eloquence, forcefulness, and a dramatic flair.

David Hamburg and I conducted a research seminar for residents throughout their last two years of residency and encouraged an open-mindedness for new data. For example, we discussed journal articles, modeling how to critically appraise research methodology, and encour-aged residents to pursue research projects. We had an occasional impact on some trainees, but the effect was limited by the prevailing psycho-analytic ideology. Although Grinker himself was often highly critical of psychoanalytic formulations, his commitment to psychoanalysis attracted many psychoanalysts as teachers in the psychiatric residency training. He also employed psychoanalytic concepts in his own research, such as "defense mechanisms" against anxiety, and in his clinical practice. Grinker considered the field of psychoanalysis as being full of interest-ing ideas that needed to be validated by testable hypotheses.

Given the culture of PPI, the interests of many friends and colleagues, and my awareness of some of my own personal problems, it was not surprising that I became interested in psychoanalytic training. I matriculated at the Chicago Institute for Psychoanalysis and completed psychoanalytic training in 1962. While I never intended to be a full-time practitioner, I did analyze patients as part of the training process and continued to do so until I left Chicago in 1974. While a number of my patients improved dramatically, others did not. I never fully understood how much of the lack of progress was due to my ineptness as compared with other plausible explanations.

The years of training at the Chicago Institute for Psychoanalysis were interesting and challenging. Some teachers were especially exciting (Franz Alexander, Joan Fleming, Heinz Kohut, Gerhart Piers, Therese Benedek). Fleming, in the process of supervising one of my analytic cases, discussed the handling of one of my analysands, in her and Benedek's book on psychoanalytic training (Fleming and Benedek 1966), as an example of learning issues. Toward the end of my analytic training I became a member of a group preparing for the final exam. While studying for our final Institute examination was the primary aim of the group, we put together several papers, two of which were published (Gedo et al. 1964; Sadow et al. 1968).

My professional experiences at PPI were valuable and exciting; my own personal maturation was also accelerated during those years. One of the most fortunate events in my life was my meeting with Edith Goldfarb, one of the psychiatric trainees who rotated through the three residency programs under the auspices of the Chicago Institute for Psychoanalysis. She was enormously attractive, brilliant, and one of the most psychologically astute people that I had ever met. After a very happy courtship, we married in June 1955. For all her talents, she was modest, kind, and very loving with me. Prior to entering medical school, as a young Yale-trained physicist, she had been selected to participate in the Manhattan Project on atomic energy at the University of Chicago. As a young researcher she worked with an extraordinary team of senior atomic physicists. She had the unique opportunity to play tennis as well as discuss scientific theory with Enrico Fermi. After the war, when she evaluated her prospects in physics as compared with other fields, she decided to become a physician, and her application to the University of Chicago School of Medicine was supported by physicists and physicians. She was accepted and did well at medical school, where she decided to become a psychiatrist. Henry Brosin was Chair of Psychiatry at that time and played an important role in her choice of specialty. Upon completion of her residency, rotating at Illinois, Chicago, and Michael Reese Hospital, Edith continued her psychoanalytic training and began an appointment with the Chicago Institute for Psycho-analysis that continued until she left Chicago to join me in Washington in 1976. I was fortunate to have a wife who was enormously talented, very loving, and very successful in her own career. She carried on clinical re-search; especially important was her involvement with Joan Fleming in psychoanalytic studies of patients who, as children, had lost a parent. She was also particularly interested in psychoanalytic education and became the Director of Training of the Chicago Institute for Psychoanalysis. Her project on supervising psychoanalytic cases was a model program of psy-choanalysis at its best without pomp, authoritarianism, or rigid ideology. She demonstrated an open-minded, subtle clinical capacity that has not always been associated with psychoanalysts. Edith was an excellent ther-apist and teacher. For me, she will always represent the very best of what psychoanalysis can accomplish.

Edith encouraged my career and I attempted to reciprocate, but I re-alized, of course, that my moving to Washington in 1974 was very difficult for her, with many considerations about her patients and her responsibil-ities at the Institute. She moved to Washington almost two years after I did and became an active teacher and supervisor in the Washington Psy-choanalytic Institute. She was also very much involved as a leader in the American Psychoanalytic Association, where she was elected a national officer and also nominated for the presidency. She continued to teach and to practice until she became ill and died in 1993, leaving me devastated.

My melancholia lasted for several years, and I was on the path to becoming a quiet retiree when good fortune and personal resilience changed everything. The good fortune involved being introduced to Marion Bennathan. She was charming, brilliant, personable, and ex-tremely attractive. She was also a formidable leader who needed some-body not easily intimidated by her remarkable capabilities. For two people in their 70s the chemistry and the social psychology merged into a love affair that overcame the barriers of years and an ocean. We married in 2000 and since then have divided our time between London and Wash-ington.

Marion is an educational psychologist who is a leader of the U.K. na-tional movement to promote nurture groups, which assist children with developmental psychosocial problems to cope better in mainstream school. Her organization, the Nurture Group Network, has succeeded in the United Kingdom and has begun to spread to other countries. Her many colleagues have welcomed me wholeheartedly to their meetings and have taught me a great deal about how understanding attachment the-ory transforms teaching practice and the ethos of schools. Marion's fam-ily and friends have also accepted me as being worthy of her.

My responsibilities at PPI increased over time, and I was appointed Assistant Director under Grinker and Hamburg. Later I became Associate Director when Hamburg left to assume distinguished leadership positions that subsequently led him to the National Institute of Mental Health, Chair of the Department of Psychiatry at Stanford, and eventually the Directorship of the Institute of Medicine. His career has been outstanding as a scientist and as a statesman.

While I had many responsibilities in clinical work at the hospital and in training programs, I was also quite active in several research projects that I had initiated. On reflection now, it is apparent that these projects played an important role in my subsequent career. I chose research projects on what became increasingly apparent to me to be major problems for the field as a whole. The research findings were interesting, as such, but their implications for how psychiatry needed to be changed became central for my career pathway.

The first project, in which I worked with Dan Offer, turned out to be quite relevant to how I perceived psychiatry as a whole. We began a study of "normal" teenagers who had been selected by interviews and objective instruments at several Chicago high schools. Dan, later joined by his wife, Margy, became involved in long-term studies of these adolescent subjects, and indeed they have recently published a significant 30-year follow-up (Offer et al. 2004). Over time, as I worked on the project, my interest in the policy implications of how we define pathology and normality became increasingly central in my thinking. Offer and I recognized that normality was defined quite differently by various groups and from different perspectives within psychiatry. The biologically oriented psychiatrists, for example, tended to utilize a classical medical model that defined psychiatric illness as involving the presence of qualitatively disturbed behavior or mental illness. Normality, in the classical medical sense, referred to the residual population not having such illness. In almost all populations the prevalence of mental illness was small compared with the overwhelming majority of "normals." No attempt was made by this group of psychiatrists to characterize this population except for the absence of an illness. The psychoanalysts, on the other hand, appeared to employ a concept that implied some degree of psychological disturbance as the rule and "normality" as the exception. Most often, this perspective was not a specifically enunciated hypothesis but could be deduced from psychoanalytic concepts and practice (Offer and Sabshin 1966). It is unlikely that many potential patients were rejected for treatment by analysts because they were "too normal." Human development involves experiencing significant problems that are seldom fully solved. All human beings tend toward utilizing some "neurotic" defenses. Such a conceptual scheme, therefore, is quite alien to the ordinary pathological or medical orientation. By the 1960s, much of the public perceived psychiatry as merely treating the "worried well" (Kirk and Kutchins 1992). Convinced that these viewpoints seriously weakened psychiatry as a medical discipline, I had begun, by the early 1960s, to believe that psychiatrists needed to reassert their medical identity. The drive to remedicalization became a central tenet of my career (Sabshin 1990).

Offer and I studied attitudes of various psychiatrists to definitions of normality. We explained the subject in several books (Offer and Sasbhin 1966, 1991), discussing how the definition of normality, especially in psychology, was also approached by a statistical average concept. Psychiatrists did not often perceive normality as "average" behavior. Offer and I also postulated the possibility of studying normal behavior over the entire life cycle to see how the concepts of what constituted normal behavior might change over time (Offer and Sabshin 1984). The Offers' work on this subject has become important in research upon the life cycle systems (Offer et al. 2004). Studies of normal behavior, adaptation to stress, and the so-called positive definitions of healthy behavior have become increasingly important in recent years. Resilience has also become popular (Charney 2004), and a broader concept of adaptive behavior may ultimately emerge from new genome studies. The psychobiology of resilience will be very important in the next decades.

Back in the 1950s and the 1960s, however, I became concerned that the implicit "universality of illness" concept, in a time of increasing accountability, would frighten away potential supporters of psychiatry and weaken its standing. The psychoanalytic implication of an almost universal prevalence of disorder was, in my judgment, an Achilles heel in the emerging managed care system. It must be emphasized that, with a few exceptions, psychoanalysts did not explicitly enunciate a theory of the universality of illness; the ubiquity of psychopathology was a product of their concept of frequent developmental problems, the employment of defenses by all of us, and the power of common unconscious conflicts. If psychiatry continued to employ these concepts, it would ultimately abdicate its place in medicine. By the 1970s psychiatry's position in medicine was already tottering and under severe challenge (Hackett 1977).

I also became concerned by the fractionation of American psychiatry among several conflicting ideologies, most of which were unsupported by scientific evidence (Strauss et al. 1964). Known as "somato-therapeutic," "psychotherapeutic," and "socio-therapeutic," each of these ideologies stressed a qualitatively distinct approach to the etiology and treatment of mental illness. Focusing on genetic and biological factors, somato-

therapists advocated biologic treatments such as medications, electroconvulsive therapy, and insulin shock therapy. Disregarding Sigmund Freud's
early work emphasizing biological formulations, the psychotherapists,
most of whom were psychoanalysts, highlighted psychological etiologies
and treatment. In contrast, sociotherapists recommended social interventions, since they perceived social, cultural, and economic factors as
the main causes of psychiatric problems. The ideologues existed in separate worlds of psychiatry, dominated particular training centers, and
employed divergent approaches. In considering how to study ideologies, I
was very much influenced by the work of Dan Levinson and his colleagues
at the Boston Psychopathic Hospital. They had been struck by two major
conflicting psychiatric ideologies at their institute, and they developed a
scale to measure the psychotherapeutic and sociotherapeutic positions
(Gilbert and Levinson 1956; Sharaf and Levinson 1957). The two deputy
directors of the Institute represented each of the ideologies in a very
powerful fashion. Milton Greenblatt was deeply interested in the sociotherapeutic processes, while Elvin Semrad was a powerful advocate for a
strong psychodynamic approach.

I was able to find resources to recruit a group of sociologists and psychologists, headed by Professor Anselm Strauss, to work at our institute
at Michael Reese Hospital.We borrowed heavily from Levinson's scales
but also postulated a third ideology, *somatotherapeutic,* which had been
adapted from a directive-organic scale discussed by Hollingshead and
Redlich (1958) that was included in their study of social class and mental
illness. Danuta Ehrlich was the chief organizer of our questionnaire study
and has published a detailed account of the entire process (Ehrlich and
Sabshin 1963, 1964). We obtained samples of several groups of psychiatrists and other mental health professionals. Some were national samples, including the American Society of Medical Psychiatrists. With this
group we were helped by its internationally famous president Ladislas
Meduna. Ehrlich constructed our scale of 185 items very carefully and was
able to obtain clear and significant differentiation of three distinct ideological groups. The conflicts in theoretical models, formulations of etiology, and therapeutic practices were very striking. It would be interesting to repeat that questionnaire study today.

Our ultimate book on ideologies in psychiatry (Strauss et al. 1964)
achieved a high degree of attention from sociologists across the world.
Some psychiatrists seemed irritated by ideological labels. However, the
lack of ideological research within the field suggests a passive indif-
ference among psychiatrists to the potentially vast implications of the
existence of these scientifically unsupported dogmas. As in the studies
on normality, my immersion in the subject ultimately translated into a

criticism of American psychiatry in the post–World War II decades. I was convinced that a field dominated by ideology had severe weaknesses and that its credibility would be decimated by disputes, quarrels, and misunderstandings. I fantasized about how to replace ideology with rational and evidence-based approaches to the diagnosis and treatment of mental illness. Helping to transform psychiatry into a reputable field based on sound scientific principles eventually became a strong personal ambition. I was ready to increase my role as a leader but needed more preparation before immersing myself in the problems of the profession.

In 1960, the position of head of the Department of Psychiatry at the University of Illinois College of Medicine became vacant with the retirement of Francis Gerty. He had also been president of the American Psychiatric Association in 1958–59. I was approached by the search committee chairman, Professor Harry Dowling, who was the head of the Department of Internal Medicine at the university. There was little hesitation on my part to become a candidate. After a number of challenging interviews, I was recommended by the search committee to the dean for appointment. The dean, Granville Bennett, was an eminent pathologist and straight as an arrow. He appointed me to become head of the Department of Psychiatry, starting in September 1961.

The medical school of this great state university was the largest in the United States in terms of the number of students. It continued to grow even larger on several sites during the days of a perceived physician shortage through the 1970s and 1980s (Council on Graduate Medical Education 1996). Under the leadership of a new, ambitious and talented dean, William Grove, the medical college reorganized into a basic science school and multiple clinical schools located in different parts of the state. To be the department chair had many attractions. It was particularly exciting for me to get to know what medical students of that generation were like. Early in my career in Illinois, I organized an informal group of students interested in psychiatry, who met with me once a week. Many of them later entered psychiatry, and some of them are now good friends.

I became deeply involved in medical education at the medical center. I was also particularly stimulated by the presence of a preeminent medical education unit in the medical school, headed by Dr. George Miller. Miller's emphasis on student learning rather than on what was taught (Miller 1961) permeated the pedagogy of most of the departments. Student examinations emphasized measurement of learning and problem-solving skills, not simply memorization of facts

The medical center had associated with it the Neuropsychiatric Institute, in which the Department of Psychiatry was located. We shared the

Institute building with the Departments of Neurology and Neurosurgery. In expanding the activities of the department, I appointed a number of new staff to the faculty. Clinical psychology was particularly improved by the recruitment of Dr. Theodore Millon, who went on to became world famous for his work on personology and taxonomy (Millon 1968, 1969, 1981, 1996). He also became a very good friend and colleague. I have had many close colleagues in clinical psychology, even when later in my career a sharp conflict about prescription privilege rights developed between the professions. I ensured that psychologists had major educational, clinical, research, and administrative responsibilities.

I also recruited the eminent psychoanalyst Dr. Merton Gill to conduct empirical research on psychoanalytic and psychotherapeutic processes. Working in an office with a two-way mirror where he could observe treatment, Gill conducted exhaustive studies upon the clinical phenomena (Gill 1963). I had also become interested in educational aspects of social psychiatry while at Michael Reese (Sabshin 1973) and taught a course to the psychiatric residents in which I led discussions on the social psychiatry of the 1960s and 70s, especially concentrating upon the work of Alfred H. Stanton, Morris S. Schwartz, W. A. Caudill (Caudill 1958; Stanton and Schwartz 1954), and Abram Kardiner (Kardiner 1978).

I continued my interest in social and community psychiatry while at the University of Illinois. Once again I was interested in conceptual questions—this time about the scope of social psychiatry—and I wanted to distinguish such interests from concerns about social issues in general. During the 1960s psychiatrists in the United States had taken public stances on several social policy issues such as the Vietnam war, poverty, and education. I had became concerned, as had many other colleagues, that acting as if we were experts on these important questions blurred our image further and that we needed to be clear on what were the proper concerns of psychiatry and what were not. Taking too broad a stance was as big an error as taking no stance. From my perspective, social psychiatry dealt with the interaction between psychiatry and directly relevant social variables. Community psychiatry was an application of social psychiatric principles to a particular population area. Community psychiatry had become increasingly important in the 1960s and 1970s as state mental hospitals markedly reduced the number of their patients (Brown 1985). Legislation supporting community treatment also was important in providing new funds for therapeutic care. My department assumed responsibility for psychiatric care in an area adjacent to our Medical Center. The program was modestly successful in its aim but would have been stronger had it been part of an overall medical involvement in the community in which all the clinical departments participated.

In the 1960s I recruited to the department three young Yale psychiatrists who had intriguing ideas about incorporating community psychiatry into public school education. Sheppard Kellam, Edward Futterman, and Sheldon Schiff developed a program in the Woodlawn area of Chicago, located on the south side of the city, more than five miles away from our Medical Center (Kellam and Schiff 1967; Schiff and Kellam 1967). The three of them spent most of their time in the community program, especially working with children. They did spend time informing me about the project and its needs. I was not able to make their project as central to the department as I would have liked. Ultimately the project was transferred to the Department of Psychiatry at the University of Chicago, which was much closer to the work.

Our community psychiatry projects both in Woodlawn and in the neighborhood adjacent to the University of Illinois involved areas with almost entirely African American populations. Several African American psychiatric residents in my program taught me a great deal about institutional racism (Sabshin et al. 1970).

The Department of Psychiatry at Illinois was involved in a wide range of activities. It had a laboratory in biological psychiatry headed by a leading neuroscientist, Dr. Leo Abood (Abood 1959). This laboratory had a distinguished history, previously having been led by Ladislas Meduna and Percival Bailey, both of whom had eminent research careers (Bailey 1956; Meduna 1955). Bailey, a neurosurgeon interested in psychiatric research, played an important role in building the Illinois State Psychiatric Institute (ISPI), which was located just a few blocks from our Neuropsychiatric Institute. Much later ISPI became fully affiliated with the University of Illinois. Frederick Gibbs, the eminent pioneer of electroencephalography (Gibbs and Gibbs 1941), also had an appointment there. Ernest Haggard and Rosalind Cartwright were important clinicians and researchers in a section on psychology. Haggard was active in studies in social isolation and conducted research on remote communities in Norway (Haggard 1954). Cartwright was an excellent researcher on sleep and dreaming (Cartwright 1978). Numerous psychiatrists, including psychoanalysts, accepted appointments in the department and did a great deal of teaching. I was fortunate during my time in Illinois to have recruited many talented residents in psychiatry, several of whom have had distinguished careers in various posts around the country.

I struggled to create an integrated department but, in actuality, did not achieve it at Illinois. The field itself was too divided, and my capacity to help in bringing it together was too limited.

I became increasingly involved in state and national activities in psychiatry. I assumed roles in the Illinois Psychiatric Society, including its presidency; I took part in Illinois State issues involving the Department of Mental Health, including serving on the Advisory Council to the Director of the State Mental Health program. Nationally, I served on several committees of the American Psychiatric Association (APA) and other organizations. I was elected to the office of Trustee on the APA's Board after a very close contest with Shervert Frazier and began to participate actively in several leadership roles. In 1972, I was appointed to the chair of the APA Program Committee, which had the responsibility of organizing APA's national annual convention program, and I played an active role in building the national convention into a much larger and educationally more effective program. In chairing the Program Committee and in a previous responsibility as Chair of the APA's Council on Research, I had an excellent opportunity to assist in the APA's commitment to scholarly research. My fantasies to change the field eventually materialized into a plan.

I spent a year at the Center for Advanced Studies in the Behavioral Sciences at Stanford in 1967–68, and that stimulated me to write and to think about how the activities I had become involved in might be integrated in my future professional life. When Alexander Schmidt, the dean of the Abraham Lincoln Medical School at the University of Illinois, was appointed director of the Food and Drug Administration in Washington, I was selected to replace him as the acting dean of the medical school. I spent an enjoyable and, I think, quite successful year in that role and might have been appointed permanent dean. Simultaneous with this, however, the eminent APA Medical Director Walter Barton decided to step down from his position, and a search committee to replace him was formed. When contacted by the committee as a potential candidate, I was faced with the choice of either continuing my work at the University of Illinois or seeking an opportunity for a special leadership position in psychiatry. The possibility for fulfilling my ambition was decisive for me.

REFERENCES

Abood LG: Some chemical concepts of mental health and disease, in The Effect of Pharmacologic Agents on the Nervous System. Proceedings of the Association for Research in Nervous and Mental Disease, Vol 37. Baltimore, MD, Williams & Wilkins, 1959

Bailey P: The great psychiatric revolution. Am J Psychiatry 113:387–406, 1956

Basowitz H: Anxiety and Stress. New York, McGraw-Hill, 1955

Basowitz H, Board FA, Chevalier JA, et al: A theoretical and experimental approach to problems of anxiety. AMA Arch Neurol Psychiatry 76:420–431, 1956

Brown P: The Transfer of Care: Psychiatric Deinstitutionalization and Its Aftermath. Boston, MA, Routledge & Kegan Paul, 1985

Cartwright RD: A Primer on Sleep and Dreaming. Reading, MA, Addison-Wesley, 1978

Caudill WA: Psychiatric Hospital as a Small Society. Cambridge, MA, Harvard University Press, 1958

Charney DS: Psychobiological mechanisms of resilience and vulnerability: implications for successful adaptation to extreme stress. Am J Psychiatry 161:195–216, 2004

Council on Graduate Medical Education: Patient Care Physician Supply and Requirements: Testing COGME Recommendations, Eighth Report (DHHS Publ No HRSA-P-DM95-3). Rockville MD, Bureau of Health Professions, Health Resources and Services Administration, 1996

Ehrlich D, Sabshin M: Psychiatric ideologies: their popularity and the meaningfulness of self-designation (abstract). Am Psychol 18:463, 1963

Ehrlich D, Sabshin M: A study of sociotherapeutically oriented psychiatrists. Am J Orthopsychiatry 34:469, 1964

Engel GL: The clinical application of the biopsychosocial model. Am J Psychiatry 137:535–544, 1980

Fleming J, Benedek TF: Psychoanalytic Supervision: A Method of Clinical Teaching. New York, Grune & Stratton, 1966

Gedo JE, Sabshin M, Sadow L, et al: "Studies on Hysteria": a methodological evaluation. J Am Psychoanal Assoc 12:734–751, 1964

Gibbs FA, Gibbs EL: Atlas of Electroencephalography. Cambridge, MA, Lew A Cummings, 1941

Gilbert DC, Levinson DJ: Ideology, personality and institutional policy in the mental hospital. J Abnorm Soc Psychol 53:263–271 1956

Gill M: Topography and Systems in Psychoanalytic Theory. New York, International Universities Press, 1963

Grinker RR (ed): Toward a Unified Theory of Human Behavior: An Introduction to General Systems Theory, 2nd Edition. New York, Basic Books, 1967

Grinker RR, Spiegel J: Men Under Stress. Philadelphia, PA, Blakiston, 1945

Grinker RR, Korchins SJ, Basowitz H,et al: A theoretical and experimental approach to problems of anxiety. AMA Arch Neurol Psychiatry 76:420–431, 1956

Hackett T: The psychiatrist: in the mainstream or on the banks of medicine? Am J Psychiatry 134:432–435, 1977

Haggard GA: Social status and intelligence. Genetic Psychology Monographs 49:141–186, 1954

Hamburg DA, Sabshin MA, Board FA, et al: Classification and rating of emotional experiences: special reference to reliability of observation. Arch Neurol Psychiatry 79:415–426, 1958

Hollingshead AB, Redlich FC: Social Class and Mental Illness. New York, Wiley, 1958

Kardiner A: The social distress syndrome of our time. J Am Acad Psychoanal 6:89–101, 1978

Kellam SG, Schiff SK: Adaptation and mental illness in the first-grade classrooms of an urban community. Psychiatric Research Reports of the American Psychiatric Association 21:79–91, 1967

Kirk S, Kutchins S: The Selling of DSM: The Rhetoric of Science in Psychiatry. New York, Aldine de Gruyter, 1992

Meduna LJ: The place of biological psychiatry in the evolution of human thought. J Nerv Ment Dis 121:1–4, 1955

Miller GE: Teaching and Learning in Medical School. Cambridge, MA, Harvard University Press, 1961

Miller JA, Sabshin M, Gedo JE, et al: Some aspects of Charcot's influence on Freud. J Am Psychoanal Assoc 17(2):608–623, 1969

Millon T: Approaches to Personality. New York, Pitman, 1968

Millon T: Modern Psychopathology: A Biosocial Approach to Maladaptive Learning and Functioning. Philadelphia, PA, WB Saunders, 1969

Millon T: Disorders of Personality: DSM-III, Axis II. New York, Wiley, 1981

Millon T: Disorders of Personality: DSM-IV and Beyond. New York, Wiley, 1996

Offer D, Sabshin M (eds): Normality: Theoretical and Clinical Concepts of Mental Health. New York, Basic Books, 1966

Offer D, Sabshin M (eds): Normality and the Life Cycle: A Critical Integration. New York, Basic Books, 1984

Offer D, Sabshin M (eds): Diversity of Normal Behavior: Further Contributions to Normatology. New York, Basic Books, 1991

Offer D, Offer MK, Ostrov E: Regular Guys: 34 Years Beyond Adolescence. New York, Kluwer Academic/Plenum, 2004

Sabshin M: Turning points in twentieth-century American psychiatry. Am J Psychiatry 147:1267–1274, 1990

Sabshin M: Theoretical models in community and social psychiatry, in Theories of Psychopathology and Personality. Edited by Millon T. Philadelphia, PA, WB Saunders, 1973

Sabshin M, Diesenhaus H, Wilkerson R: Dimensions of institutional racism in psychiatry. Am J Psychiatry 127:787–793, 1970

Sadow L, Gedo JE, Miller J, et al: The process of hypothesis change in three early psychoanalytic concepts. J Am Psychoanal Assoc 16:245–273, 1968

Schiff SK, Kellam SG: A community-wide mental health program of prevention and early treatment in first grade. Psychiatric Research Reports of the American Psychiatric Association 21:92–102, 1967

Schlessinger N, Gedo JE, Miller J, et al: The scientific style of Breuer and Freud in the origins of psychoanalysis. J Am Psychoanal Assoc 15:404–422, 1967

Secord PF, Dukes WF, Bevan WW: Personalities in faces, I: an experiment in social perceiving. Genetic Psychology Monographs 49:231–279, 1954

Sharaf MR, Levinson DJ: Patterns of ideology and role definition among psychiatric residents, in The Patient and the Mental Hospital. Edited by Greenblatt M, Levinson DJ, Williams RH. New York, Free Press of Glencoe, 1957

Siegel S: Certain Determinants and Correlates of Authoritarianism. Provincetown, MA, Journal Press, 1954

Stanton AH, Schwartz MS: The Mental Hospital: A Study of Institutional Participation in Psychiatric Illness and Treatment. New York, Basic Books, 1954

Strauss A, Schatzman L, Bucher R, et al: Psychiatric Ideologies and Institutions. New York, Free Press, 1964

Wallerstein RS: The future of Psychotherapy. Bull Menninger Clinic 55(4):421–443, 1991

4

Reflections During the Search

Walter Barton was the third medical director of the American Psychiatric Association (APA) and served from 1963 to 1974. When he announced his retirement, a search committee was established to seek a successor. The committee was chaired by Howard Rome, with Bernard Holland as Vice Chairman; Henry Brosin, James Johnson, Henriette Klein, John Looney, James Sussex, Harold Visotsky, Charles Wilkinson, and Paul Wilson were also involved. Perry Talkington, the current president, and Alfred Freedman, the president-elect, served ex officio. More than half of the committee had careers in academic psychiatry, with five departmental chairs. Almost all had a good deal of experience in the governance of the APA as president, speaker of the assembly, and council chairs and in other major roles. There was one African American and two directors of private psychiatric hospitals. It was a committee of the 1970s heavily emphasizing education, but with what would now be insufficient minority membership—for example, only one woman—and no primary researcher and no trainees.

Appropriately the search committee was very respectful to Walter Barton; he had been a most able, distinguished leader. Quite naturally they agreed that they should find a somewhat younger leader who would represent some new directions to the field. They achieved this consensus quickly and then invited applicants. I was intensively questioned about my own interests and ideas about how I would make any changes in the staff or in the functioning of the medical director's office. Emphasizing my research on ideology and interests in psychopathology and normality, I expressed my deep concerns about the profession. Committed to transforming psychiatry into a respected scientific field, I advocated major alterations in the field and expressed my desire to recruit a new able generation of young physicians into the APA.

Despite my membership on the Board of Trustees and on the Program Committee of the APA, I acknowledged that I had much to learn about the history, staff, and organizational structure of the APA. Nevertheless, I unabashedly stated my concerns about the field's lack of public and governmental agency support and argued for a commitment to establishing psychiatry's scientific and professional prestige.

I made it clear that the presence of several ideological factions among my psychiatric colleagues disturbed me. I also stated my conviction that the public had little respect for psychiatric diagnosis or treatment. With the growth of insurance system payments for medical illness, the distrust of psychiatric diagnosis and therapeutic recommendations had become a serious flaw. I anticipated increasing pressure on psychiatrists and emphasized my hope that the APA would become a central focus to combat this distrust. I was especially critical of the concept of "universality of psychopathology." It seemed to imply that no one was so well that he or she did not need some psychiatric help. I spoke about this as vulnerability for the field which needed major correction. Explaining my research on ideology, I described my vision of a more unified scientific profession that included reliable diagnoses and treatment guidelines that are based on empirical evidence.

The members of the search committee knew a good deal about my role as chair of the APA Scientific Program Committee, and they understood that the Annual Meeting had begun to contribute to improvement for the profession. I had begun a "New Research" component of the annual program and was eager to publicize the component's scientific activities at the Annual Meeting. I also had become interested in supporting other organizations holding their annual meetings in conjunction with the APA. My activities, in the context of the Annual Meeting, were a good reflection of my administrative style, as, of course, were aspects of my work as a departmental chair. The search committee also reviewed my role as a member of the APA Board of Trustees, and I think that my contributions to the Board were a strong element in my ultimate selection.

My position in academic psychiatry was also quite significant for the search committee. In the two decades after World War II, academic psychiatry had become a more influential component of the APA; its educational activities were paramount. The number of residents entering psychiatry had begun to increase rapidly, and an interest in residency training and certification was rising. I had participated in several educational conferences conducted by the APA and, indeed, had been a leader in the APA's educational work. I also had served as chair of the Research Council. I believe that the search committee was impressed with the fact that my image as a psychiatric educator and researcher would be helpful to the new psychiatry.

The opportunity to become medical director of the APA was not something that occurred very often. I had not been preparing myself explicitly for being the medical director, but during the search process I realized that my work had prepared me for just that opportunity. I asked the search committee if it might be possible for me to visit with staff and components of the organization and then to meet with the search committee again. That I requested such a procedure indicating that a learning period might be useful was a wise thing to do. Walter Barton had done a very good job in many aspects of leading the staff. His work on hospital systems, state programs, the evolution of community services, and the development of components to reflect the best in those systems had been first rate. Much planning had been accomplished. On the other hand, government affairs activities had been a relatively low-priority activity. While there were two staff members involved in a small office of government issues, this capacity was not nearly at the level needed by the organization if it were to become a genuine participant in the real world of seeking support for psychiatry and mental health. I became knowledgeable and acutely aware of the differences between serious engagement and pro forma exercises that characterized the APA at that time.

By the time I was selected by the Search Committee and the Board of Trustees, I was perceived as an advocate for sophisticated involvement with governmental agencies. It is difficult to realize that at that time, there was considerable opposition to our professional organization conducting lobbying work. It was seen as crass and undignified. By the time that I was on board as medical director, the opposition had begun to weaken. I worked very hard to confront the opposition, and I was successful in being able to point out that the best way to influence the government was to increase the scientific image of the field and of its practitioners. Indeed, I envisaged a government affairs office that would understand the principle that the profession would be elevated if science replaced ideology. I proposed many ideas to the search committee about how we might accomplish that goal.

During the early 1970s, the organization had held several legislative and government affairs conferences, but they consisted primarily of listening to long reports rather than of efforts at training members to become effective spokespersons for the profession. I changed that pattern, because by the middle of the 1970s my concern with the public image of psychiatry had grown. Films and newspaper stories had become increasingly negative in their portrayal of psychiatry and psychiatrists (Gharaibeh 2005). In the immediate post–World War II era, patients and professionals had been handled in a much more positive manner. In the movie *Spellbound* Ingrid Bergman plays a most sympathetic psychiatrist working with Gregory Peck as a suspected killer with amnesia. In *Snake Pit,* the plight of psychiatric patients was presented quite sympathetically, as was the psychotherapeutic work of the therapist played by Leo Genn. In the 1940s and 1950s, the psychiatrist was almost exclusively portrayed as a psychoanalyst. Indeed, in *Spellbound* the most experienced psychiatrist at the hospital looks like a replica of Sigmund Freud. During the 1940s, 1950s, and 1960s psychiatrists in films were magically incisive, brilliant psychoanalysts (Gabbard and Gabbard 2006).

By the time I became medical director of the APA, however, the negative portrayals had begun to outnumber the positive. Newspaper stories about psychiatry began to focus on problem areas. Crimes committed by recently discharged mental patients had always produced a special anxiety. Eliminating the possibilities of such crimes would mean that it was almost impossible to discharge a patient who had previously demonstrated violent behavior. Public attitudes toward mental patients often demonstrated old prejudice about mental illness ("these people should be locked up and the keys thrown away"). Often, when juries found a prominent defendant "not guilty by reason of insanity," there was criticism of the decision presented in newspaper editorials and other public denunciations. In effect, a critical public believed that psychiatrists were against appropriate punishment for criminal acts and insufficiently concerned about public safety.

Antipsychiatry had developed with many faces and shapes (Dain 2000), and when I became medical director, I realized that this trend was going to become even more important for the field as a whole. Before I left Chicago, one of my friends told me about a Scientologist leader who lived in the suburbs of the city. I arranged for a meeting with her, and we had several interesting conversations about reducing friction between their movement and psychiatry. I was prepared to follow this up with continued discussions during my first year at the APA, when an issue of the Scientology newspaper viciously attacked psychiatry. After that, negotiations with Scientologists were never really an option.

Among the antipsychiatry psychiatrists, Thomas Szasz caused me much anguish. He repeatedly wrote articles and books, such as *The Myth of Mental Illness* (Szasz 1972), saying that there was no such thing as a psychiatric illness; primarily such disorders were a figment of psychiatry's imagination. In a way, his criticism was facilitated by the lack of a genuine diagnostic system in psychiatry like the *Diagnostic and Statistical Manual of Mental Disorders* (DSM). Before coming to the APA as medical director, I had begun to criticize some of his positions. Ultimately, psychiatry's assumption of a more scientific status diminished his arguments considerably.

R. D. Laing, a British psychiatrist, working originally at the Tavistock Institute in London, the prestigious center of psychoanalytic study and practice, also developed radical theories of mental illness. He saw psychosis as an attempt to express distress and therefore capable of being a transforming experience for the sufferer. He particularly saw the family— for example, the "schizophrenogenic mother" (Fromm-Reichmann 1948)— as being deeply involved in the etiology of mental illness, a view expressed in *Sanity, Madness and the Family* (Laing and Esterson 1964). Again, as with Szasz, Laing's theorizing and practice could flourish in the absence of an accepted, evidence-based diagnostic system.

I was particularly interested in the APA becoming much stronger in both education and research. At the University of Illinois, I had been fortunate in having as a colleague Dr. George Miller, who had organized an excellent Department of Medical Education (Miller 1961) (see Chapter 3, "Implicit Preparations for a Leadership Role in Psychiatry"). I had also been a member of the psychiatry examination committee of the National Board of Medical Examiners in Philadelphia and had become very impressed with the thoughtfulness of the board. As chairman of the Committee on Instruction at the University of Illinois College of Medicine, I had numerous opportunities to think more deeply about the nature of teaching and learning and the preparation of examinations. The development of an excellent education system for medical students was very high on my agenda. I think that I helped to improve the educational scene at Illinois, but I knew that our psychiatric education was insufficiently balanced. The educational task at this very large medical school was immense. At that time, the University of Illinois had more medical students than any other school in the country. Psychodynamic psychiatry had been heavily emphasized in the department. I resolved to handle psychiatric education in a different way when I went to the APA.

By the 1970s, psychiatric education had become very important. Since World War II, the number of departments of psychiatry that had become independent, rather than being a "division" within the Department of Internal Medicine had grown quite rapidly. Almost every medical school in the country included a psychiatry department. In many schools, psychiatry had begun research programs also, but education was the primary function for a long time.

Psychodynamic psychiatry, based on psychoanalytic principles, had become very popular. In most medical colleges, an introductory course sponsored by the Department of Psychiatry was taught in the first year, an introduction to psychiatric evaluation was introduced in the second year, psychopharmacology was part of the second year pharmacotherapeutic education, and a clerkship in clinical psychiatry was part of the major rotations of time that medical students spent in the clinical years. During the early 1970s, the psychopharmacological revolution began with the advent of the use of chlorpromazine and reserpine. Rapidly, hundreds of new agents were introduced, and by the 1980s, the use of drugs had become a center of psychiatric treatment and education.

At the beginning of the new era of pharmacotherapy in psychiatry, I published a paper about how tentatively the drugs had been accepted at Michael Reese Hospital, with its strong psychotherapeutic ideology (Sabshin and Ramot 1956). Later, of course, for very important reasons, psychopharmacology outpaced psychotherapy and social forms of psychiatric treatment. During this period it became increasingly evident to me that many of my colleagues advocated specific modes of treatment and strongly opposed what seemed to me to be plausible alternatives. In many ways this developing viewpoint was an important initial step in my thinking about therapeutic ideologies.

The impact of psychiatry's weaknesses in nosology had also become apparent to me while working at Michael Reese Hospital. I realized that diagnoses were ambivalently provided as a label to help in obtaining insurance reimbursement for patients. The psychodynamic formulation was much more important to the clinicians. By the time I came to the APA, I was determined to play a role in facilitating a much more comprehensive nosology. The most important issue involved changing psychiatric practice to an evidence-based system. The need to be able to highlight the nature of the patients' problems with as specific a diagnosis as possible would be very important and would help to shape a more appropriate type of treatment. That therapeutic guidelines would also need to be evidence based was part of my fantasy about work that might be accomplished at the APA.

Even before I came to the APA I had become determined to organize a first-rate Office of Research. For equally important reasons, I became interested in coordinating our education activities into an Office of Education. It was particularly fortunate that Dr. Carolyn Robinowitz joined the APA staff as director of a new Office of Education and took on many leadership posts within the APA and, indeed, in psychiatry as a whole. It was also important that we were later able to recruit a director for the Office of Research, Dr. Harold Pincus, who also, as discussed in Chapter 11 ("Psychiatric Research"), would become a major national leader.

While at the University of Illinois, I had become interested in international psychiatric activities. During the search process for the medical directorship at the APA, I became even more aware how much American psychiatry could learn from what was happening abroad. Many advances in psychiatry in the late 1960s and early 1970s had originated in other countries and had been transported to the United States. Certainly the generation of psychoanalysts from Central Europe who came to the United States played a powerful role. The development of the early psychopharmacological agents had also occurred in other countries (e.g., France in the case of thorazine). I had begun to realize that the United States also had much to contribute in international psychiatry. At the University of Illinois, we had an Agency for International Development (AID) contract with Chiang Mai University in Thailand, and I had had the opportunity to be involved in the training of several Thai psychiatrists who returned to Thailand to take on responsibilities there. Indeed, one of the Illinois trainees, Dr. Chamlong Disayavanish, became chair of the Department of Psychiatry at Chiang Mai University. Several visits to his department were particularly instructive for me. Once again, the importance of cross-cultural psychiatry shaped my thinking. Chamlong would spend one month each year as a Buddhist monk, and his religious concepts very much affected his practice of psychiatry.

During those same years I became interested in the World Psychiatric Association and attended many international meetings. I realized that the APA had the possibility of being a larger player in international affairs for psychiatry, and I began to think of how the association might function in this important area. From the beginning I knew that there were special problems in international work. For some of my colleagues, the pleasure of travel exceeded their scientific interest in international questions. Early on, I knew that serious conceptual enquiries needed to replace "junkets," but I understood that gaining acceptance for serious international work was not going to be simple.

One of Dr. Barton's major impacts at the APA had been his strong leadership in the areas of hospital psychiatry, administrative psychiatry, and new systems of community care (Barton 1962, 1987). The development of the journal *Hospital and Community Psychiatry* and the Institute of Psychiatric Services was an excellent illustration of the organization's leadership in this area. Dr. Donald Hammersley, who later became a deputy medical director of the APA, was also very active in the journal and in service delivery systems. Robert (Robbie) Robinson was a very significant staff leader of the APA during the 1960s and 1970s. He had diverse responsibilities, including work on public affairs in the 1970s. Along with Ray Glasscote, he organized the Joint Information Service, which was a major area for APA publications. In addition, he edited *Psychiatric News*, which was a main communications bimonthly newspaper for the APA membership. Both Robbie and Ray had some concern about my appointment. They wondered whether their priorities would be changed too much.

Robbie Robinson adapted to my appointment with a very strong effort as the Director of Public Affairs. Before my arrival, he wrote with Dr. Barton a very thoughtful paper on current criticisms of psychiatry. Indeed, both Barton and Robinson raised questions about the propensity of psychiatrists for "self-flagellation" in public. Robinson said, "If we are to improve our public image, we need to study our own behavior" (quoted in Barton 1987). I agreed with this opinion, but I thought that much of the self-criticism involved strong ideological splits among psychiatrists. In his book on the history of the APA, Dr. Barton noted that at the time of my appointment, "Psychiatry has been under siege, suffering loss of prestige, status, and income. Often it has appeared that operations by the staff are more bail-out than steering a course. Survival demands a quick response and a most political orientation" (Barton 1987, p. 257).

I very much agreed with Robbie Robinson's concern about psychiatry's declining status in its public image. The decline of the public portrayal of psychiatrists in films was of particular concern to me. In the period following World War II, psychiatry was frequently depicted as a positive profession working hard to try to be helpful to patients. In the movie *The Snake Pit* (1948), the psychiatrist was the film's hero, struggling to humanize the therapeutic milieu. By the time I came to Washington, psychiatrists were rarely portrayed as film heroes. *One Flew Over the Cuckoo's Nest* was released in 1975. The Golden Age had vanished.

I was very fortunate in that Walter Barton was strongly supportive of my appointment and stated this opinion often to our staff. When I received the news that I had been selected as medical director, we set a date for me to move to Washington in September 1974. While my appointment rather naturally caused anxiety in some quarters of the staff, I felt that I was very well received by an overwhelming majority. I had sought out numerous contacts during the selection process and continued to do so all through the period leading up to my arrival. I was quite fortunate also with the medical director's staff. Phyllis Kristianson had been the special assistant to Walter Barton, and Carol Davis had been the executive assistant. Both were repositories of APA history and understood how the organization conducted its business. They both taught me a great deal about the APA. Phyllis Kristianson stayed on to help in the transition and then retired to join her husband, John, in South America for a foreign service post. Carol Davis, who succeeded Phyllis, remained in that position until my retirement and stayed on for several years after my retirement in a different role. Almost her entire adult life had been spent working very productively for the APA. She is still a good friend.

The APA Board of Trustees approved the recommendation of the search committee, that I be approved as medical director. In so doing, they indicated their recognition that change in scope and direction should take place. My academic role resonated with the new leadership within the APA. I think that it was important that I had formal psychoanalytic training, but also that I had expressed some criticisms of psychoanalysis and indicated that I would be in favor of some changes in that area. That I had conducted research and had served as chair of the APA's Research Council was received quite positively; my interest in both social and biological psychiatry was also an asset. While I did not then use the term *biopsychosocial*, popularized by George Engel in 1980, in effect, my approach called for an integration of multiple systems. My preference learned from Roy Grinker was to use the term *transactional* to express the relevant constellation of all the variables over time.

Departing from Chicago was not easy. I had lived there for twenty-one years. Most of my friends and colleagues lived there. Most importantly, my wife, Edith, was affected tremendously by the decision to move to Washington. She shared my pleasure in the new appointment, but she knew that it would be very hard to work out her relationships with patients adequately. Indeed, she spent an additional eighteen months in Chicago after I left so that she could make sure that each of her patients could be followed up appropriately. She had major responsibilities at the Psychoanalytic Institute and, along with other staff at the Institute, tried to make sure that there would be adequate continuity to her work there. I was very grateful to her, but I regretted causing a major disruption in her career.

Leaving the University of Illinois involved separation from the Department of Psychiatry and from the Dean's Office at the Abraham Lincoln Medical School. There were many departure parties, and I was treated very warmly by my colleagues and staff. One special party at the Dean's Office was held under the rubric of "Milton Shabskin Is Departing from the Dean's Office; we invite you to a party in his honor." The good humor, even with the countless frustrations at having to spell my last name and its being routinely misspelled, was a good sign of the mixture of feelings about my departure. My administrative assistant at the department, Elaine Engstrom, had been with me throughout my tenure at

Illinois. I respected her knowledge and loyalty, and I knew that she would facilitate the transition to a new leader. Her commitment to the department and her knowledge about it was admirable.

Since my departure, there have been three heads of the Department of Psychiatry. The most recent chair, Dr. Joseph Flaherty, had been a resident during my tenure. He has outdone my short period as acting dean of the medical school with his appointment as the full-time permanent dean. Psychiatry has come a long way at the University of Illinois.

REFERENCES

Barton WE: Administration in Psychiatry. Springfield, IL, Charles C Thomas, 1962

Barton WE: The History and Influence of the American Psychiatric Association. Washington, DC, American Psychiatric Press, 1987

Dain N. Antipsychiatry, in American Psychiatry After World War II: 1944–1994. Edited by Menninger RW, Nemiah JC. Washington, DC, American Psychiatric Press, 2000, pp 277–298

Engel GL: The clinical application of the biopsychosocial model. Am J Psychiatry 137:535–544, 1980

Fromm-Reichmann F: Notes on the development of treatment of schizophrenics by psychoanalysis and psychotherapy. Psychiatry 11:263–273, 1948

Gabbard GO, Gabbard K: Psychiatry and the Cinema, 2nd Edition. Washington, DC, American Psychiatric Press, 1999

Gharaibeh NM: The psychiatrist's image in commercially available American movies. Acta Psychiatr Scand 111:316–319, 2005

Laing RD, Esterson A: Sanity, Madness and the Family. London, Penguin, 1964

Miller GE: Teaching and Learning in Medical School. Cambridge, MA, Harvard University Press, 1961

Sabshin M, Ramot J: Pharmacotherapeutic evaluation and the psychiatric setting. AMA Arch Neurol Psychiatry 75:362–370, 1956

Szasz TS: The Myth of Mental Illness: Foundations of a Theory of Personal Conduct. London, Paladin, 1972

5

Clarifying the Mission

When I was appointed medical director of the American Psychiatric Association in 1974, I had a number of specific proposals for improving and expanding the effectiveness of the organization. In some cases I had specific suggestions about how to accomplish these changes. I did not, however, have a clear overall strategy about the integration of all the diverse plans with the means to carry them out over a long time span. If I had attempted to persuade the search committee that recommended me for the medical directorship to the APA Board that I already possessed a comprehensive plan to change American psychiatry systematically, I believe that I would have been given a diagnosis rather than the job. Giving such an impression would have been based on my appearing to have made specific decisions with insufficient evidence and experiences, along with a touch of grandiosity. My genuine wish to understand more about how the governance system really worked and the history of the APA was appreciated. While I knew a good deal about a few areas, there were many parts of a complex system about which I was grossly ignorant. The history of the APA is extraordinarily complex, and I still find myself learning about it while I write this book.

While I was not authorized to be chief executive officer, that being part of the president's role at the time, I was clearly expected to be more than a chief operating officer. From the very beginning, I recognized that there were problems inherent in this somewhat ambiguous role definition. (The position was clarified at last in 2004 when Medical Director Jay Scully had CEO added to his title.) The timing, pace, and intensity of how I managed the expectations of policy leadership were central to how I was able to adapt to the new position. Errors by being too aggressive or too passive were continuously possible. How we, president and medical director, managed that relationship was particularly important for my success or failure. Dealing with successive presidents, with varying executive styles, was the ultimate administrative challenge. Some presidents micromanaged intensively; others told me to take over and let them know when I needed help. I did not ask for a change in the job description, but I was determined to lead whatever the formal and personal constraints.

After about two years on the job, the plans for change were becoming clearer in my mind. Some ideas about the *Diagnostic and Statistical Manual of Mental Disorders* (DSM) had begun to be formulated just before I came to the APA, as is discussed in Chapter 10 ("Evidence-Based Diagnosis and Treatment"). The awareness of how the DSM and Practice Guidelines could radically affect the image of the field and its scientific status struck me as a powerful insight during my second year in office. The interaction of a new medical and scientific identity for psychiatry coalesced with plans to build coordinated Offices of Research, Education, Government Relations, Public Affairs, and Business Administration. This made sense in thinking how to achieve a newly clarified mission. Everything depended on the agreement of the Board, the Assembly, and a clear majority of the membership that large-scale change was necessary and desirable. In each segment of the effort, other APA leaders played a major role in conceptualizing and implementing the plans. The medical director needed to comprehend the integration of the mission's diverse elements and lead in the organized implementation of the effort to make it work. In retrospect, the new mission that was started in the 1970s did indeed have long-range implications. The current plans for psychiatry to be reimbursed in parity with other medical disciplines can be traced back to the radical steps begun thirty years ago. The progress made can be seen in this excerpt from a recent lead editorial in the *New York Times*, "Fairness for Mental Health" (2007):

> After a decade of small-bore measures and frustrating stalemates, it looks as if Congress may be ready to require that insurance coverage for mental illness and substance abuse be provided on the same terms as coverage for physical ailments. So-called parity legislation would be a boon to the millions of Americans who suffer from mental illness or addiction and find it hard to afford treatment. . . . The Senate and the House should move aggressively to pass this much-needed legislation and send it to President Bush for his signature.
>
> Neither the Senate nor the House versions would require employers or health plans to cover mental illness[,] but if they do provide such cover-

age, the financial terms and treatment limits would have to be the same for medical and surgical benefits....The Bill is backed by Senators Ted Kennedy, Democrat of Massachusetts, and Pete Domenici, Republican of New Mexico, both long term champions of equal treatment for mental health....Given that President Bush has endorsed the idea of mental health parity and that both houses seem poised to enact it, the prospects look good for ending the long stalemate.

Without the changes begun in the 1970s psychiatry, no editorial supporting parity would have been conceivable; in all likelihood we would be very far away from being treated as a major medical speciality, especially in a managed care system that demands objective data. In a way, the medical director of the APA has had an opportunity to observe long-term consequences of decisions more readily than most of the officers in the association. Long tenure helps in managing comprehensive planning, but it also can be abused. To have been at the helm of an organization for 23 years granted me a unique vantage point. Of course, historians are professionally skilled in retrospectively explaining the rationale for the changes. My perspective, however, as a participant, differs from some of the historical descriptions currently available. This book permits my memories to become part of history.

At the beginning of my tenure I was fortunate in being able to draw on the experience I had gained in several of the organizational leadership posts that I had previously held in the APA. In order to be effective in long-term planning, however, I needed to become much more familiar with many governance issues and all of the basic problems facing the field. I also needed to be aware that there were aspects of the administrative responsibilities about which I was significantly less knowledgeable and at which I needed to become more skilled. At the beginning I did not have sufficient capacity in being a hands-on leader in improving the fiscal status of the APA. My experiences as a department head and an acting dean were useful but not pertinent enough for a membership association. I knew from the beginning that the APA needed to have improved strength in business administration and in the capacity to obtain new resources to reach ambitious goals. A fiscal plan was essential. Fortunately I had some skills in seeking new sources of revenue. I was not an expert on the nuances of APA governance and constitutional processes. I needed much help in understanding how a large voluntary organization functioned and might be changed. I knew that much depended on the skills of the staff to carry out the tasks.

At the beginning I also did not know a great deal about the full complexity of the APA's state and sub-state organizations and District Branches, with its 74 local groups, including 3 in Canada. During my first two years in office I spent a great deal of time in learning about the organization. Fortunately there were many willing teachers and I was a motivated pupil. In addition to the staff at the national office, the staff at the District Branches were particularly good instructors. Several of them had devoted many years to the branches and were extremely knowledgeable about the state of psychiatry in their area. I began to visit District Branches all across the United States and Canada, paying particular attention also to the seven area councils (see Appendix 10, this volume).

The APA encompasses both a national executive and a legislative system with a state and regional organizational structure. The medical director needs to understand the long-term interactions and the way in which these parts function. The nationally elected officers have the difficult task of being elected by a secret mail ballot. The APA began a new system of contested national elections in 1973. In those years, a spirited group of young psychiatrists under the vigorous leadership of Fuller Torrey was very active. Calling themselves "The Concerned Psychiatrists," they supported particular candidates for APA elected offices, including me in my successful race in 1973 for APA Trustee at Large. Their primary intent was to refocus psychiatry upon the chronically mentally ill, but they advocated many other new policies. Taking to heart their mentor's dire predictions about the field of psychiatry (Torrey 1974), these young psychiatrists made suggestions that have been genuinely helpful for a new psychiatry. Since the time of the "Concerned Psychiatrists" there have not been formally organized national electoral constituents in the APA. Nevertheless, elections have been quite lively, and campaign statements have served as an excellent indicator of professional concerns.

The medical director needed to be scrupulously neutral in the election process. Dr. Barton had been very much hurt when some members wrongly implied that he might have influenced close presidential contests, as in one instance when there was a difference only of three votes between the two candidates. Yet, while the medical director had to remain strictly neutral, he also needed to be able to assess where the heterogeneous constituencies might stand on a variety of issues both currently and in the future. The "area" geographical structure (see Appendix 10, this volume) also played an important role in policy formation, and there were significant differences among these areas. For example, Area 1, New England, and Area 5, Southern States, demonstrated disagreements about the pertinence of specific social issues, the role of psychoanalysis, and ways of coping with the insurance reimbursement systems. The Assembly of District Branches was organized in the 1950s with particularly strong leadership efforts by Daniel Blain, the first medical director of the APA, and Robert Garber, who had been both speaker of the assembly and president of the APA, and it has had extensive discussions, debates, and conferences about its fundamental powers and responsibilities.

The ultimate decision-making power of the APA lies in its Board of Trustees; over the years, however, the Assembly has sought active participation in most decision-making functions, including the power to require a reconsideration of specific Board decisions. At one stage of APA history, in 1979, there was a membership vote on a constitutional change that would have given the ultimate decision-making power to the Assembly. In actuality, a small majority of the voters favored the recommendation, but the two-thirds level required for constitutional change was not achieved. At the time I was quietly pleased with the outcome since I had many questions about how a group as large as the Assembly could carry out executive responsibilities. It seemed awkward and possibly very expensive to administer. Later I realized that at the American Medical Association, its massive House of Delegates does indeed have the final authority, operating in conjunction with its Board of Trustees.

Since the vote on the APA constitution in 1979, the Board–Assembly relationship has on the whole stabilized. Much effort has been made to coordinate the work of the Board and the Assembly with many joint activities—for example, a joint reference committee and a joint commission on government relations. Deputy Medical Director Henry Work assumed many of the coordinating functions. At his suggestion a formal office to link the activities of the Board and the Assembly was established. Jeanne Robb carried out that coordinating function for many years in an extremely dedicated and competent fashion. Occasionally substantial differences occurred and rumblings of discontent were audible, but there were no disagreements fundamental enough to have brought about a constitutional crisis.

The specific composition of the membership of the Board and the Assembly have had important changes in the half century of their interaction. After World War II, the prime career affiliation of APA Board leadership shifted toward the academic psychiatric community. As a previous departmental chair, I was probably more familiar with professionals in this community than with those in other areas of work. The hospital superintendents, the great barons of psychiatry who led the APA before World War II, were gradually replaced, mainly by department chairs, as presidents of the APA. The chairs of the most prestigious departments, by and large, perceived the APA Presidency to be an honor, and this opinion persisted well into the 1980s.

By the turn of the twentieth-first century an interesting change had occurred. Most psychiatric department chairs were not seeking to become officers of the APA in the way that many of them had done in the previous four decades. There have been marvelous exceptions, but the change was palpable. Rather, they sought leadership roles in the Society of Biological Psychiatry, the American College of Neuropsychopharmacology, and several other groups. Elsewhere, I have described the impact of the changing American psychiatry upon choices of academic department heads. For a variety of reasons the research-oriented chairs no longer perceived leadership roles in psychiatric practice or even in education as a particularly prestigious part of their curricula vitae. What a far cry from the immediate postwar period.

It also should be noted that the Board of Trustees' composition began to be more similar to the Assembly's leadership by the 1980s. Elected Area Representatives on the Board often had previously served as Assembly leaders. Both the presidents of the Association and the Assembly speakers were leaders in improving the status of psychiatric practitioners and their patients. They were pleased that scientific principles had reduced the power of professional ideology, and they worked hard to capitalize on psychiatry's changed image. They paid precise attention to the economic implications of psychiatric policies. Of course, there have been exceptions; in recent decades some presidents have been particularly interested in providing broad leadership in the full "biopsychosocial" implications of the field. On the Assembly side most current speakers are also leaders in psychiatric practice; the Assembly is a powerful reservoir of advocates for parity and in fighting discrimination against psychiatric patients (see Appendix 2 for a list of the Speakers of the Assembly). Relatively few speakers have been chairs of academic departments of psychiatry. Heads of private psychiatric hospitals and directors of psychiatric sections of general hospitals have been particularly prominent in serving as Speakers of the Assembly. The Assembly includes articulate practitioners who work diligently to achieve the best possible support for psychiatric patients. Many are particularly knowledgeable about economic health care policies. Their meetings have been lively with spirited debates, articulate advocates, and carefully monitored parliamentary procedure.

No District Branch has been more visible in the history of the Assembly than the Washington group. Its location in the District of Columbia makes it not surprising that the U.S. Senate and the House of Representatives seem to be somewhat like two additional local legislative bodies for the Washington District Branch. Just as California psychiatrists in the California District Branches pay attention to legislative activities in Sacramento and Georgia psychiatrists follow closely what happens in Atlanta, the Washington psychiatrists pay close attention to "The Hill" as if it were their local authority. More than any other District Branch its action papers have often involved suggestions for federal legislation and regulation.

Confrontation was inevitable. At times there have been sharp conflicts between the APA Joint Commission on Government Relations and the Washington Psychiatric Society (the Washington District Branch). Some of these conflicts were quite intense and required intervention by the Board of Trustees, which generally tended to support the Joint Commission. Occasionally, it should be noted, there was some tension between the APA staff and the Washington Psychiatric Society on the specific language of legislation, which required some careful negotiation. Quite significantly, the Washington Psychiatric Society had been represented in the Assembly by strong advocates of psychoanalysis for well over a quarter of a century. More than any other group in the APA they have fought the changing direction of American psychiatry. Occasionally they behaved like an opposition party. Psychoanalysis was always most popular in big cities, where there was at least one Psychoanalytic Institute. This was true in Washington, but there were other, special reasons why psychoanalysis was particularly powerful in the District. During the "halcyon days" after War World II, the fact that a significant number of federal government employees had excellent health insurance for many years had an important impact on practice patterns. A large number of intelligent, psychologically minded individuals held government positions, and many were quite sensitive to psychiatric issues. The presence of nationally prominent psychiatric hospitals and other centers with strong psychoanalytic leanings facilitated the utilization of psychodynamic psychiatry. Many veterans received treatment in the Washington, D.C., area, and psychodynamic psychotherapy was the preferred method.

Whatever the underlying factors, psychoanalysis had powerful supporters in the APA Assembly, including the Washington group. They fought very hard to maintain the power of psychoanalysis within American psychiatry. Occasionally they found themselves in conflict with other District Branches and the APA Staff leadership. For many years they were somewhat ambivalent to both Jay Cutler, who became the APA's director of government affairs, and me. This persisted until Harold Eist became president (1996–97) of the APA and made a special point of supporting me at the local district branch. After my retirement, I became an elder statesman rather than a bête noire. This book, however, may stir up some old memories.

In the 1970s, during the work on the third edition of DSM (DSM-III; American Psychiatric Association 1980), a significant part of the opposition to the acceptance of this edition of the manual came from criticism by the Washington Psychiatric Society. Its members were by no means alone in this criticism, but they did provide some strategic leadership by raising important questions and recommending modifications. They also were particularly strong in fighting any federal legislation that continued to demonstrate discrimination against psychiatric patients. Their goals for combating bias were laudatory; any compromise that involved acceptance of something less than full parity was strongly criticized by them. Their arguments were often presented with an aura of righteousness that was occasionally persuasive. After the weakening of psychoanalytic reimbursement, they became strong advocates of maintaining psychotherapeutic benefits. Our Government Affairs office needed to make careful assessments of what was practically possible, and in the real world, shrewd compromises were necessary. For passionate advocates, compromise is never easy. The analytic group in the Assembly fought very hard against the major changes in the 1970s, but it finally was overwhelmed by the large majority who sought change. Subsequently, the Washington Psychiatric Society and most of its allies shifted strategy to become the most vocal spokespersons for psychotherapy, confidentiality, and parity. Historians will need to decide whether we would be as close to parity as we are now if their earlier strategy had prevailed. An objective description of the history of psychiatry in the District of Columbia would be very interesting.

The Board of Trustees met six times a year, including two brief ceremonial transition sessions during the Annual Meeting. The budget process was particularly important, and on occasion special fiscal decisions were necessary. When the APA purchased new office property, we required a mandatory assessment from each member to assist in covering the cost. Whatever the problems affecting the membership, the assessment was remarkably successful, with almost all members making the required payment.

By the 1990s, the largest part of the APA income was coming from its publications, its research contracts, and the earnings from the Annual Meeting. During the early postwar years, the APA's income had come almost exclusively from the members' dues. The transition from a "members club" to a more business-like mammoth organization had many consequences. The APA could be effective in many areas not previously accessible, but it no longer was a "Mom and Pop" shop as some might have preferred it to continue to be. For many there was a nostalgic fondness for the good old days.

During the 1970s the Board's regular meetings were supplemented by an Executive Committee of the Board that assumed some of the Board's work. Ultimately, largely because of complaints by those Board members who were not members, the Executive Committee was terminated. In many areas of APA governance, participatory democracy was preferred to administrative efficiency.

With the expansion of membership—which, for example, grew from 20,856 in 1974 to 40,978 in 1997 (see Appendix 5 for membership totals from 1873 to 2007)—and the sheer complexity of the organization, the agenda of the Trustees' meetings became overloaded. By 1972, it was realized that less time was available for policy discussions, and it was decided to hold a special summer meeting each year that would be devoted to such policy discussions. The APA Summer Policy Meetings discussed a wide variety of topics during a 20-year span. The president of the APA determined each year's agenda, usually after requesting proposals for discussion items from the members of the Board and later from the Assembly officers. I was also often asked for suggestions. Repeatedly I requested discussion of the DSM process, the Practice Guidelines, and the building of a strong Government Affairs office. This was a particularly significant opportunity for my proposals to be discussed, and I had many openings to influence APA policies.

Most of my presentations at the District Branch level have not been published, but the themes I reiterated were of an accountable, evidence-based psychiatry. Each year, the *American Journal of Psychiatry* published my Annual Report to the Assembly, and these reports included descriptions of my plans. Surprisingly some of my strongest papers on the need for organizational change in the APA were presented at international sessions such as those in Auckland, Madrid, and Prague. Comparisons of the organizations in various countries seemed of great interest to international audiences. They also provided me with an opportunity to try out some new ideas on generally supportive audiences. The staff of the APA were acutely aware that I was deeply committed to getting across the theme of the profession becoming accountable. Two papers typical of what I presented during this time are included in Appendix 1. The content of these papers, which includes evidence-based therapeutics and professional accountability, demonstrates what I hoped to accomplish.

In addition to the Board of Trustees and the Assembly, the governance system included a "third estate": a system of councils, commissions, committees, and task forces that included hundreds of members who, during one weekend each fall, held their discussions at a meeting in Washington, D.C. Some of the components had additional meetings during the year, but their combined fall meeting was a glittering event. Among its features was the midyear summation of issues by the APA president. These components contributed importantly to the intellectual vigor of the APA, and their recommendations were reviewed, and most often approved, by the Assembly and the Board. A joint reference committee was established to review topics emanating from the components before they were finally presented to the Board. Appendix 14 provides a diagram that illustrates the relationship between the governance bodies. The Joint Reference Committee was composed of members of the Assembly and the Board. The medical director was also a voting member of this committee; the one instance in which he was given the right to vote. Somehow that privilege seemed more than symbolically important to me; it suggested that my voice in the APA was heard officially, as well as in the many other settings where I was allowed the privilege of the "the floor." I was essentially secure in my capacity to be effective, but my pleasure in having a vote on the Joint Reference Committee strongly suggested some less-than-conscious anxiety on my part.

Clearly the APA governance structure was exceedingly cumbersome but nevertheless turned out to be prudent and democratic. There were many checks and balances and great opportunities for membership participation. By the time I left the APA, I was convinced that its structure would serve as a barrier to a recurrence of ideological domination of the organization.

One major change in the APA governance system was brought about by the inclusion of trainees in psychiatry into the decision-making processes of the APA. During the immediate postwar period, the organization had been strongly patriarchal and that psychiatrists at the resident stage could serve on the APA Board would then have been hardly imaginable. Currently the younger members of the APA are exceedingly active; often they are particularly effective as spokespersons.

Residents are elected as full voting members of the Board and the Assembly; their active participation is now not merely encouraged but confidently expected. With over 50% of psychiatric residents being women, it is not surprising that many of the elected are female. Their opinions on recruitment into psychiatry, the organization of psychiatric services, questions of gender equality, and future directions for psychiatry are valuable. They often are very perceptive about emerging problems and their solutions. It is also very interesting to see which sessions at our Annual Meeting are particularly well attended by younger members. Recent decisions to include representatives from other psychiatric organizations in the Assembly have also been a creative way to enroll their direct participation in APA decision making. Voting rights in the Assembly have been meaningful.

No one knows the role of the APA in leading American psychiatry better than the staff working at national headquarters or at the District Branch level. The APA's capacity to retain employees for long periods has been excellent. This retention of staff has built up a body of committed colleagues whose advice to me and to officers about reorganization—about making an even more effective system of governance—has been of central importance. Not all of my efforts to clarify the APA's mission and to change the field have turned out as expected. The mission has been clarified, but many new problems have appeared. The American health system, including psychiatric care, provides efficient treatment for many people but insufficient attention for a significant minority.

There is still much more to be accomplished in the next stage of American psychiatry's goals. Deep in retirement, I am still clarifying the mission.

REFERENCES

American Psychiatric Association: Diagnostic and Statistical Manual of Mental Disorders, 3rd Edition. Washington, DC, American Psychiatric Association, 1980

"Fairness in Mental Health." New York Times, March 24, 2007

Torrey EF: The Death of Psychiatry. Radnor, PA, Chilton, 1974

6

En Route to Equity

*T*here is a very long road from the worst care of the mentally ill to the very best treatment. Through most of human history mental health care has hovered around gross stigma, dehumanized care, punishments, demonization, and derision. Over time, the chains of mental patients began to be removed, punishment was reduced, and the concept of illness began to replace blame and heresy. This worldwide pattern of gradual episodic progress has been replicated in the shorter history of mental health care in the United States, with occasional periods of increasingly humane treatment followed by lapses into "warehousing" and mistreatment. A short period of "moral" care, in which "Yankee" patients were treated with dignity, occurred in the middle of the nineteenth century (Barton 1987; Bockoven 1963). This was followed by a long period during which pessimism dominated, especially in periods of heavy immigration, when massive state mental institutions were constructed, primarily for the poor. The ending of World War II brought a relatively short wave of hope, including genuine concern about the casualties of war. The creation of institutions for the care of veterans reflected new interest in their treatment and was accompanied by the emergence of many new academic psychiatric departments, which were often linked closely to veterans' hospitals. Psychoanalysis began to flourish and tended to be the most popular symbol of American psychiatry for about three decades. The most severely ill psychiatric patients, however, remained institutionalized. Concern for their welfare, and disenchantment with ideological formulations, increased among some quarters of American psychiatry during the 1960s (Grob 1991).

By the 1970s, a new period emerged in which there was great interest in reassertion of a medical identity for psychiatry and a commitment to scientific progress. This focus was especially prominent in studies of the precise symptomatology of illness, of its various ideologies, and of its treatment and, ultimately, prevention. These new professional goals were laudable, but they needed to be accepted by the nation's political, social, and economic decision-making systems if real change were to be made.

Early in my career as medical director, it seemed obvious that the American Psychiatric Association should become a major catalyst for a new evidence-based psychiatry. It needed to lead the field's reform by demonstrating its commitment to diagnostic reliability, to evidence-based treatment, and to active participation in the new realities of health care financing. A multipronged approach was necessary. In Chapter 9 ("Forensic Psychiatry"), I describe how DSM-III (American Psychiatric Association 1980) and the Practice Guidelines became the central focuses of a new, empirically oriented field. To take advantage of this new scientific direction, we needed an increased staff able to make our new direction visible to decision makers. To effect widespread changes in the field, we needed a professional staff to act as continual liaison with various government agencies and to negotiate with insurance companies. A professional staff would ensure that the APA's message was consistent, forceful, and intelligent rather than episodic and qualitatively variable.

Persuading the APA leadership of the need for an effective professional staff was not simple. Several APA officers resisted what they conceived to be "grubby" lobbying that was below the dignity of a truly professional association. Speaking before state legislatures was laudable; William Menninger, for example, a distinguished public figure and co-founder of the Menninger Institute, spoke compellingly before many such bodies, but day-to-day contact and personal negotiations with politicians were considered by many to be demeaning. Perhaps overwhelmed by the strength of the antipsychiatry movement, some leaders were pessimistic that a costly investment in lobbying national and state agencies would yield tangible benefits for the profession. Having insufficient knowledge of the actual tax laws, some APA leaders incorrectly argued that the APA's tax-exempt status forbade lobbying. However, the proposed budget for lobbying activities was a relatively small proportion of APA's income and allowed lobbying with specific restrictions. There were many opponents, but the motivation to change rapidly grew stronger and prevailed.

During my first year as medical director I presented the case for an Office of Government Affairs at the Board, the Assembly, and at many District Branches. I also talked about the need for other new offices such as Public Affairs and Economic Affairs, but I acknowledged we needed more time and funds to organize all of these programs along with simultaneous building of the Office of Research and Office of Education. Fortunately, the arguments against the Office of Government Affairs weakened quickly during my "honeymoon" period when I gained support from the Assembly of District Branches and several articulate officers. The argument for active advocacy and publicity was effective. Our governance bodies agreed to support a search committee for a Director of Government Affairs on whose recommendation I would be authorized to make an appointment. It was also agreed that we would take whatever budgetary steps were necessary to support the Office, including raising membership dues, terminating some lower-priority activities, and beginning serious planning about new sources of income. These plans were also related to the development over time of other high-priority offices and programs. It was vital that other sources of income be obtained, and ultimately the success of these efforts (e.g., publications, research contracts, advertising) would make it possible to succeed in many of our ambitions. Although the issues were complex, there was powerful agreement to seek a Director of Government Affairs.

When our search committee, chaired by John McGrath, recommended the appointment of Jay Cutler in 1975, I was delighted. Jay and I hit it off from the start. I was fascinated by his work on health policy for U.S. Senator Jacob K. Javits of New York, for whom I had a great deal of admiration. He was an articulate, progressive Republican leader who had attracted a first-rate staff. Jay was Minority Counsel and Staff Director of the Human Resources Committee in the Senate. I was convinced that Jay was the right person to deal with government officials in a capable, professional, knowledgeable, and effective manner. Jay clearly thought that I was able and willing to back him on the tactics and the resources required to strengthen governmental support of psychiatry. Our compatibility was important, and it lasted. From the beginning, Jay also agreed that the scientific image of the field was poor and needed marked improvement if we were to become able to be convincing to critical decision makers. Jay was a powerful and shrewd advocate for an evidence-based psychiatry. He understood that without it, the opposition would be overwhelming. We recognized a broad definition of government affairs with legislative and regulatory activities at national and state levels as our highest priorities. In addition, there were many responsibilities involved in working with the executive branch of the federal government. The National Institute of Mental Health (NIMH), as discussed in Chapter 11 ("Psychiatric Research"), was of crucial significance, and both Jay Cutler and I envisaged a strong alliance with that institution. Department of Defense affairs, such as the Civilian Health and Medical Program of the Uniformed Services (CHAMPUS), veterans' health questions, Social Security support, and overall health policies were all important for us. Dealing effectively with federal governmental agencies was essential for the progress of a new American psychiatry.

To accomplish our goals at the state level, we had to ensure close coordination with our Assembly. Each state needed a government affairs program. Financing of local mental health activities depended strongly on state resources, but the provision of some national assistance would be necessary. Our Office of Government Affairs needed to be vigorous in coordinating national, regional, and state activities. Jay also supported my plans to strengthen public affairs as a high priority area. He was very active in making his plans visible and comprehensible to our leadership and our membership, and he was quite successful in achieving their overwhelming approval. In fact, some of those who had been most skeptical about my high priority for Government Affairs complained that we should have acted earlier when they saw what Jay achieved.

By 1980 a complex new system of practice regulations and constraints about reimbursement for medical care had been enforced across the United States. To deal with this new system, the APA was required to undertake the organization of complex but practical involvement with a number of federal and state agencies. The APA began to think of itself not as a small family shop completely dependent on the beneficence of others, but as a genuine participant in formulating plans and policies. Finally, we learned that in the American political system, pleading for fairness is insufficient. We needed to engage the real world of decision making in a systematic and intelligent fashion.

Jay Cutler was assertive, tough, candid, and sensitive about what it took to be successful. He knew when it was necessary to negotiate and when to compromise in achieving our primary goals. He was occasionally harshly criticized by members who failed to understand that government affairs work often involved a protracted series of infinitesimal steps, and who expected unrealistic results. Some of our members advocated for programs that were flawed with inherent weaknesses. For example, Jay and I were criticized for our concerns that reimbursement for psychodynamic psychotherapy and psychoanalysis would be harshly curtailed unless sufficient data were presented to lawmakers about its efficacy. Representatives of the Washington (D.C.) Psychiatric Society in the Assembly, for many years considered the voice of psychoanalysis in the APA (see Chapter 5, "Clarifying the Mission"), had difficulty accepting that decision makers were unimpressed and unconvinced by the data presented. Why could we not persuade the legislators that they were wrong? The Washington Psychiatric Society and others pushed very hard within the APA to seek better reimbursement for psychodynamic psychotherapy. One of the first areas in which these struggles occurred involved insurance programs for federal employees. These issues were, of course, particularly important in the District of Columbia, where the decline in reimbursement for psychotherapeutic care caused severe problems. Objective outcome studies, which may have been more palatable and convincing to decision makers, were not prominent in psychoanalysis. Rather than attempting to provide scientifically based data to increase reimbursement for psychoanalysis, advocates tended to blame regulatory bias for their reimbursement woes. Some bias most certainly existed, but the frailty of the evidence at the time severely limited APA's success in obtaining reimbursement for psychotherapy.

Another factor strongly contributing to the declining reimbursement for psychotherapy was its rapid "demedicalization." By the 1980s, an enormous number of non–medically trained "therapists" had emerged in private practice. Thus, claiming that psychotherapy was a reimbursable medical procedure became increasingly problematic. Many clinicians were psychologists or social workers, but other practitioners with much less training also joined the field, claiming to practice psychotherapy. Since all groups claimed to be "therapists," many patients made no distinction between minimally trained clinicians, psychiatrists, and therapists with master's or doctoral-level training. Because psychoanalysis in 1991 began to accept nonmedical candidates on an equal basis, its medical status declined further. Jay Cutler recognized the impossibility of retaining psychotherapy as a medical procedure. This realization that psychotherapy was not exclusively a medical discipline caused consternation for many APA members. An era of American psychiatry in which psychotherapy dominated psychiatric practice was coming to an end.

The battle to remedicalize psychiatry was often bitter, but it opened the way for a scientific psychiatry with long-term goals of parity and equity with other parts of medicine. Since the constraints on psychotherapy reimbursement in the 1970s and 1980s, a much more intensive effort for evidence-based psychotherapies has been undertaken (Clemens 2002), and the implications for combining psychotherapy and pharmacotherapy by psychiatrists have also become important for the future of psychiatry (Karasu 1982; Riba and Balon 2005).

The detailed accomplishments of the APA's Office of Government Affairs could fill several volumes. Ten thousand small steps accompanied by periodic major victories have characterized the period from the 1970s to the present. We are now close to parity with the rest of medicine, but the achievement of full equity will take much longer. Equity for psychiatry in a health care system that requires large profits for the private insurance firms will not be easily accomplished, but psychiatry has come a long way from the progressive steps first taken in the 1970s.

Listing the APA's accomplishments in three decades of presenting its message to governmental officials could easily trivialize the hard work spent in preparation of research data, the skills of persuasion, the formal testimony, and the political support by our potential allies. I have selected a few examples that I believe are representative. We have particularly relied on some legislators who have experienced mental illness in their own family and were willing to discuss this in public, such as Senator George McGovern and Governor Michael Dukakis. Many of those without any personal contact or experience in the field were potentially vulnerable to false statements about the untreatability of psychiatric patients. This was a constant struggle! Activities designed to correct public perceptions were vital in making politicians more open to listening to our arguments. Jay recruited an exceptional staff to take leadership at all levels of governmental activities. In Appendix 8, I have listed members of the Joint Commission on Government Relations, whose members have had a tremendous impact on public acceptance of psychiatry.

To make government affairs a successful enterprise, our Office of Government Affairs began a series of long-term projects to broaden the number of participants and to publicize our messages. Annual meetings of APA leadership groups were initiated and focused alternately on state and national issues. These meetings featured training for presentations to legislators, in which witnesses were taught to stay calm when the audience appeared inattentive to what they were saying. Participants were also taught how to convey cogent information when they visited senators and congressmen. Many elected public officials attended our Government Affairs conferences; some were very strong allies, and their congressional staff provided advice that was particularly useful. Nuances of pending legislation were discussed in detail, and many APA leaders became informed about the decision-making process and skillful in testimony. Finally, we had a substantial leadership cadre able to work with government agencies. The will to change was augmented by success in building the road.

An annual national Mental Illness Awareness Week was authorized by joint congressional resolutions and presidential proclamation. Special events were held across the country and produced good publicity about out professional goals. The activities in Washington were particularly important. I remember Herbert Pardes, who was then director of the NIMH, addressing a large gathering of congressional staff at a meeting organized by the APA about research and policy questions in the field, and his presentation stimulated a very lively discussion on principles for action. We were accepted as significant and intelligent advocates. Many congressional staff became staunch allies.

From the very beginning our Office of Government Affairs (now Department of Government Relations, or DGR) understood the importance of alliances with other groups for influencing government consideration of mental health objectives. Coalitions like the ad hoc Group for Medical Research, the Fairness Coalition (for parity), and the Mental Health Liaison Group were often chaired by APA staff. After a rocky start, our relationship with the National Alliance on Mental Illness (NAMI, formerly the National Alliance for the Mentally Ill), discussed elsewhere (see Chapter 1, "Post–World War II Scene in American Psychiatry"), has become increasingly close since the early 1980s . Their current president (in 2007), Dr. Suzanne Vogel-Scibilia, is a psychiatrist who recently received a special commendation from APA President Pedro Ruiz (see Plate 14). The DGR has also been central to the APA's relationship with the American Medical Association (AMA), an alliance that has become stronger in recent years. Psychiatrists are now much more visible in AMA leadership roles. The recent election of Jeremy Lazarus (Speaker of the APA Assembly 1997–98) as the Speaker of the AMA House of Delegates is an outstanding example. DGR staff, in conjunction with Medical Director Jay Scully, assisted in the coordination of our liaison with the AMA. The ties to NAMI and the AMA are vital for the APA and are clearly a product of the changing of American psychiatry. Our pre-1970s stance would not have permitted such alliances.

The professionalism of the DGR's role in legislative affairs is also well illustrated by the development of the APA Corporation for the Advancement of Psychiatry (APACAP). This entity was set up as a separate corporation after much Board discussion in January 1981 to create a political action committee. We needed to organize such a separate group to be able to provide fiscal support for the election of specific candidates for national and state elections whom we thought would be sympathetic to our legislative positions. Some of our members balked at becoming so involved in the political world. Would we became too attached to one political party and alienate the other? Would this become a way to support or oppose social issues not directly related to psychiatry? From my perspective the APA has been careful to maintain its political bipartisanship and has not become involved in advocating issues that transcend our competence.

The passage of the Mental Health Systems Act (Public Law 96-398), which was signed into effect by President Jimmy Carter in October 1980, was the culmination of a presidency with very strong involvement in mental health issues. This legislation had been recommended by a very active Presidential Commission on Mental Health, which advocated a comprehensive community mental health system and much stronger services for the chronically mentally ill, the elderly, children, and many other vulnerable people (U.S. President's Commission on Mental Health 1978).

This act was a good example of particularly important legislation that reflected more positive support for psychiatry. Another example was the 1996 federal Mental Health Parity Act (MHPA), which changed the 1974 Employment Retirement Income Security Act (ERISA) law that had made it difficult to impose mental health benefits for employees. The MPHA prohibits group health plans from imposing limitations on mental health coverage that are more restrictive than those imposed on medical and surgical coverage (Sundararaman and Redhead 2006).

Medicare has been particularly important in helping many elderly patients and others in payment of their medical costs (Crosby 1966; Gibson 1966; Hess 1966; Hudson 1966; Rome 1966). Efforts to end discrimination by Medicare coverage for psychiatric care have been undertaken for well over a quarter of a century and, indeed, are still taking place today. When in 1982 a prospective payment methodology was introduced, Dr Joseph English (who later would become president of the APA, 1991–92) led an APA Task Force that fought hard and succeeded in bringing about psychiatry's exemption from prepayment restrictions that would have been extraordinarily hurtful to psychiatric patients (English et al. 1986). While Medicare and Medicaid have been vital for providing better health care, equity for the psychiatrically disabled must remain a long-term high priority goal.

The determined efforts by psychologists to be permitted to prescribe medication has required special attention by our DGR staff. The introduction of DSM-III had reduced psychologists' role in employing their tests to suggest a diagnosis. They needed to broaden their range of activities. Another factor was they had greatly expanded their work in psychotherapy, for which reimbursement, with the introduction of managed care, was becoming ever more difficult to obtain. Led by Pat DeLeon, one time president of the prestigious American Psychological Association and advisor to Senator Inouye (D-Hawaii), the claim was that psychologists were as well fitted as many physicians to prescribe drugs: as Robert Resnick, another past-president of the American Psychological Association, wrote, "85% of all prescriptions for psychotropic medications are written by non-psychiatric physicians who get 4 to 6 weeks of training. I'm sure we could do a better job" (Resnick 1992).

On the surface psychiatrists' resistance to these proposals may appear to be simply a protectionist stance. When looked at closely, however, the psychologists' proposals argue against the fact that psychiatrists are truly physicians; this is a frontal attack on the basic definition of medical education. Medical training involves learning multiple basic sciences that are subsequently integrated with clinical diagnosis and treatment choices. Pharmacology is taught in conjunction with other basic sciences (i.e., physiology, biochemistry, pathology) and then linked to clinical medicine.

In spite of this, in 1991 the Military Health System set up a Psychopharmacology Demonstration Project to train military psychologists to prescribe psychotropic medications at military hospitals and clinics. The project closed in 1997 after training 10 psychologists; when costs of training and of supervision by psychiatrists were taken into account, the program was considered not to have been cost effective (U.S. General Accounting Office 1999). The termination of this project was a bitter defeat for those psychologists who had sought national support for prescription privileges.

Some states have nevertheless considered legislative proposals that would permit some clinical psychologists to prescribe, and two, Louisiana and New Mexico, have adopted such proposals. Many states have considered the proposals and have turned them down. It will be important to follow the way this type of legislation is implemented.

Psychopharmacology has become much more complicated in recent years, and mastering this medical procedure would be much more difficult for nonphysicians. In spite of this, efforts by psychologists continue, and training programs in psychopharmacology have been developed in academic psychology departments. Not all psychologists favor the attempts to achieve prescription privileges. Some have been particularly critical of overmedication without adequate psychotherapy. Others acknowledge privately that psychologists cannot practice medicine. Nevertheless, the conflict has soured some of the many areas of close cooperation between the two professions.

The problem of nonphysicians, such as optometrists and podiatrists, asserting medical practice rights has emerged for many medical disciplines, and the AMA has developed a committee structure to deal with this significant issue with active participation by the APA. It is important to understand that the way psychiatry was practiced from the end of World War II to the mid-1970s rendered the field vulnerable to this incursion by psychologists into medical practice. Our demedicalization invited allegations by Pat DeLeon and other psychologists that psychiatrists were paying insufficient attention to the use of medication and some were incompetent to prescribe (DeLeon and Wiggins 1996). It is the remedicalization of psychiatry that allows the APA to work closely with the AMA in countering the organized efforts by some psychologists. The battle is still lively.

Since the 1980s the APA's Office of Government Affairs (now Department of Government Relations) and Office of Public Affairs (now Office of Communications and Public Affairs) have developed fundamental arguments to use at national and state government offices to support legislation and to have an impact on public attitudes. These include evidence that

- Over 20% of adults in the United States suffer from mental illnesses or substance abuse each year.
- Individuals with mental illness still face blatant health insurance discriminations.
- The costs to society of untreated and undertreated mental illnesses are high and have been well documented.
- Parity in mental illness coverage could help states to save money.
- Advances in medical science have yielded successful and cost-effective treatments in recent decades.
- Equitable coverage of treatment for mental illness is affordable.
- Equitable coverage for mental illness results in minimal cost increases, as demonstrated in states with parity laws.

These are powerful arguments and are far removed from ideological pronouncements. They are well supported by data and have had an impact on many American citizens. These principles, however, continue to require much education, elaboration and reiteration. The APA's Office of Communications and Public Affairs and our Division of Advocacy overall play an important role in popularizing understanding of these principles.

Opposition to psychiatric practice continues to come from several different sources. There are active antipsychiatric groups such as the Scientologists, who dispute each of the seven principles listed above. Carrying picket signs with provocative messages such as "Psychiatry kills," Scientologist protesters attempt to destroy the public image of psychiatry. Libertarian groups oppose government efforts to establish treatment programs, claiming that involuntary psychiatric hospitalization is a cardinal violation of patients' civil rights. Insurance agencies have occasionally employed antipsychiatric rhetoric in questioning equitable coverage of psychiatric illnesses. Methodological weaknesses in psychiatric research efforts become special targets of these groups; the errors will be widely cited and generalized to the entire field; antipsychiatrists will employ almost any argument to hold down psychiatric costs. The

general public is no longer against psychiatry, but old myths and prejudices are still present and can be resurrected by a variety of events, such
as crimes committed by previously hospitalized patients, allegations by
Scientologists, and malpractice charges against psychiatrists. Publicized crimes committed by an expatient released from a psychiatric hospital always expose the vulnerability of psychiatry. Many will ask the
logical question of why the hospital discharged such a dangerous person. The problem often involves patients who failed to obtain adequate
follow-up treatment and discontinued their medication. It is also true,
however, that some of these horrible acts are committed by patients being treated; mistakes are made, and in some cases we simply do not know
enough about what triggers violent behavior. We are also under considerable pressure from groups who are antihospitalization and demand
justification about why patients remain in a psychiatric hospital. These
pressures are often quite intense.

Occasionally an act occurs when a psychotic person commits a crime
that causes strong negative reactions against psychiatry. When John
Hinckley Jr. attempted to assassinate President Ronald Reagan and was
later found not guilty of a crime by virtue of his insanity, there was a national outcry, which led to pressure to restrict the use of the insanity defense, as discussed in Chapter 9 ("Forensic Psychiatry"). Psychiatry today remains vulnerable to such tragic events, which often expose what
we do not know and how near the surface of national consciousness once-
overt stigma still lurks. To work against this stigma and to improve public education, Jay Scully, Medical Director, in 2003 unified the Office of
Government Relations and Office of Communications and Public Affairs,
along with the Office of Healthcare Systems and Financing, to create a
new Division of Advocacy under the overall leadership of Gene Cassel.
Studies of diverse national samples demonstrate greater sophistication
and comprehension about mental illness than ever before (von Sydow
and Reimer 1998). There also is greater awareness about the role of
psychiatrists. Most of the general public is also somewhat clearer that
psychiatric problems can be understood as disorders like other medical
conditions. When celebrities discuss their own mental illnesses, they
help to teach that such disorders can be alleviated. The "treatability" concept has begun to replace the terrible fears of inevitable deterioration
and long incarceration if one has any mental illness.

A survey carried out for the APA Office of Communications and Public
Affairs gave encouraging insight into the present state of public knowledge and attitudes. Respondents to the interview-based survey believed
by a ratio of 3:1 that the way American adults think about psychiatrists
has changed for the better in recent years. They also thought that mental

illness is understood to be serious, even if less so than high-profile physical illnesses; that stigma associated with mental illness is slightly in decline; that medical qualifications for treating mental illness are considered to be important; and that there is still reluctance to seek help for fear of stigma and costs (American Psychiatric Association 2005–2006).

Just as many psychiatrists have learned to be effective spokespersons in government affairs, the same thing has happened in public affairs. For many years Harvey Rubin, Chair of the APA Public Affairs Committee in 1985, conducted a widely popular radio program about psychiatric illness. What he said was very effective and widely appreciated. Newspaper and magazine stories about psychiatric research and new treatments have also frequently been quite positive. When an attack is made on psychiatric treatment results by an expatient, a playwright, a Scientologist, or even a serious researcher, the profession needs capable public responders.

Currently our ability to respond is much stronger. During my tenure as medical director, I brought John Blamphin into the APA to head our staff activities on public affairs. He worked with a joint membership commission in helping to create a much more positive climate of public opinion about mental illness. He recognized the complexities of public opinion by various segments of the population in different parts of the country, by different age groups, and by other population entities. Attitudes toward mental illness improved considerably under his leadership.

Nevertheless, as the less-encouraging responses on the APA survey demonstrate, there is still much to be done in educating the public, and continued long-term work will be required to have further impact on public attitudes. Many people support good mental health care for others but think that they themselves and their family could not possibly be affected by mental illness. When these people choose their own insurance coverage, they often select options that provide very limited or no mental illness coverage. I am convinced that the general public is also insufficiently aware of the range of biopsychosocial factors that are involved in the etiology of mental illness. They are also not generally aware of the new evidence-based cognitive treatments or the renaissance of a better-documented psychodynamic psychotherapy.

In addition to the important role of psychiatrists as spokespersons in promoting public understanding of psychiatric illness, the support of celebrities is very important. In 2005, well-known actress and mother Brooke Shields was criticized by actor and outspoken Scientologist Tom Cruise for taking paroxetine during her struggle with postpartum depression—an experience that she chronicled in her best-selling book

Down Came the Rain: My Journey Through Postpartum Depression. In an articulate rebuttal published in the *New York Times* (Shields 2005), the Princeton-educated Shields suggested that even negative statements in the press could be beneficial for promoting psychoeducation. "If any good can come of Mr. Cruise's ridiculous rant, let's hope that it gives much-needed attention to a serious disease." Quoted by national broadcast and print media, APA leaders also responded swiftly and forcefully to Cruise's "rants" (see Hausman 2005). Two years later, Shields was the featured speaker in a well-received "Conversations" event hosted by the American Psychiatric Foundation during APA's 2007 Annual Meeting.

Health care economics has emerged in the last three decades as an immensely important subject in our dealing with government officials. Experts on economic aspects of mental health care have had vital roles in several Presidential Commissions on health policy. They also have been important in the collection and organization of data providing the basis for parity and equity for mental illness.

The APA organized an Office for Economic Affairs under the able leadership of Sam Muszynski. Ultimately that office was reorganized and became the Office of Healthcare Systems and Financing and, later, part of the Division of Advocacy. The twenty-first century argument against equitable support for psychiatric coverage has often been based on economic grounds. Simply stated, inclusion of full coverage for psychiatric patients has been resisted because it would be too costly. As noted in the principles stated earlier, the projected costs for parity would be relatively small and the savings from an equitable program could exceed the costs. Politicians have not been particularly receptive to arguments about lowering costs in the long term. They tend to focus on the not-too-distant future. Fortunately in recent years new spokespersons are becoming more effective in pointing out long-term consequences. The data from the APA's economic affairs staff have been crucial here and will be particularly important in reinforcing the message in the next several decades. More psychiatrists have become particularly knowledgeable about the economics of psychiatric care. Strong new alliances with health economists would be a positive step for psychiatry and could be important in shaping future legislation.

Psychiatry in America is well on the road to a new parity with the rest of medicine. There are many pitfalls and special problems in the way that health care policies are implemented. Opponents of equity for psychiatric care are still very powerful. Had not psychiatry changed radically in the last three decades, there would have been little chance for nondiscrimination. The field should clearly establish its long-term goals for equity, and its spokespersons should recognize the vital importance of evidence-based practice in bringing us this far along the road. They should also recognize that a powerful advocacy effort will be required for reinforcing the political, social, and economic success of the new psychiatry.

REFERENCES

American Psychiatric Association: Diagnostic and Statistical Manual of Mental Disorders, 3rd Edition. Washington, DC, American Psychiatric Association, 1980

American Psychiatric Association, Office of Communications and Public Affairs. Unpublished national survey, 2005–2006

Barton WE: The History and Influence of the American Psychiatric Association. Washington, DC, American Psychiatric Press, 1987

Bockoven JS: Moral Treatment in American Psychiatry. New York, Springer, 1963

Clemens NA: Evidence-based psychotherapy. J Psychiatr Pract 8:51–53, 2002

Crosby EL: Psychiatric implications of Medicare: the role of the modern hospital. Am J Psychiatry 123:181–190, 1966

DeLeon P, Wiggins JG: Prescription privileges for psychologists. Am Psychol 51:225–229, 1996

English JT, Sharfstein SS, Scherl DJ,et al: Diagnosis–related groups and general hospital psychiatry: The APA Study. Am J Psychiatry 143:131–139, 1986

Gibson RW: Psychiatric implications of Medicare: the role of the psychiatrist and his helpers. Am J Psychiatry 123:191–195, 1966

Grob GN: From Asylum to Community: Mental Health Policy in Modern America. Princeton, NJ, Princeton University Press, 1991

Hausman K: Cruise finds himself at sea after antipsychiatry tirade. Psychiatr News 40(15):7, 2005

Hess AE: Medicare and mental illness. Am J Psychiatry 123:174–176, 1966

Hudson CL: Psychiatric implications of Medicare: the role of the medical profession. Am J Psychiatry 123:177–181, 1966

Karasu TB: Pharmacotherapy and psychotherapy: toward an integrative model. Am J Psychiatry 139:1102–1113, 1982

Resnick R: Psychologists' crusade for Rx privileges not likely to abate. Clinical Psychiatry News, October 1992, pp 1, 15

Riba MB, Balon R: Competency in Combining Pharmacotherapy and Psychotherapy: Integrated and Split Treatment. Washington, DC, American Psychiatric Publishing, 2005

Rome HP: Psychiatric implications of Medicare: introduction. Am J Psychiatry 123:173–174, 1966

Shields B: War of words. The New York Times, July 1, 2005

Sundararaman R, Redhead CS: Mental Health Parity: Federal and State Action and Economic Impact. Report for Congress. Washington, DC, Congressional Research Service, August 8, 2006

U.S. General Accounting Office: Prescribing psychologists (GAO/HEHS-99-98). Report to the Committee on Armed Services, U.S. Senate, June 1999

U.S. President's Commission on Mental Health: Report to the President from the President's Commission on Mental Health, Vol 1 (040-000-00390-8). Washington, D.C., U.S. Government Printing Office, 1978

von Sydow K, Reimer C: Attitudes toward psychotherapists, psychologists, psychiatrists, and psychoanalysts: a meta-analysis of 60 studies published between 1948 and 1995. Am J Psychother 52:463–488, 1998

Wallerstein RS: The Psychotherapy Research Project of the Menninger Foundation: an overview. J Consult Clin Psychol 57:195–205, 1989

7

International Affairs

*I*nternational affairs have been an important part of the history of the American Psychiatric Association, despite being perceived by many members to be of low priority. I have been a strong proponent of international activity by the APA. Whether it is recognized or not, all psychiatrists are internationalists, and the field of psychiatry is international. I have enjoyed acknowledging this point in overseas presentations by beginning talks with a phrase such as "I speak here today as a foreign psychiatrist like most of you in this audience." Too often, however, American psychiatrists perceive international psychiatry as comprising "foreign psychiatrists and us." Perhaps a remnant of an isolationist America, these attitudes persist despite American psychiatry's prominence on the world stage in the twentieth century.

Isolationist America in the first half of the twentieth century changed dramatically into an international superpower in most scientific areas, as well as in foreign policy. American psychiatry exerted its influence in world psychiatry in the biological, neuroscientific, and psychopharmacological areas. Although initially conceived to transform the practice of psychiatry in America, DSM-III (American Psychiatric Association 1980) and DSM-IV (American Psychiatric Association 1994) had a powerful and unexpected effect on the global practice of psychiatry. A central feature of American influence in the late twentieth century, DSM-III and DSM-IV have been adopted worldwide. Psychiatrists from all over the world now come in large numbers to the APA Annual Meeting (see Chapter 13, "A Changing Membership"); their greatest current interest appears to be about psychopharmacological developments. Will this neuroscientific dominance of American psychiatry continue for several decades, or will new developments in Europe, Asia, Africa, and South America begin to play a role in changing psychiatry again? Many American psychiatrists look forward to a more balanced psychiatry in which we in the United States are able to learn more from the rest of the world while continuing to play a teaching role.

In this chapter I describe the impact of the rise of American psychiatry, but I also discuss problems that have resulted from this international dynamic. Can a truly biopsychosocial psychiatry help to restore a balanced international perspective? Can anything change the neuroscientific hegemony of the United States while maintaining the new scientific standards of the twenty-first century?

From the end of the war until the mid-1970s, the major trends in American psychiatry were largely products of European origin. Since then, American psychiatry has become a major world leader in nosology, practice guidelines, and basic research in psychopharmacology. It has also become particularly strong in neuroscience. Selected aspects of the story of these substantial changes are discussed in this chapter as perceived during my active participation in some of the decisions. Explaining some of the processes, aspirations, and the people involved in these changes is the main goal of this chapter. Occasionally I will diverge by discussing international topics that have had special meaning for me.

Before World War II, few foreign-born psychiatrists working in the United States had a powerful impact on the practice of psychiatry there. One notable exception, Swiss born Adolph Meyer, served as a major catalyst in preparing the field for a new psychiatry (Meyer 1948, 1950). Weir Mitchell had, in 1894, criticized the research and academic status in psychiatry in this country and presaged the changes of the latter part of the twentieth century (Mitchell 1894). Despite these and other exceptions, pre-war leadership in psychiatry in the United States was mostly home grown.

World War II weakened the political leadership of isolationists, some of whom had opposed American involvement in the war. With its entry into the war the United States became a world power and, later in the century after the "Cold War," the only superpower. With the postwar emigration of many Austrian, German, and Central European psychiatrists to America, psychoanalysis became a central focus of American psychiatry. Indeed, analysis achieved a level of influence far beyond that in any other country in the world. The effects upon psychiatric training and practice were profound. In addition, the effect on culture and the arts, such as theatre, novels, and cinema, was even more powerful and lasting. The stereotypical analyst was that of a "foreign"-looking gentleman speaking with a Central European accent. Cartoonists often depicted analysts as bearded figures sitting behind a couch. The therapeutic impact of psychoanalysis in the United States, as discussed in Chapter 8 ("Psychoanalysis"), was primarily on large cities. While there was an important influence upon academic training, the main location of therapeutic work and teaching was at independent Psychoanalytic Institutes. The academically sponsored Psychoanalytic Institutes at Columbia University and the University of Pittsburgh, plus the special situation of the influential Menninger Clinic in Topeka, were exceptions. Almost all the institutes' staff were full-time practitioners, with nonpractitioner researchers being rare. Most of what was called "research" involved narrative reports of clinical work; objective hypothesis testing was almost unknown. Academic psychiatric centers often appointed analysts as part-time teachers for medical students and supervisors of residents in psychotherapeutic education. Shorter (1997) attributes much of psychoanalytic influence in the United States to its special acceptance by Jewish women.

It is true that most of the immigrant psychoanalysts were Jewish, and so were many of the early generation of patients. The composition of analytic patients became more culturally diverse as psychoanalysts migrated to cities in the American heartland and beyond, such as Atlanta, Denver, Dallas, Houston, Cincinnati, Minneapolis–St. Paul, Pittsburgh, Seattle, and Topeka. The penetration of Freud's ideas into America was a phenomenal example of a profession being dazzled by a remarkable group, largely of European transplants. Perhaps still longing for familiar Viennese coffee houses, these expatriates nevertheless transformed the practice of psychiatry in their adoptive land.

Social and biological aspects of psychiatry also had important stimulation from outside America. For several decades Marxists were major critics of psychoanalysis, advancing social and economic explanations for mental illness. That fierce old Marxist ideology is almost all forgotten today in America. Social psychiatry, as developed in Germany, France, Italy, and the United Kingdom, has had a declining influence in the United States for several decades but has persisted in Europe much more strongly. The Berlin journal *Social Psychiatry and Psychiatric Epidemiology* is heavily oriented toward European work. The late-century rise of biological psychiatry in the United States has also reduced the research in cross-cultural psychiatry, which had peaked in the 1970s and 1980s. This field of work is still of strong interest to minority psychiatrists (Griffiths et al. 1999), but in general the search for equity in treatment has taken precedence over the search for alternative social theories of the etiology of mental illness.

The work of Abram Kardiner was particularly important in helping me to understand how diverse cultural pattern of human development had an important impact in shaping behavioral patterns (Kardiner 1939, 1945; Kardiner and Ovesey 1951). Transcultural psychiatry, taught by "progressive" analysts seeking new hypotheses, is less apparent in American psychiatry today.

International social and cultural psychiatry as a special field is exemplified by Norman Sartorius, who personifies internationalism more than any other psychiatrist of our generation. His leadership at the World Health Organization (WHO) and the World Psychiatric Association (WPA) has been exceptionally important. His work symbolizes what I hope will become an international trend later in this twenty-first century. Sartorius's mastery of many languages, his observational skills and perceptiveness in discovering unexpected behavioral patterns in ordinary settings, and his mastery of nosology are unique. For several decades he has traveled widely and spoken to more diverse psychiatric groups than any other person. His personal observations are full of plausible new hypotheses that at some point should be the subject of major research (Sartorius 1975). As language skills and world travel become more common, it is likely that a larger number of psychiatrists will develop some of the skills that Sartorius demonstrates today. Then, perhaps, a new era of international research might be achieved and hypothesis testing methodology may become much more prominent in international social psychiatry.

The WPA, founded in 1950 by the eminent French psychiatrist Jean Delay, has played a major role in improving international psychiatric communication. By sponsoring World Congresses and many regional meetings, it has provided a vital educational service and has been extraordinarily helpful to progress in psychiatry in developing countries. I was elected to its Executive Committee in 1983 and have had the good fortune to work with many distinguished psychiatric leaders such as Professors Pierre Pichot, José López-Ibor, Felice Lieh-Mak, Costas Stephanis, Jorge Costa deSilva, Ahmed Okasha, and Norman Sartorius, all of whom have been presidents of the WPA during my time in that organization.

Biological psychiatry and classification of mental illness in the United States during the postwar era were heavily dependent on German, French, and Swiss work. Nevertheless, during that period, nosology in America was weaker than in all major world psychiatric centers. Emil Kraepelin, Wilhelm Griesinger, Eugen Bleuler, Jean-Martin Charcot, and Pierre Janet still exerted an influence, but Sigmund Freud and his American emissaries became much more central to psychiatric education and practice in the United States. By the 1970s, this influence was in decline, and what followed was an avalanche of biological, phenomenological, and nosological research that led to new forms of diagnosis and practice that had a worldwide impact. Much brilliant neuropsychiatric research is conducted in Europe, but the pharmaceutical-industrial research complex of the United States exerts the greatest influence. Biological researchers in the United States have become important figures in world psychiatry. Their visibility is not so much in organizational leadership but in their books, articles, presentations, and consultation roles. For many psychiatrists outside America, international psychiatry is mostly defined as learning as much as possible about what the Americans are doing.

The APA opened its Office of International Affairs after my arrival. I had already served on the APA's Council of International Affairs and was determined that the APA should became more active worldwide. My primary emphasis was not on how such an office would be important for APA's fiscal status; nevertheless, I must acknowledge that the very existence of the office, in conjunction with the APA's new world leadership role in science, the APA's many new books, and the increased popularity of our Annual Meetings with many foreign registrants, contributed mightily to the organization's financial success. I recognize that my statement about underestimating the fiscal implications of international affairs will be hard to accept by some critics. I wanted the world to learn about important changes in American psychiatry, but I did not anticipate that the effort would be so successful financially.

The formal establishment of an Office of International Affairs at the APA in 1982 was a product of many events and much determination, and its accomplishments far exceeded my expectations. We had participated in some international activities prior to my medical directorship in that a Council on International Affairs had been formed and had been chaired by important leaders of the APA. Some international study trips were made available for members to join, but we could not offer these in a systematic way at the time without staff to coordinate such functions. In addition to the Council, several officers of the APA had been active in international organizations, and world psychiatric leaders were often well known in the United States. By the early 1970s, international activities had begun to increase. Howard Rome, Past President of the APA, was elected president of the WPA and had become a strong force for the future direction of APA's international work. Indeed, the choice of Hawaii for the WPA's World Congress in 1977 was based on the principle that the World Congress was usually held in the home country of the WPA President.

The organization of the Congress was extremely fortunate for the future development of international activities by the APA. As the major psychiatric association in the home country of the WPA president, the APA took full responsibility for organizing the meeting. A major concern for the WPA and the APA at that time was the growing number of allegations that abuse of psychiatry had been occurring and was continuing in the Soviet Union. Hawaii was chosen as the Congress site, in part because it was thought by some that the Soviets might be more willing to come to Hawaii rather than attend a meeting on the mainland of the United States. Hawaii, of course, was also a particularly attractive venue because of the natural beauty of the state.

Instead of continuing the practice that the WPA had followed in previous years of contracting with professional congress-organizing companies, the APA hired two multilingual individuals, Rosa Torres and Rosely Stanich, to implement the program while the APA's Meetings Management Department, headed by Kathleen Bryan, organized the logistics. I had been the Scientific Program Committee Chair for the APA Annual Meeting held in Hawaii in 1973 and was soon to be appointed medical director, and, thus, there was experience and another reason for choosing Hawaii as the venue for the World Congress.

This was also the time when the first serious allegations about the abuse of psychiatry in the Soviet Union were made and there was great interest in holding a special session on such abuse during the World Congress. Gerald Sarwer-Foner was the chair of the Congress Program Committee. His broad experience in Canadian psychiatry, including his educational leadership, was important in selecting an excellent program.

Shervert Frazier, another major psychiatric leader in the United States, was the WPA Organizing Committee Chair and agreed to schedule a forum to discuss the issue of abuse. There was much hope that the Soviet Union would send representatives to be part of this discussion, which they did. I will never forget meeting the ten Russian delegates at the registration desk, where I saw how they opened a suitcase filled with American currency to pay their registration fees. This was my first meeting with Professors A.V. Snejnevski and Marat Vartanian, which became very important later when I worked with them about specific allegations of abuse.

Jack Weinberg was the president of the APA for 1977–78, and in this role he served as the Delegate to the General Assembly meeting of the WPA, held during the World Congress. It was particularly poignant that Jack had been born in Ukraine, having immigrated to the United States as a child with his parents. He led the discussions of the charges made against the Soviets for their alleged abuses of psychiatry by putting dissidents into mental hospitals to suppress their dissent. Other key American psychiatrists, including Walter Reich and Paul Chodoff, were also very much involved in this work. The forum and subsequent General Assembly debate yielded a resolution condemning the All-Union Society of Psychiatrists and Neuropathologists for these alleged abuses of psychiatry and also creating a review committee mechanism for WPA member societies to bring allegations of psychiatric abuse against any country, to which the member societies of the respective countries were expected to respond. The APA and many other member societies subsequently brought allegations against the Soviets, who chose not to respond.

That meeting was a turning point for the APA's international activities. In particular, it helped to begin Ellen Mercer's formal activities for the APA in international work. She had had considerable international experience before coming to the APA, including living and working in Taiwan and Laos, and I was very fortunate to be able to recruit her to work in my office after she spent eight months in the Office of Professional Affairs, headed by Henry Work. In planning for the Hawaii Congress, Ellen had her first and intense exposure to international psychiatry.

Concern about the use of psychiatry to suppress dissent became a significant part of the early stages of APA's international work. We felt that organized international psychiatry had an important role to play in monitoring such abuses and helping to bring such practices to an end. Over the years, many members incorrectly perceived that our international activities were related only to this issue, which was, in fact, not the case.

Another extremely important event facilitated the APA's involvement in world psychiatry when, in 1979, arrangements were made for a delegation of Chinese psychiatrists to visit the United States. As recently as 1977, the Chinese had been invited to attend the Hawaii WPA Congress and declined to participate. In their statement to us, they made the remarkable comment, "We have no need for psychiatrists in our country." By 1979, however, an extraordinary visit by seven Chinese psychiatrists occurred. The group was organized by a Sri Lankan/American psychiatrist, David Ratnavale, and included Professor Xia Chen-yi and others. They first visited selected psychiatric departments around the country and ended with participation in the APA's Annual Meeting in Chicago. The success of that visit was an important facilitator for additional international activities by Ellen Mercer, who undertook this work while continuing her medical director's office responsibilities for 5 years until formal establishment of the Office of International Affairs.

Having the Chinese psychiatrists at the APA Annual Meeting drew a great deal of attention from our membership. Professor Xia, the head of the delegation and head of the Institute on Mental Health in Shanghai, spoke briefly at the opening session of the meeting, ending his talk by stating that he hoped that "the friendship between our two countries will flow as freely as the Mississippi and Yangzi Rivers." I assigned Ellen Mercer the responsibility of helping the Chinese during this meeting, and she did it in a way that prompted them to write many letters of appreciation to her and the APA. Because of this work, she formed an active relationship with the staff of the Chinese Embassy in Washington, who asked her to coordinate other visits of physicians. These very bright and accomplished psychiatrists had been so isolated from international colleagues that they were greatly relieved to find that someone was available to help them through the challenges of attending such a large meeting, where they met hundreds of psychiatrists from the United States as well as other countries. These contacts served them well throughout the years, and some of them returned at other times, at the invitation of APA members, with their visits coordinated by Ellen. Over the years, she worked with three generations of psychiatric leaders in China and forged a very close working relationship with the Chinese Medical Association staff. Because of those relationships, she was able to arrange for collaboration for many APA members going to China as well as for other organizations, such as the International Association for Child and Adolescent Psychiatry and Allied Professions, for whom she organized a study tour in 1986.

In 1980, APA leadership visited China at the invitation of the Chinese Medical Association. We enjoyed their excellent hospitality and participated in many scientific discussions. We made numerous visits to psychiatric hospitals, where we often saw patients lying in their beds apparently reading the works of Mao Tse-tung. Ten years later while visiting in Western China, our local guide was highly critical of Mao; times had indeed changed. Chinese psychiatry had become increasingly sophisticated by the end of the century.

Over the years, the Office of International Affairs built a broad network of psychiatrists all around the world—a network used by many APA members and patients for referrals, collaborative research and education, and service. Among many other things, Ellen Mercer, working closely with the American Psychiatric Press and the APA Membership Department, arranged for returned or slightly damaged books and journals to be sent to developing countries. The first DSM-III sent to Ethiopia was hand-carried by an Ethiopian/American psychiatrist traveling for the World Bank. He returned with photographs of this prized book being in a locked glass cabinet and accessible only to those who wanted to use it in that one room of the psychiatric hospital there. We stocked their library, as well as many others around the world, without ever requiring them to purchase a book or journal. This kind of good will had extremely broad ramifications as psychiatrists in these countries entered the world stage. Building international good will for the United States became an important function for the Office of International Affairs.

Before my arrival at the APA, we had a category of membership called "Corresponding Members," by which psychiatrists from other countries could join at no fee but also with few benefits. We gradually changed this designation into an "International Member" category, by which, for a small membership fee, psychiatrists could join us and receive many discounts on our services and products, including the registration fee at Annual Meetings. The Office of International Affairs wrote and distributed a newsletter to those members and to others that kept them informed of our overall activities and how they could participate. This effort was part of my attempt to "internationalize" the APA, in part by facilitating more interaction with other APA departments, committees, and members.

In 1989, there were 1,255 visitors from other countries, including Canada, at the APA Annual Meeting. After the Office of International Affairs took over the responsibilities for these visitors, the number increased astonishingly to more than 8,000 by the time the Office was closed ten years later. Over the years, the Office organized an International Scholars Program with support from Mead Johnson Pharmaceuticals, which brought five speakers to each APA Annual Meeting for a number of years. The speakers included Victor Frankl, Sir Martin Roth, Jorge Luis Borges, Ambassador Shimon Shamir, Justice Richard Goldstone, and many other renowned psychiatrists, literary figures, and academics. Later, the Office organized a hospitality suite for international visitors, generously funded by Pfizer, Inc., which provided a friendly and convenient meeting place for those coming from abroad. There were numerous services provided by the Office at those times, and it was a main attraction of the meeting. International psychiatrists continue to remind me how much they appreciated that suite. It symbolized that they were truly welcome.

For several years in the late 1990s, the Office arranged a fellowship program for young psychiatrists from developing countries; this was another popular program bringing together psychiatrists from countries such as Libya, Egypt, Ghana, Ethiopia, China, Rwanda, Romania, Russia, and Bangladesh.

In the early 1980s, the APA had the opportunity to sponsor a very innovative program that was brought to us by an APA member, William Davidson, who was the founder and director of the Institute for Psychiatry and Foreign Affairs and chair of the APA Committee on Psychiatry and Foreign Affairs, established in 1977. This program, known as the "Psychological Aspects of the Middle East Peace Process," was funded by the U.S. Agency for International Development, the U.S. State Department, and the National Institute of Mental Health (NIMH), the latter under the leadership of Herbert Pardes. The APA Committee on Psychiatry and Foreign Affairs and the APA Office of International Affairs organized small meetings, for a period of 5 years, bringing together Israelis, Egyptians, and Palestinians to discuss impediments to peace. This process, which was called "track two" diplomacy, increased the understanding of key figures involved in mainstream diplomacy among states. Meetings were held in Washington, D.C., Switzerland, Austria, and Egypt, where psychiatrists, academics, politicians, diplomats, and foreign service personnel came together under isolated and protected circumstances to learn ways of working together. While the meetings were totally off the record, they produced positive results in Israel, Egypt, Gaza, and the West Bank of Israel. Ellen Mercer was responsible for managing the grants, with the help of our Accounting Department, finding locations for the meetings and organizing them, and for the main communication with the Middle Eastern participants, in conjunction with the Committee. This was the most innovative international program taken on by the APA, and I am proud to have supported and facilitated it along the way.

The APA offered many services for our U.S. members as well as for those from abroad. For some years, we held biannual scientific meetings in other countries: Australia and New Zealand, Mexico, France, Italy, Germany, China, Kenya, Barbados, Philippines, Ireland, and South Korea. In 1992, we organized a bilateral exchange with the psychiatric associations in Poland, Hungary, and Czechoslovakia and, with outside funding, took twelve American psychiatrist leaders to share the latest developments in their respective psychiatric subspecialties. We served in a formal consultant role to Saudi Arabia, where a number of our members were sent for weeks at a time, and with Sri Lanka, where we worked closely with the then–Sri Lankan Ambassador to the United States and David Ratnavale on the improvement of services there. We formed an International Program Development component that would provide a fee for service to other countries, calling upon the expertise of our membership, but, unfortunately, the potential of this component was not fully realized before the Office of International Affairs was discontinued in 1999. The initiative had come from the APA Committee on International Education under the leadership of Normund Wong, Robert Leon, and others. Also at the initiative of that Committee, the Office of International Affairs put together a directory, the *International Psychiatric Directory*, that proved to be a good resource of information from 103 different countries (American Psychiatric Association 1993).We had committees and task forces on many important issues. One such committee, with psychiatric representation from the U.S. military and the State Department, examined problems faced by Americans living overseas. In 1986, this group organized an important conference in Washington with the American Bar Association. Another component that is even more timely today was the Task Force on Terrorism, chaired by L. Jolyon West, in the late 1980s (American Psychiatric Association 1982). While international medical graduate members of the APA were represented through the Council on National Affairs and Office of Minority and National Affairs, there was some overlap in activities with this important constituency of the APA (see Chapter 13, "A Changing Membership," for further discussion of this particular group).

Our relationship with Canadian psychiatrists has always been special, since many Canadians are members of the APA. There are three district branches in Canada, and they have been vigorous participants in the Assembly as well as in APA's international affairs. Ray Freebury from Ontario has been a leading spokesperson on questions of psychiatric abuse. During my tenure as medical director, I attended the Canadian Psychiatric Association's Annual Meeting every year and enjoyed both good hospitality and a Canadian education.

With all of the collaborative activities undertaken by the Office, we were also very involved with ethical and human rights issues. Our Committee on International Abuse of Psychiatry and Psychiatrists and the Committee on Human Rights were actively following specific cases and individuals around the world, notably in the U.S.S.R., Chile, Cuba, and South Africa. The Office, on behalf of these committees, wrote literally hundreds of letters asking for information on specific cases and never received a response. We joined with the Committee on Human Rights (now Physicians for Human Rights) and the American Psychological Association in a 1985 mission to Chile under the Pinochet regime, funded by the MacArthur Foundation. The Medical Society of Chile had taken very courageous positions against torture and had invited this delegation, which included APA Past President Lawrence Hartmann and Ellen Mercer. Their report was riveting and resulted in testimony before a Congressional committee. Dr. Hartmann continues to be a driving force in the area of human rights in his current role as chair of the APA's Council on Global Psychiatry (2007–08). The APA Board of Trustees spoke out against the activities of psychiatrists such as Radovan Karadzic, whose "brutal and inhumane actions as the Bosnian Serb leader" we condemned: "These actions deserve condemnation by all civilized persons, but psychiatrists issue that condemnation with particular offense, urgency, and horror because, by education and training, Dr. Karadzic claims membership in our profession."

In the early 1970s, there were allegations of abuse of psychiatry in South Africa during the apartheid system of government. Many psychiatric facilities were run there by the Smith-Mitchell Corporation, which invited the APA to send a delegation to investigate these allegations. Drs. Alan Stone, Jeanne Spurlock, Charles Pinderhughes, and Jack Weinberg went there as the APA delegation. While they did not find evidence of direct political abuse of psychiatry, as was the case in the U.S.S.R., they did find huge discrepancies in the treatment of patients in the facilities for blacks compared with those for whites. They wrote a strong report that condemned this practice, and I had the difficult role of hand delivering this report to the South African Health Ministry on a trip I took to South Africa in 1975. The minister and his staff were quite harsh with me and denied all the charges, but I stood my ground. Years later, after the end of apartheid, the South African Society of Psychiatry was effusive in its praise of the APA's visit. The APA continues to advocate that psychiatrists uphold high ethical standards, as evidenced by its position statement regarding psychiatrists' participation in the interrogation of detainees (American Psychiatric Association 2006).

In 1988, the APA joined together with the American Association for the Advancement of Science (AAAS) for another human rights mission to South Africa, but the applications for visas were denied. Not long afterward, as the system of apartheid was slowly being dismantled, a trip with the AAAS was possible, and Larry Hartmann represented the APA. In 1996, Mary Jane England went to South Africa as president of the APA and furthered our collaborative relationships with the Society of Psychiatrists of South Africa.

Ellen Mercer established a good working relationship with the president of the Cuban Psychiatric Association, Dr. Ricardo González Menéndez, who, in 1994, arranged for visas for a group of individuals to travel to Cuba and look into allegations of abuse of psychiatry there. The delegation was to include Ray Freebury, from Canada, and Carola Eisenberg, M.D., Chair of the Committee on Abuse of Psychiatry; Carlos Sluzki, M.D., Chair of the Committee on Human Rights; and Ellen. Both Drs. Eisenberg and Sluzki are originally from Argentina. After all of the arrangements were made, however, the trip was cancelled by then–APA President Jerry Wiener, M.D., because of objections of some of our Cuban American members who felt that such a delegation should not go without a Cuban American representative. Later, when efforts were made to take a trip that overcame earlier objections, visas were denied.

Under the leadership of Past President Lawrence Hartmann, the APA established the Human Rights Award, which still exists today, to honor individuals and organizations who have stood up for human rights around the world. Recipients of that award included the Committee on Scientific Freedom and Responsibility of the AAAS; the Geneva Initiative on Psychiatry; Jack Weinberg; Inge Kemp Genefke and the International Association for Treatment of Torture Victims; Semyon Gluzman; Richard Mollica; and others.

By far the most publicized of our human rights activities, however, were those related to the Soviet Union, since it was our profession being used in a nonmedical and coercive fashion. We supported Soviet psychiatrists and others who opposed the abuse of psychiatry, such as those involved with the Moscow Working Commission to Investigate the Abuse of Psychiatry. We especially worked on behalf of psychiatrists Semyon Gluzman and Anatoly Koryagin. Dr. Gluzman was forced to serve seven years in a labor camp and three years in Siberian exile in the late 1970s and early 1980s for refusing to diagnose a famous Soviet General, Petr Grigorenko, as being mentally ill when he spoke against the human rights abuses in the U.S.S.R. Dr. Koryagin was imprisoned for six years for his work on the Moscow Working Commission. He was released earlier than his sentence required because of international pressure from the APA and many other organizations around the world. The APA Office of International Affairs arranged for him to participate in the APA Annual Meeting to an enormous standing-room-only crowd only a month after his exile from the U.S.S.R. to Switzerland. Dr. Gluzman subsequently visited the APA on many occasions after the fall of the Soviet Union.

Historic trips were made to the U.S.S.R. in 1989 and 1990, facilitated by the U.S. State Department, funded by the NIMH, and organized, in part, by the APA. Because of international pressure on the U.S.S.R., the Soviets were no longer a part of the WPA; the NIMH had long refused to have joint research or collaboration with Soviets because of the alleged abuses of psychiatry; and the long-ranging meeting of the U.S. Commission on Security and Cooperation in Europe did not end until an agreement was made with the Soviets for a full on-site investigation of the charges that had plagued them for so many years. Through the U.S. State Department's Office of Human Rights, the Soviet Ministries of Foreign Affairs and of Health agreed to allow an unprecedented invitation, to include psychiatrists, specialists in mental health law, and human rights specialists, to come to the U.S.S.R. to examine patients and former patients in psychiatric hospitals and to visit special psychiatric hospitals, run by the Ministry of the Interior. In 1989, a small group of people, led by a State Department representative with Loren Roth as the psychiatric team leader, visited Moscow to negotiate the terms of this agreement. Ellen Mercer participated in both trips and wrote a detailed account of the negotiations. The larger mission took place some months afterward, with the psychiatric team undertaking extensive examinations of alleged political prisoners, with the help of three Russian émigré psychiatrists and State Department interpreters. There was also a hospital visit team, led by Harold Visotsky, that visited two special psychiatric hospitals in Chernyahovsk and Kazan, respectively, and two general hospitals in Lithuania. The final report of the mission was published in NIMH's *Schizophrenia Bulletin* (United States Delegation to Assess Recent Changes in Soviet Psychiatry 1990).

My activity in the WPA increased over the years as I served as a member of its Executive Committee until 1989. During my tenure, the APA Office of International Affairs organized two WPA Regional Symposia in the United States: one in New York in 1981 and another in Washington, D.C., in 1988. We participated in many regional symposia in other parts of the world, and this proved to be a valuable opportunity for increasing our international network. In addition, we had a chance to learn from and teach our colleagues living in other countries, and to increase our international membership and participation in the APA Annual Meetings. For me personally it was an outstanding learning experience. With my support, Ellen Mercer served as the Secretariat for the WPA Ethics Committee, under the leadership of Costas Stefanis of Greece. In addition, at my encouragement, she took a contract, with funds donated to the APA, for two years leading up to the World Congress in Madrid.

My role in the WPA was complicated at times, as I worked to uphold the goals and resolutions of the APA while at the same time being an independent member of the Executive Committee, not formally representing the APA. I deliberated whether I ought to make an effort to seek nomination for the presidency of the WPA. Ultimately I decided against seeking the nomination because of a possible conflict of interest with my role in the APA.

We also collaborated with a number of other international organizations, such as the WHO, the World Federation for Mental Health, the Pacific Rim College of Psychiatrists, Geneva Initiative on Psychiatry, the Inter-American Council of Psychiatric Organizations, as well as many psychiatric organizations in other countries. One important function of our Office of Research, which is elaborated upon in Chapter 11 ("Psychiatric Research"), was the work on the *Diagnostic and Statistical Manual of Mental Disorders* (DSM) and the *International Classification of Diseases* (ICD) published by the WHO. Our Office of International Affairs was a valuable participant in many APA staff functions and was much appreciated by other APA offices.

The Council on International Affairs suggested policy to the APA Board and Assembly and was led by many distinguished APA leaders: Alfred Freedman, Jack Weinberg, Fritz Redlich, Harold Visotsky, Eugene Feigelson, Pedro Ruiz, and Jeffrey Geller. The activities of the Council became much more proactive after the establishment of the Office of International Affairs, which provided strong staff support, and this activity continued through my tenure at the APA.

In addition to the activities mentioned above, we had a formal consultation with the Department of Mental Health in Saudi Arabia and arranged for APA members to spend weeks at a time in that country helping them improve their mental health system. We were active in the Arab Federation of Psychiatrists and the Inter-American Council of Psychiatric Associations. All of these activities were interrelated with events such as the APA Annual Meetings and played a key role in dramatically increasing attendance at our conferences. Psychiatrists worldwide experienced the APA as a welcoming place where they would have the opportunity of meeting colleagues from all over the world. I do believe that the APA has sponsored many outstanding conferences in the psychiatric world, and as these became accessible to the world community, the APA benefited in many ways, including scientifically and financially. Our members and their patients also benefited, since the Office of International Affairs made more than 250 personal patient referrals a year when individuals were moving or traveling abroad.

While we were active in organizations such as the WPA, WHO, and the World Federation for Mental Health, I believe that we were primarily respected for our scientific and academic knowledge, our ethical stand on human rights, our generosity to those less fortunate, and our welcoming approach to psychiatrists from all over the world. I remain proud of what we accomplished and regretful that the Office of International Affairs was disbanded two years after my retirement from the APA. The hundreds of letters received from around the world after this action was taken attest to the fact that the Office would be greatly missed.

The termination of the Office of International Affairs by my successor at the end of 1999 caused me much private concern. I perceived this action as a bitter personal defeat, and for several years I limited my contact with the APA until Jay Scully was appointed medical director. I do not fully understand the reasons for the decision to close the Office, but it occurred during the time of efforts to streamline the APA and reduce the expenses on "low priority" items. If this was part of an economy drive to abolish what were perceived as costly, less important, areas, it misunderstood the effects of the office on many income streams. Some members of the APA leadership rated international affairs as a low priority because such efforts did not appear to deal with the great practice pressures experienced by our members under the new managed care system. Most often these critics had little understanding of the fiscal benefits derived from an organized system of international relationships. They had even less understanding of what our Office of International Affairs meant for our reputation in the world. It is conceivable that some of the critics believed that American psychiatry was so popular worldwide that we could carry on successfully without the Office. Since his appointment in 2003, Jay Scully has helped to restore a "Global Council" and has restructured staff responsibilities for international work. He fully recognizes its multiple areas of importance for the APA and is in the process of finding support for resuming even broader activities.

Two of APA's past presidents are currently members of the WPA's Executive Committee. Pedro Ruiz and Alan Tasman have followed in the footsteps of several past presidents and officers who have recognized the importance of international affairs for all of us. Howard Rome, Alfred Freedman, George Tarjan, Larry Hartmann, and Jack Weinberg provided exemplary leadership. All of our elected officers recognize that our highest current APA priorities are to achieve parity and equity for our patients and our colleagues. To be a devoted teacher and a continuous participant in learning about international psychiatry does not contradict this role. It is more important to the goal of equity than some of our members have understood. An American psychiatry that is respected and admired across the world and that is able to perceive and absorb creative new ideas will be more likely to achieve equity than will an organization that functions as a self-absorbed isolated trade union.

REFERENCES

American Psychiatric Association, Committee on International Affairs: An International Psychiatric Directory. Edited by Mercer ER, Mesner L. Washington. DC, American Psychiatric Association, 1993

American Psychiatric Association, Task Force on Terrorism and Its Victims: Ethical dimensions of psychiatric intervention in terrorist and hostage situations: a report of the APA Task Force on Terrorism and Its Victims. Am J Psychiatry 139:1529–1530, 1982

American Psychiatric Association: Diagnostic and Statistical Manual of Mental Disorders, 3rd Edition. Washington, DC, American Psychiatric Association, 1980

American Psychiatric Association: Diagnostic and Statistical Manual of Mental Disorders, 4th Edition. Washington, DC, American Psychiatric Association, 1994

American Psychiatric Association: Position statement: psychiatric participation in interrogation of detainees, in American Psychiatric Association Operations Manual. Arlington, VA, American Psychiatric Association, May 2006

Griffiths EEH, Gonzales CA, Blue HC: The basics of cultural psychiatry, in The American Psychiatric Press Textbook of Psychiatry, 3rd Edition. Edited by Hales RE, Yudofsky SC, Talbott JA. Washington, DC, American Psychiatric Press, 1999, pp 1463–1492

Kardiner A: The Individual and His Society: The Psychodynamics of Primitive Social Organization. New York, Columbia University Press, 1939

Kardiner A: The Psychological Frontiers of Society. New York, Columbia University Press, 1945

Kardiner A, Ovesey L: Mark of Oppression: A Psychosocial Study of the American Negro. New York, WW Norton, 1951

Meyer A: The Commonsense Psychiatry of Dr. Adolf Meyer. New York, McGraw-Hill, 1948

Meyer A: Collected Papers of Adolf Meyer. Edited by Winters EE. Baltimore, MD, Johns Hopkins Press, 1950

Mitchell SW: Address before the fiftieth annual meeting of the American Medico-Psychological Association, held in Philadelphia, May 16th, 1894. J Nerv Ment Dis 21:413–437, 1894

Sartorius N: Mental health evaluation worldwide: an interview with Norman Sartorius. Interview by Susan Salasin. Evaluation 2(2):12–16, 1975

Shorter E: A History of Psychiatry: From the Era of the Asylum to the Age of Prozac. New York, Wiley, 1997

United States Delegation to Assess Recent Changes in Soviet Psychiatry: Report of the U.S. Delegation to assess recent changes in Soviet psychiatry. Schizophr Bull 15 (4, suppl):1–79, 1990

8

Psychoanalysis

When psychoanalysis burst forth in American psychiatry, alternative theoretical constructs were weak. It filled a large void with its imaginative albeit speculative formulations. It dealt in a courageous fashion with topics that were often taboo. Undoubtedly as a result of psychoanalysis many people were helped to understand themselves better. But what proportion of patients were helped and what proportion were not remains frustratingly obscure. Scientific evidence about therapeutic outcome is still weaker than advocates claim.

Today, the clinical practice of psychoanalysis does not fit easily into an American managed care medical system. It did not fit any better in the maelstrom of Soviet socialist reality or in most of the so-called Third World. It must be acknowledged, however, that in the United States it found a warm welcome in some very special environments. Most often this occurred in places where artistic creativity, imagination, and somewhat more liberated sexuality flourished. During the 1950s and 1960s, psychoanalysis became very popular in Hollywood and Manhattan, both of which had many of the fundamental attributes for an analytic-friendly culture. Communities with high interest in the arts, many university towns, and even some large cities in the United States still support the practice of psychoanalysis.

The theoretical and scientific foundations of psychoanalysis depended originally on Sigmund Freud and a small group of colleagues. Beginning with the first presentation of psychoanalytic formulations, there were devoted adherents but also bitter opponents. The struggle has continued throughout most of the history of psychoanalytic growth and maturation. Until recently, psychoanalysis resembled the stereotype of an ideology rather than a science (Strauss et al. 1964).

When Freud accepted an invitation to visit America in 1909, he was at the peak of his creative powers and the psychoanalytic movement achieved a foothold in this vast country. After World War II the institutional and organizational support for the intellectual work of psychoanalysis was established. In addition to activities at older and newly formed psychoanalytic institutes, theoretical and scientific work in psychoanalysis found a special positive reception in several American psychiatric departments, in psychological research centers, and in humanities departments. While there was continuous opposition to psychoanalytic theoretical formulations during this time, there also was widespread interest.

By the 1970s when constraints began to be placed upon clinical practice, criticism of psychoanalytic research methodology and its theories began in earnest and have continued up to the present. In recent years, however, the leadership of a new generation of psychoanalyst theorists and work on neural correlates of analytic processes, mentalization, and hypotheses derived from attachment theory have slowed the momentum of the dismissal of the basic principles of psychoanalysis.

Exceptions to the usual settings receptive to psychoanalytic clinical practice and theoretical work occurred, and psychoanalysis became strong in some communities that were totally unlike Hollywood, Greenwich Village, or Clark University, in Worcester, Massachusetts, where Freud gave his famous "Clark Lectures" in 1909 (Rosenzweig 1994).

The growth in Topeka, Kansas, of a psychoanalytic institute, along with a psychoanalytically oriented hospital and a large training and research facility, requires a special explanation (Crank 1994). I believe that the exceptional skills and talents of Karl and William Menninger, their children, and others in the family played a key role in organizing a home for psychoanalysis in a modest-sized middle American town. One special point involved the conceiving of a famed hospital facility built far away from the big-city world. The "asylum" functions were useful in the therapeutic care of many well-known individuals. This was a truly "national asylum" (Winslow 1956). Ultimately, toward the end of the twentieth century, a variety of pressures and new possibilities led to the transfer of the entire facility to Baylor University in Houston, Texas. The Menninger training program had included the largest psychiatric residency facility in the country, where many significant leaders in psychoanalysis were trained. Its powerful leadership has had a major impact on shaping postwar psychiatry and psychoanalysis (Robbins 1963; Robbins and Wallerstein 1956).

Freud had been wary of the fate of psychoanalysis in America, and, of course, he was right in anticipating the ultimate weakening of its support. Psychoanalysts, in general, have tended to be wary about societal acceptance of their principles. The forces of repression are ubiquitous, and defensive operations warding off anxiety tend to prevail. Even more important, it began to be realized that, brilliant and stimulating as it was, psychoanalysis lacked an adequate scientific base and that sooner or later that Achilles heel could not be ignored (Eysenck 1953). Nevertheless, psychoanalysis was accepted by many American psychiatrists during the postwar period and became a powerful force in their field. By the beginning of the twenty-first century, the scene had changed considerably. Psychoanalysis is much less influential in psychiatry (Scully et al. 2000; Wallerstein and Weinshel 1989). It retains a foothold in the humanities, in the arts, in philosophy, in mental health groups, and in privately funded therapeutic arrangements. Psychoanalytic Institutes continue to function, and some have flourishing programs with extensive community services.

There are, however, many reports about the demise of psychoanalysis. Shorter (1997), in his lively history of psychiatry, refers to the period of psychoanalytic dominance of American psychiatry as a "hiatus." In my opinion, his interpretations are somewhat tendentious and inaccurate, but it has to be acknowledged that analysis does not have the popular status it once achieved.

The question of whether there can be a new adaptation by psychoanalysts to cope with the reality of professional, political, and scientific life in America is now at a crucial point. Would even stronger efforts to objectify therapeutic work and the evaluation of psychoanalytic treatment weaken the magical aura of its core processes? Would the creative and imaginative thinking of many analysts be hindered by scientific monitoring of their work? Is the essence of analysis more like an artistic process than like the more measurable and predictable requirements of a medical "treatment"? There are risks, of course, in asking these questions. Paradigm shifts have occurred in some fields when comparable questions were asked and answered.

Most psychoanalysts abhor the way managed care has dominated the American therapeutic system. The "golden age" of psychoanalysis in America was not hampered by petty systemic constraints upon reimbursement (Gabbard 2004). Psychoanalytic treatment today is primarily funded by out-of-pocket payments by patients or their relatives. In order to be "fully analysed" today one must be fairly well off, even though most analysts now spend a considerable amount of time in offering psychodynamic psychotherapy on a once- or twice-a-week basis rather than the classic five hourly sessions a week offered in the "golden age." The insistence on the classic routine of a minimum of four sessions a week for treatment to be truly psychoanalytic has begun to be modified.

Psychoanalytic leadership in America is now working hard to seek a more positive public image and at least some reimbursement from government and private health insurance. For years, in my opinion, such efforts have been hampered by the lack of a specific diagnostic system, by inadequate outcome results, and by, in some cases, a rigid belief that "outsiders" are incapable of evaluating analytic procedures. Of course, bias against analysis has also played a significant role, but that has not been the sole problem. American psychiatry coped with analogous concerns by committing itself to a research agenda that has helped the profession to come closer toward achieving parity with other medical disciplines both in its scientific status and in its reimbursement. As Robert Michels (1994) asks, can psychoanalysis also adapt by developing its own scientific niche?

For many years I was concerned that there was powerful resistance by most analysts to the acceptance of a serious research agenda for the profession as a whole (Sabshin 1990). At times it almost seemed that analysts who advocated specific research activities were caustically advised to seek additional therapeutic help. That depreciation of research is no longer dominant.

During the last two decades a shifting of attitudes seems to have begun. Leadership of the American Psychoanalytic Association has recognized the public image problem and has begun serious efforts in lobbying and public relations. I have been particularly impressed by the work of Glen Gabbard, who epitomizes the changing course of American psychoanalysis. His textbook on psychodynamic psychiatry (Gabbard 2004), his discussions of the meaning of neurobiology for analysis, and his advocacy for a robust change in American psychoanalysis are important. Gabbard's public statements, most recently in *Psychiatric News* (Arehart-Treichel 2007), that research on neuroimaging is the "cutting edge" work necessary to ensure the future of psychoanalysis are powerful commentaries that were not often enunciated by a previous generation of psychoanalysts.

Freud himself was passionately involved in studying the relationship between neurophysiology and psychology as evidenced in his "Project" (Freud 1895[1950]). As Eric Kandel (1998, p. 458) describes it, "When Sigmund Freud first explored the implications of unconscious mental processes for behavior, he tried to adopt a neural model of behavior in an attempt to develop a scientific psychology. Because of the immaturity of brain science at the time, he abandoned this biological model for a purely mentalistic one based on verbal reports of subjective experiences."

I have seen very little evidence until recently that most analysts understood these theoretical constructs. Today, a sea change is beginning at least among psychoanalytic leadership. This change has also been evident in presentations of psychoanalytic work at recent APA Annual Meetings. For example, the Annual Meeting in San Diego in 2007 included the symposium "New Models of Psychodynamic Psychotherapy for Borderline Personality Disorder," to which eminent psychoanalysts such as John Gunderson, Otto Kernberg, and John Clarkin contributed (American Psychiatric Association 2007). The symposium featured a paper by Bateman and Fonagy (2007) entitled "Is Mentalization More Effective Than Structured Supportive Psychotherapy for BPD?" In this paper the authors described a project in which patients were assessed by consensus criteria and treated for an agreed-upon time, and outcomes were compared with those in a control group. Such approaches could indeed be a sign of positive changes in psychoanalysis's attitude to research (Allen and Fonagy 2006).

In his important paper "A New Intellectual Framework for Psychiatry," Eric Kandel (1998), Nobel laureate for his work in neurobiology, made significant suggestions for psychoanalysis. Kandel argues powerfully that analysts should align themselves with the major new directions in neurobiology: "It would be unfortunate, even tragic, if the rich insights that have come from psychoanalysis were to be lost in the rapprochement between psychiatry and the biological sciences" (p. 467). Even while Kandel is criticizing the weak research stance of psychoanalysis, his admiration for analysis is quite visible. He continues, "The future of psychoanalysis, if it is to have a future, is in the context of an empirical psychology, abetted by imaging techniques, neuroanatomical methods, and human genetics. Embedded in the sciences of human cognition, the ideas of psychoanalysis can be tested, and it is here that these ideas can have their greatest impact" (p. 468).

Kandel's proposal has been important for psychoanalysis, and a number of analysts have hailed its possibilities. Kandel differs from Shorter (1997) and many others, such as Wilson (1993) and Paris (2005) in *Fall of an Icon: Psychoanalysis and Academic Psychiatry,* in hoping that analysis will have a "renaissance." In his book *A History of Psychiatry,* Shorter (1997) entitles one of his chapters "From Freud to Prozac" and discusses the psychoanalytic influence as a regrettable hiatus in the history of American psychiatry. I agree with Kandel rather than Shorter, but I would add several concerns about this renaissance. I make these suggestions as a psychiatrist interested in seeing new studies jointly conducted by analysts and psychiatrists. If this is not feasible I hope that psychiatrists can take the lead in seeking new research possibilities by formulating new basic hypotheses derived originally from psychoanalysis.

The key distinction I wish to emphasise is the difference between confirming that psychoanalytic treatment has an impact on cerebral structure and the willingness to test psychoanalytic hypotheses by diverse research methodologies. I am delighted that Glen Gabbard and other major leaders in psychoanalysis are now seeking to demonstrate that the mental processes altered by analytic treatment can be reflected by changes in neurostructure (Beutel et al. 2003). I look forward, however, to the time when we can understand even more about what specifically induces the structural change, how long it lasts, and what the alteration of cerebral structure signifies.

Perhaps most important to my concerns is how willing analysts might be to acknowledge that many psychoanalytic formulations are composed of underlying hypotheses that have not been adequately tested. I believe that Freud, despite his strong assertions when challenged, fundamentally understood this point, but I do not observe clear acknowledgment of its validity by newer generations of psychoanalytic leadership. For example, the basic continuity or discontinuity of relationships between childhood experiences and adult behavior still requires long-term hypothesis testing. The relationship between defense mechanisms and normal adaptation opens up many profound questions that need to be formulated in genetic, environmental, and biological hypotheses that will require multilevel research. The fundamental implications of dreams, of the process of free association, of transference and countertransference, of basic regulatory and inhibitory functions, of the universality of the Oedipus complex, of the lifetime course of variations in human sexuality, and many other questions need to be formulated into biopsychosocial hypotheses tested by a variety of techniques. I agree with Paris (2005) when he states, "While philosophers still argue about the precise boundaries of science, however, there is a consensus about its essence. Hypotheses must be tested with measurable data. No theory of the mind, and no method of treating patients, can survive without empirical testing" (p. 150).

Would the acknowledgment that a substantial portion of psychoanalytic theory consists of hypotheses that still require basic confirmation render psychoanalysis more vulnerable to its sizeable number of detractors? Would current efforts to seek better reimbursement for psychoanalytic treatment be weakened by frank discussion of the need for fundamental research ? Could the opposite effect be more likely? I am well aware that some analysts would say, "Starting with Freud we have always acknowledged our field as consisting of formulations of unverified hypotheses. Why depreciate ourselves now in this more hostile environment?" I disagree that psychoanalysis has made it clear that its theoretical constructs are largely based on untested hypotheses; the delineation of a long-term hypothesis testing agenda by psychoanalysts is particularly notable by its absence. Other analysts have taken the position, sometimes implicitly, that the methodology to test analytic formulations is not yet available and would therefore end in frustration. Still others have pointed out that a research agenda could be fruitful but that support from funding agencies would not be available, especially at a time of widespread bias against analysis.

From my perspective, clear advocacy of a long-term research agenda would be a progressive and helpful step for American psychoanalysis. This agenda could not be carried out by analysts alone, and the need for genuine interdisciplinary research should be clearly acknowledged. New alliances with biologists, behavioral scientists, psychologists, and academic psychiatry would be necessary. This cooperation would not be easy to accomplish for several reasons. Psychoanalysts have tended to believe that non-analysts could not deal adequately with the complexity and the frightening implications of unconscious processes. Some will react to my suggestions as arrogant intrusion. At least equally important today would be that potential research allies would need to be persuaded that the research was important and could actually be conducted. Funding for such research would be difficult in today's research climate, but acknowledging the need would be a progressive act.

For all the problems in conducting research in psychoanalysis, there are already good examples of long-term research agendas emanating, at least in part, from psychoanalytic hypotheses. John Bowlby's enunciation of the importance of attachment for human development is a superb example of change in psychoanalytic thinking. His *Maternal Care and Mental Health* (Bowlby 1951), commissioned by the World Health Organization, a work spurred by concern for the number of children orphaned in the aftermath of World War II, was widely recognized as changing child care practice in all its aspects. His monumental three-volume work *Attachment and Loss* established his reputation and the concept of attachment beyond doubt (Bowlby 1969, 1973, 1980).

At first, his research was scorned by leading analysts, who derided his utilization of animal behavioral data about infant–mother bonding (A. Freud 1960/1969). That criticism tells us a great deal about an older, rigid, closed system of psychoanalysis. Today, with new understanding of attachment theory and new psychoanalytic leadership, there is strong support for its significance and much investigation of its implications for future mental health (Emde 2005). Peter Fonagy's important research in this field and in its clinical ramifications (Fonagy 2001) increases my confidence in a more flexible and scientific psychoanalysis.

For psychiatry, testing psychoanalytic hypotheses would require several complex steps. Biological imaging and genetic research on psychoanalytic processes are beginning and, one hopes, will continue. Ultimately the predictive power of biological variables will reach its limits in explaining the etiology and the treatment of mental illnesses without integration with social and psychological variables. Of course, social and psychological processes have their impact ultimately on the central nervous system, but they cannot be studied only by measurement of neurochemical processes. They need to be formulated in appropriate terminology. This distinction is of considerable importance for research purposes and for basic definitions of the range of psychiatric concerns. Even with the growing recognition of neuropsychiatric linkages with psychiatric conditions I believe that special interest and competence in the psychological and social variables will continue to distinguish the psychiatrist from his neurological colleagues. As Kandel (1998) predicts, the fields of neurology and psychiatry will overlap more in the future, but I fear that his advocacy of a merger between psychiatry and neurology into a neuroscientific specialty would fundamentally weaken attention to psychosocial variables.

There is reason to be concerned, as Paris (2005) acknowledges, that psychiatrists might lose their skill in talking to patients. That danger is present today and needs to be tackled at many levels. One hopes that interest in psychosocial subjects and techniques will motivate a new generation of psychiatrists to test many social and psychological hypotheses including some that will be derived from psychoanalysis.

These questions should interest academic psychiatric centers in the future, especially when the ultimate limitations of pharmacological treatment for various mental illnesses become more apparent. Advances in cognitive and interpersonal therapy should also overlap with psychodynamic psychotherapy, and their new applications should be reviewed by academic psychiatry. Combined psychotherapy and pharmacotherapy may become the mode rather than the exception!

From my perspective, Kandel's "renaissance" of psychoanalysis is now becoming more evident. The *Psychodynamic Diagnostic Manual* (PDM; Alliance of Psychoanalytic Organizations 2006) is a step in the right direction but is still limited by its avoidance of any aggregate data about mental illness and epidemiology. Freud was always concerned about the unreliability of conducting studies on therapeutic outcomes as well as about epidemiological studies. In a letter to August Stärcke in 1912, he wrote,

To compile statistics, as you propose, is at present impossible. Surely you know that yourself. To begin with, we work with much smaller numbers than other doctors, who devote so much less time to individuals. Then the necessary uniformity is lacking which alone can form a basis of any statistics. Should we really count together apples, pears and nuts? What do we call a severe case? Moreover, I could not regard my own results in the past twenty years as comparable since my technique has fundamentally changed in that time. And what should we do about the numerous cases which are only partially analysed and those where treatment had to be discontinued for external reasons?" (Jones 1955, pp. 124–125)

Freud's concern about statistics is still a large problem for many analysts, but new methods to deal with most of his questions have now been developed.

Today, focusing upon the individual should not preclude an interest in aggregate data. To understand why some disorders are quite prevalent and others are not could be very useful in basic understanding of the disorders themselves and ultimately finding methods to reduce their occurrence. The PDM does not acknowledge clearly enough how research can lead to discarding old formulations. The few examples that are cited primarily involve changes of clinical opinion rather than changes due to research findings. It is therefore limited by the absence of a long-term research agenda on the study of psychodynamic hypotheses relevant to psychiatric diagnoses. Nevertheless, the PDM is a long overdue step that needs to be followed up. Its formulations and the articles included in the manual are filled with many potential hypotheses in addition to historical reiteration.

Interesting developments in the field of neuroanalysis can also update Freud's "Project" using twenty-first century concepts. The international neuroanalytic conferences and publications are an indicator of potential changes in psychoanalytic research. I would be most interested to read publications on the subject of changes in major psychoanalytic formulations as a result of neuroanalytic investigations. Willingness to discard old hypotheses would be a sign that science has truly replaced ideology. Confirmation of analytic hypotheses by these new methods would be a powerful step in a psychoanalytic renaissance. It is my judgment that the long-term future of psychoanalysis in America hinges on its willingness to develop and support a genuine scientific agenda.

REFERENCES

Allen JG, Fonagy P (eds): Handbook of Mentalization-Based Treatment. Hoboken, NJ, Wiley, 2006

Alliance of Psychoanalytic Organizations, PDM Task Force: Psychodynamic Diagnostic Manual. Silver Spring, MD, Alliance of Psychoanalytic Organizations, 2006

American Psychiatric Association: 2007 New Research Program and Abstracts, American Psychiatric Association 160th Annual Meeting, San Diego, CA, May 19–24, 2007. Washington, DC, American Psychiatric Association, 2007, p 53

Arehart-Treichel J: Scientists search brains for evidence of transference. Psychiatr News 42(5):14, 2007

Bateman A, Fonagy P: Is mentalization more effective than structured supportive psychotherapy for BPD? Paper presented at the 160th Annual Meeting of the American Psychiatric Association, San Diego, CA, May 19–24, 2007

Beutel ME, Stern E, Silbersweig DA: The emerging dialogue between psychoanalysis and neuroscience: neuroimaging perspectives. J Am Psychoanal Assoc 51:773–801, 2003

Bowlby J: Maternal Care and Mental Health. Geneva, World Health Organization, 1951

Bowlby J: Attachment and Loss, Vol 1: Attachment. London, Hogarth Press, 1969

Bowlby J: Attachment and Loss, Vol 2: Separation: Anxiety and Anger. London, Hogarth Press, 1973

Bowlby J: Attachment and Loss, Vol 3: Loss: Sadness and Depression. London, Hogarth Press, 1980

Chessick RD: The Contemporary Failure of Nerve and the Crisis in Psychoanalysis. J Am Acad Psychoanal 29(4):659–678, 2001

Crank HH: The early years of psychoanalysis in Topeka: and a modest proposal. Bull Menninger Clin 58(1):9–14, 1994

Emde RN: A developmental orientation for contemporary psychoanalysis, in The American Psychiatric Publishing Textbook of Psychoanalysis. Edited by Person ES, Cooper AM, Gabbard GO. Washington, DC, American Psychiatric Publishing, 2005, pp 117–130

Eysenck HJ: What is wrong with psychoanalysis? in Uses and Abuses of Psychology. London, Penguin, 1953

Fonagy P: Attachment Theory and Psychoanalysis. New York, Other Press, 2001

Freud A: Comment on Bowlby's paper "Grief and Mourning in Infancy and Early Childhood" (1960), in The Writings of Anna Freud, Vol 5. New York, International Universities Press, 1969, pp 167–186

Freud S: Project for a scientific psychology (1895[1950]), in Standard Edition of the Complete Psychological Works of Sigmund Freud, Vol 1. Translated and edited by Strachey J. London, Hogarth Press, 1966, pp 281–397

Gabbard GO: Long-Term Psychodynamic Psychotherapy: A Basic Text. Washington, DC, American Psychiatric Publishing, 2004

Gabbard GO, Gabbard K: Psychiatry and the Cinema, 2nd Edition. Washington, DC, American Psychiatric Press, 1999

Jones E: The Life and Work of Sigmund Freud, Vol 2. New York, Basic Books, 1955

Kandel ER: A new intellectual framework for psychiatry. Am J Psychiatry 155:457–469, 1998

Michels R: Validation in the clinical process. Int J Psychoanal 75(pt 5–6): 1133–1140, 1994

Paris J: Fall of an Icon: Psychoanalysis and Academic Psychiatry. Toronto, University of Toronto Press, 2005

Person ES, Cooper AM, Gabbard GO (eds): The American Psychiatric Publishing Textbook of Psychoanalysis. Washington, DC, American Psychiatric Publishing, 2005

Robbins LL: The contributions of psychoanalysis in psychiatric hospital treatment. Intensive Care Nurs 12:232–238, 1963

Robbins LL, Wallerstein RS: Psychotherapy Research Project of the Menninger Foundation, I: orientation. Bull Menninger Clin 20:223–225, 1956

Rosenzweig S: The Historic Expedition to America (1909): Freud, Jung, and Hall the King-maker, 2nd, Revised Edition. St Louis, MO, Rana House, 1994

Sabshin M: Turning points in twentieth-century American psychiatry. Am J Psychiatry 147:1267–1274, 1990

Scully JH, Robinowitz CB, Shore JH: Psychiatric education after World War II, in American Psychiatry After World War II: 1944–1994. Edited by Menninger RW, Nemiah JC. Washington, DC, American Psychiatric Press, 2000, pp 124–151

Shorter E: A History of Psychiatry: From the Era of the Asylum to the Age of Prozac. New York, Wiley, 1997

Strauss A, Schatzman L, Bucher R, et al: Psychiatric Ideologies and Institutions. New York, Free Press, 1964

Wallerstein RS, Weinshel EM: The future of psychoanalysis. Psychoanal Q 58:341–373, 1989

Wilson M: DSM-III and the transformation of American psychiatry. Am J Psychiatry 150:399–410, 1993

Winslow W: The Menninger Story. Garden City, NY, Doubleday, 1956

9

Forensic Psychiatry

Some of my younger colleagues complain bitterly about the current legal constraints hampering their practice. To them forensic psychiatry has many negative connotations. Their teachers had told them about a halcyon time when the threat of litigation against psychiatrists was almost nonexistent. It was a time when malpractice allegations were minimal. For some of this older group who had dealt with very sick patients, it was much easier to employ legal mechanisms to compel a patient to enter a state hospital when it seemed appropriate: others, who practiced dynamic psychotherapy or psychoanalysis, were respected by the public and there was no *Osheroff* decision (Osheroff v. Chestnut Lodge 1985) threatening legal action if medication was not employed.

These complaints against forensic regulations are symbolic of some of the conflicts experienced by practitioners today and require thoughtful responses. First of all, it must be reiterated to a new generation of psychiatrists, who sometimes do not understand that the flourishing of psychiatry in America has absolutely depended on its place in a democratic society whose laws protect all of our rights. Without such laws, there is little utility of psychiatry except to support the State, which was what happened, tragically, in the U.S.S.R. and in Nazi Germany. It is also important to note that for most Americans with severe mental illnesses, the postwar years were not halcyon times. The number of people housed in our state hospitals was immense, and pessimism about their potential recovery had replaced the more optimistic "moral therapy" of the middle nineteenth century (Bockoven

1963). Throughout history there have been occasional bursts of therapeutic optimism about the care of the insane. (Moral treatment was one
such gentle approach, but it was ended when a large number of recent immigrants began to replace our "Yankee" patients in the 1860s.) The freedom to practice psychiatry under rational regulations ultimately depends
on political protection.

American medicine advanced remarkably through the latter half of
the twentieth century. Its costs, however, sky-rocketed, and regulation
of its expenditures was required. Many of us are critical of the overall
current health system, but all of us recognize that some equitable way to
control costs is necessary. Furthermore, the practice of medicine in a democracy requires a scientifically based regulatory system that restricts
the use of therapeutic techniques that are scientifically demonstrated to
be less effective or have been proven to be potentially dangerous. The increasing complexity of medical practice requires careful and even more
detailed scrutiny.

American psychiatry made a decision to replace its postwar ideological stances with an evidence-based system of diagnosis and treatment.
This decision was made at a time of growing economic constraints on all
of medicine. Opting for a rational empirically based diagnostic system
was a necessary path for achieving parity. It also was a step that stimulated the growth of a massive forensic system to regulate the employment of the new science and the new economic accountability.

Forensic psychiatry has had a long and significant history in American psychiatry. The thirteen founders of the American Psychiatric Association (APA) in 1844 were all experienced in dealing with the definition
of insanity; the *American Journal of Insanity,* precursor of the *American
Journal of Psychiatry,* included many articles on forensics. In the latter
part of the nineteenth century and the first half of the twentieth century,
there was some decline of interest in forensic psychiatry. Protecting the
rights of the many recently immigrated psychiatric patients was not a
very high priority (Bockoven 1963). The rapid growth of forensic psychiatry in the last quarter of the twentieth century and its achievement of
formal approval as a subspecialty in 1992 were significantly influenced by
the requirements of the new scientifically based practice and the new
economic forces regulating treatment and its reimbursement.

I am not a forensic psychiatrist and have never been in a courtroom
as an expert witness. Working at the APA, however, has brought me into
contact with many lawyers and forensic leaders in the field from whom I
have learned a great deal.

In first thinking about this chapter, my focus was upon the legal implications of mental illness and its treatment, and I wanted to use a sub-

title such as "From *Durham* to *Osheroff*," which seemed to fit in with my overall theme of the changes in American psychiatry. In retrospect, I realized that the decisions which those names signify were not as clear-cut as I had thought.

The 1954 decision by Judge David Bazelon in *Durham v. United States* had special personal meaning for me. Before I came to Washington as medical director of the APA, I was introduced to Judge Bazelon by my friend and colleague, Dr. Harold Visotsky. Harold had become a psychiatric leader in Illinois and nationally at a very early age and had been "adopted" by the judge as someone to share his concerns about psychiatry. When Visotsky introduced me to Judge Bazelon, the Judge took me into his fold also. For several years I had the extraordinary privilege of lunching occasionally with him and some of his friends, including Supreme Court Justices and other high-level government officials. The Judge told me of his disappointment about the psychiatric follow-up to his *Durham* decision. In this case he had stated that "a defendant might be found to be not responsible for a crime if it could be proved that the act was a product of mental illness." He had hoped that psychiatrists would have followed up actively on the implications of this ruling. He indicated that his decision had been influenced by the prevailing psychiatric and psychoanalytic zeitgeist that emphasized how relevant unconscious determinants were involved in the committing of criminal acts and that psychiatrists could uncover these causes and their effects.

In 1961, Judge Bazelon received the Isaac Ray Award from the APA and gave a lecture in which he said, "I really cannot say it too strongly—that psychiatrists have a great opportunity under a liberal rule like *Durham*—an opportunity to help reform the criminal law and also to humanize their own work and increase its relevance." That was indeed a powerful opportunity for psychiatry, but the field was not ready to take advantage of it.

Although Karl Menninger proclaimed, in his *The Crime of Punishment* (Menninger 1968), that the *Durham* decision was more revolutionary than the Supreme Court's decision on desegregation, in fact, Judge Bazelon, like many of his psychiatric sources, had failed to perceive the weakness of his judgment. He lacked awareness of the status of psychiatric research of his time; he relied too heavily on the prevailing psychoanalytic theory that implied more knowledge than could be proved about the "behavioral products" of unconscious conflicts.

The *Durham* decision resulted in more acquittals by reason of insanity, but legal arguments continued with lawyers wanting a tighter definition of what constituted a mental disease. There was little agreement among psychiatrists about this, with one group even suggesting that "sociopathic" patients could not be held accountable for their acts (Reisner et al. 2004). In 1972 the *Durham* standard was overruled by the *Brawner* decision, which states that "a person is not responsible for criminal conduct if, at the time of such conduct, as a result of mental disease or mental defect he lacks substantial capacity to either appreciate the wrongfulness of his conduct or to conform his conduct to the requirements of the law" (United States v. Brawner 1972).

For me the *Durham* decision stands as an important historical reflection of the lofty aspirations of postwar American psychiatry. While DSM-III (American Psychiatric Association 1980) began to provide a diagnostic rationale not available at the time of Durham, we still are a long way from accurately predicting specific "products" of mental disorders. I regret not having had a chance to discuss with Judge Bazelon how close and how far we are today from seizing the opportunity he offered us.

Ultimately the rights of psychiatric patients and psychiatrists depend on a rational judicial system that respects the principle of liberty and justice for all. Throughout human history, however, discrimination against the mentally ill has been the rule rather than the exception. During the last 200 years a slowly evolving period of enlightenment has been taking place, but in many parts of the world gross abuse of psychiatric patients has continued to flourish. The World Psychiatric Association (WPA) has dealt with many serious allegations of abuse during the late twentieth century, and there is strong evidence that abuse continues to occur today.

In the United States the rights of psychiatric patients did not emerge full-blown with the adoption of the Declaration of Independence and the Constitution. Gross discrimination against the mentally ill, accompanied by stigmatization and incarceration, dominated psychiatric practice until the latter part of the twentieth century. Deinstitutionalization of the mentally ill began to be massively applied in the 1970s, although it is questionable whether the primary motivation for this change was the liberty of the patients or the high costs of and poor reimbursement for patient care in the state hospitals (Grob 1991).

Forensic psychiatry in the United States began to grow rapidly in the latter part of the twentieth century (Halleck 1968, 2000). At first it was primarily involved with the issues of involuntary hospitalization and the courtroom decisions concerning the relationship of the presence of "insanity" and guilt. By the end of the twentieth century forensic psychiatry had become a subspeciality approved by the American Board of Medical Specialties and the American Board of Psychiatry and Neurology in 1992. It had grown from a small group of pioneering leaders to several thousand practitioners who deal with burgeoning fields of malpractice, disability assessment, mental competency, criminal offenders, and civil liberties. These psychiatrists are experts in providing assistance to legal systems, to prosecutors, and to defendants coping with questions of a wide variety of forensic issues. Often they are superb teachers of psychiatrists and many others concerned with the law. The best practitioners of this aspect of psychiatry value their clinical psychiatric base as a foundation for their forensic roles. I am particularly grateful to Dr. Robert Simon, who has taught me a great deal about the importance of a sound practical knowledge of such clinical competence for the highest level of forensic practice (Simon and Gold 2004).

Forensic psychiatry during its entire history has played an important role in shaping American psychiatry, but it has also, in turn, been shaped by the changes in American psychiatry. I will attempt to discuss this linkage by focusing upon a few of the transactions between the legal system and psychiatry in the context of these changes in the field.

As noted earlier, many older psychiatrists look back nostalgically at the immediate postwar period. This is not surprising when the intensity and magnitude of today's regulatory controls are compared with the relative freedom and the power then to make decisions. Historically, psychiatrists were given the right to hospitalize a patient in order to treat (Stone 1974), and there was little challenge to their authority. The postwar "glow" facilitated this power for psychiatrists. Equally important was the widespread belief that if we could find the unconscious conflicts and motivations precipitating the criminal acts, treatment would be possible, as had been demonstrated by the generally positive results of treating soldiers with traumatic neuroses in World War II (Roche 1958).

The powerful role that psychoanalysis assumed in American psychiatry during the post–World War II years raised important issues that had major legal implications. For many people the strict adherence of the psychoanalyst to the principle of confidentiality made it permissible for them to utilize "free association" during treatment. Anxiety about revealing reprehensible thoughts, let alone criminal acts, stifled free association. Even without the external guarantee, the capacity for free association is hampered by many internal constraints. Later, as statutory exceptions to the therapist's right to maintain confidentiality were enunciated in court decisions (on the grounds of dangerousness to self and others, intent to commit a criminal act, questions of competency, information required by other therapists), absolute confidentiality could not be assured. By and large, however, the overwhelming majority of psychiatrists and psychoanalysts adhered to the rules of confidentiality but several public exceptions, however, caused problems for the profession. There are times when the rights of society for specific information are in sharp conflict with the rights of confidentiality, which are central to the ethical code of psychiatrists.

Sexual misconduct by psychiatrists and psychoanalysts also received wide publicity and weakened public confidence. Significantly, in several films that attempted to portray psychiatrists and analysts in a positive manner, as discussed in Chapter 8 ("Psychoanalysis"), the analyst has a "romantic" relationship with his or her patient, as in the film *Prince of Tides*, with Barbra Streisand. Ingrid Bergman's attachment to her amnesic patient, Gregory Peck, in *Spellbound* is distinctly unethical; it seems that the story requirements superseded ethical concerns, even though, most interestingly, the studio hired a prominent analyst to advise on many of its productions (Farber et al. 1993). Sexual misconduct by prominent therapists has been a major concern in all the "mental health" professions. In many ways the ethical, and in some cases legal, violations by analysts were particularly painful. The ethical standards of psychoanalysis were an essential part of its practice, and violation of these standards contributed to public image problems. In several Woody Allen films conversation about bizarre sexual behavior of analysts takes place as if that were to be expected.

As psychiatry began to change in the 1970s, dramatic modifications occurred in forensic psychiatry and in its impact on practice. Perhaps the best symbol of the late-century change for clinical practice was the case of Dr. Raphael Osheroff, a nephrologist who in 1982 sued a psychiatric inpatient facility, Chestnut Lodge (Klerman 1990), for inadequately treating him with psychotherapy alone for his severe depression. He claimed that even after seven months of intensive psychotherapy, his condition had deteriorated to the point of psychosis. Dr. Osheroff's condition allegedly improved only after he transferred to another facility, where he was started on psychotropic treatment and discharged after three months of treatment. Until this landmark case, Chestnut Lodge was generally respected as the place where Harry Stack Sullivan and Frieda Fromm-Reichmann pioneered the treatment of severe mental illness with psychotherapeutic techniques. For many years, Chestnut Lodge remained one of the few private psychiatric hospitals in the United States that attempted to treat schizophrenia and other disorders largely on psychodynamic principles (Hornstein 2000). For the first time, the efficacy of psychotherapy was judged against medical treatment not only in the scientific arena but in a court of law. Although settled out of court, the case still stands out powerfully to me as an indication of how times had changed. Employment of long-term psychotherapy alone became limited in the presence of empirical evidence favoring the employment of antipsychotic medication. For me, the *Osheroff* case symbolizes the changing directions of American psychiatry in a powerful and succinct fashion. Ideology was trumped by empirical evidence in an American court.

The new wave of psychopharmacology that dominated American psychiatry in the last quarter of the twentieth century was accompanied by an ever-growing list of legal precautions and precedents regarding their use. Although some of these safeguards were similar to those in other parts of medicine (e.g., appropriate dosage, careful monitoring for toxicity, patient's informed consent), many special issues needed careful monitoring for psychiatric patients. While the right to refuse treatment has implications for all of medicine, the limits of that right have required special attention for psychiatric patients.

As a logical follow-up to *Diagnostic and Statistical Manual of Mental Disorders* (DSM), the APA began to publish Practice Guidelines for the disorders listed there (Zarin et al. 1999). As some critics of the DSM had predicted, the DSM and the guidelines became the "bible" for many plaintiff attorneys against psychiatrists who were alleged to have failed to make a correct diagnosis and/or failed to employ appropriate treatment. In the courtroom, attorneys began to employ the DSM classifications and the guidelines in many circumstances, and some acted as if these were fully validated standards and sought penalties against those who did not use them properly. This occurred frequently despite the fact that the authors of the DSM had chosen the term "guidelines" to indicate the current state of somewhat limited reliability and to sound a cautionary note about the manual's use. The danger of misuse is a problem in the early phases of a new nosology, especially when associated with a fiscal system in which payment for therapeutic care hinges on a reliable diagnosis and a reasonable treatment plan.

With the DSM and the Practice Guidelines, however, the scientific status of psychiatry has progressed dramatically and the efforts for an even more evidence-based practice will continue. The judicial system has taken notice of the scientific advances in the field, which puts increased pressure on practitioners to pay attention to the forensic aspects of their work.

For the practitioner, the managed care system is also very demanding forensically. Many important legal issues now fill new and thicker volumes of forensic psychiatric textbooks. Today, the enormous panoply of biological psychiatry requires careful regulation in protecting the rights of psychiatric patients and /or their guardians. Psychiatrists need special knowledge and new skills to protect themselves from suit. They require written records to prove compliance with regulations, such as informed consent. With the *Tarasoff* decision, which calls for mental health care providers to disclose certain kinds of information provided by the patient that would be useful to protect others, they must balance conflicting aspects of treatment (Tarasoff v. Regents of the University of California 1976). Indeed, current forensic psychiatry requires an increasingly sophisticated balancing between the rights of patients and the rights of society.

One event that had a major impact upon forensic psychiatry occurred on March 30, 1981, when John W. Hinckley Jr. attempted to assassinate President Ronald Reagan and wounded three others (Border 1981) in a disturbed attempt to impress a movie actress with whom he was obssessed. The assailant pleaded not guilty by reason of insanity, and his trial was under the jurisdiction of the American Law Institute (1955). He was acquitted and found not guilty by reason of insanity, and committed to St. Elizabeth's Hospital in Washington, D.C., where as of 2008 he remains; he has, however, controversially been given the privilege of extended unsupervised visits with his family ("Hinckley Wants More Visits" 2006). There was a tremendous public outcry against the initial court decision, with much condemnation of psychiatric imprecision and bias (Halpern 1982; Slater and Hans 1984). Many antipsychiatric movements in the United States took advantage of the verdict to deride our field and weaken its status. But many psychiatrists were also unhappy with the decision. The APA Council on Psychiatry and Law recommended several changes in the American Law Institute procedure, including a deletion of a section which seemed to reduce penalties. As a matter of fact, Congress supported recommendations similar to those of the APA, but many states shifted from the American Law Institute rule to the old more controlling McNaughton proviso based on the trial of Daniel McNaughton in London in 1843. In attempting to murder prime minister Sir Robert Peel, by mistake he shot his private secretary instead. The ruling in the case was that persons cannot be held responsible for a crime if they were laboring with a deficit of reason based on disease of the mind such that they did not know the nature and quality of the act or, if they did know it, they did not know that what they did was wrong. This decision has been utilized in many countries for over 150 years and still has current salience.

Despite all the progressive changes in American psychiatry since 1843, the profession and our patients are still vulnerable to regressive legal, political, and social censure when the public is once again outraged by criminal acts committed by released psychiatric patients. Decisions to release these patients obviously should be conducted with great care. Occasionally the decision is made somewhat quickly, especially in underfinanced or poorly administered institutions, but even when the greatest care is employed predictions of future violence are imprecise. Becoming too strict about discharge is also criticized by some as illustrating the "authoritarian," controlling bias of psychiatry; occasionally the same groups criticize the profession as being both too liberal and too restrictive. Psychiatry needs to maintain the search for better ways to predict violence more accurately but we also require a way to work with the relevant communities to understand the current limits of predictability. If reasonable attempts are made to balance the needs of the patient and those of society, the public will understand better but the vulnerability remains. It is a conundrum.

While I was writing the paragraph above in April 2007, a horrifying massacre of 27 students and 5 faculty members by a Virginia Tech student was taking place (Shuchman 2007). The murderer is said to have been seen in a mental health clinic, and I find myself anxious that the clinic's failure to institutionalize him will lead to new constraints. It is hard to be rational in the face of such a tragedy. A few days after the massacre, I noted a newspaper column about it. The writer, a mental health professional, wrote about "our wobbly" mental health system. For him, the murders were a reflection of our defective mental health system. He may be right, but the column seemed to me a call for impulsive action. I still react with fear of regressive policies enacted in the heat of our horror.

Forensic issues occasionally transcend international boundaries; the WPA has developed a careful procedure to investigate allegations of psychiatric abuse in one country by another country's psychiatric society. Perhaps the most prominent allegations were those made by the APA and the Royal College of Psychiatry (United Kingdom) about abuse in the Soviet Union. These two psychiatric organizations alleged that several political dissenters in Russia had been falsely diagnosed as mentally ill so that they could be incarcerated in mental institutions. After severely resisting the validity of these allegations, the All-Union Society of Psychiatrists and Neuropathologists, the major psychiatric association of the U.S.S.R., resigned from the WPA (see Chapter 7, "International Affairs"). Years later, after political changes in the U.S.S.R., an extensive investigation of the abuse was held under the leadership of Loren Roth, one of the most distinguished American forensic psychiatrists. In this process he was strongly supported by Darrel Regier, who at that time worked at the National Institute of Mental Health, which also supported the mission.

During this investigation patients were interviewed carefully and assessed; while it was difficult to ascertain the clear presence of abuse, helpful recommendations were produced to protect the rights of psychiatric patients in Russia ("Report of the U.S. Delegation" 1989). The Russian Society of Psychiatrists has since regained its membership in the WPA.

Several Soviet psychiatrists who opposed the abuse had been imprisoned during the most difficult periods in the Soviet Union. Some, such as Anatoly Koryagin, have become international celebrities after long periods of harassment (see Chapter 7). The number of active psychiatric protesters was quite small, which highlights the power of an authoritarian state.

Abuse has been stated to occur in many countries. Political allegations have been made recently about practices in China, notably confinement of members of the Falun Gong group to secure mental hospitals. In the United States, the American poet Ezra Pound was kept in a psychiatric hospital, supposedly because of his pro-Fascist beliefs during World War II. Today psychiatric leaders are still very much involved in protesting the psychological abuse of prisoners, as did APA President Steven Sharfstein after his visit to Guantanamo Bay Prison (Sharfstein 2005; see also Janofsky 2006).

As American psychiatry has changed to become more evidence-based, its ethical and legal principles have expanded, and patients are much more protected from many kinds of abuse. There are still gross disparities in the decency and effectiveness of psychiatric care among the world's nations. Hwoever, even the most democratic societies must recognize that their scientific base, their economic support for psychiatric patients, and their public's understanding and legal understanding of mental illness will need to continue to adapt and to change.

Forensic psychiatry and all of its ramifications have had a tumultuous history during the latter part of the twentieth century. In America, psychiatry has been profoundly affected by the nation's legal systems, both state and federal, and these systems have helped to create a generation of legal scholars who have had much to say about changing American psychiatry. They have helped to formulate new boundaries and new directions for the field. The appointment of Alan Stone in 1972 as Professor of Law and Psychiatry at Harvard Law School was a prescient symbol of the importance of scholarly transactions between the two professions. The APA was fortunate that Stone chose to seek leadership of the organization; he was elected president of the APA in 1979. He was, in fact, a major leader before his presidency and has continued to be active in many important concerns, such as the alleged abuse in China, long after his presidency.

It may be his regard for strict legality that caused Alan Stone to become concerned that in the changes I helped to achieve in American psychiatry, I had become very powerful in the APA. Subsequent to his presidency he wrote a note to each newly elected president to warn them about my assumption of too much power. I have not seen a copy of this letter, but several presidents told me about it. Jay Scully, the current medical director, has now officially been given the power of Chief Executive Officer of the APA. I assumed some of those powers at least implicitly.

The only other time when the power of my position received special public attention was at the delegates' meeting of the WPA, when its eminent president Pierre Pichot noticed my presence at the back of the room and commented somewhat ambiguously, "There is the person who runs this organisation, and he is standing at the back of the room. Mel Sabshin is not a delegate, but he is important in determining what we do." Like Stone's comment, this statement had a few kernels of validity. Pichot, like Stone, was quite astute, and he has been a major historian and world leader in psychiatry. He, like Stone, remains a good friend.

There have been many other leaders bridging the worlds of law and psychiatry. I had the good fortune to be able to bring Joel Klein to the APA as its counsel in 1975. He was a brilliant and forceful scholar of the close relationship between legal practice and major issues for psychiatry. His subsequent career in the U.S. Department of Justice and as Commissioner of Education in New York City demonstrates his special creativity and broad talents. At a crucial time in the changing of American psychiatry, we were fortunate to have his insights.

Forensic psychiatry is a very active part of today's American psychiatry. In its full complexity, the current legal system demonstrates the strengths and some of the weaknesses of psychiatry's status. Our science, our education, and our therapeutic practices are still in transition. By the middle of the twenty-first century, I hope that part of Judge Bazelon's visionary concepts may be fulfilled. Court decisions may pay even more attention to an evidence-based psychiatry.

REFERENCES

American Law Institute: Model Penal Code, 4.01(1): Mental Disease of Defect Excluding Responsibility (Tentative Draft No 4). Philadelphia, PA, American Law Institute, 1955

American Psychiatric Association: Diagnostic and Statistical Manual of Mental Disorders, 3rd Edition. Washington, DC, American Psychiatric Association, 1980

Bockoven JS: Moral Treatment in American Psychiatry. New York, Springer, 1963

Border DS: Reagan wounded by assailant's bullet. The Washington Post, March 31, 1981

Durham v United States, 214 F2d 862 (DC Cir 1954)

Farber S, Green M: Hollywood on the Couch: A Candid Look at the Overheated Love Affair Between Psychiatrists and Moviemakers. New York, William Morrow, 1993

Grob GN: From Asylum to Community: Mental Health Policy in Modern America. Princeton, NJ, Princeton University Press, 1991

Halleck S: American psychiatry and the criminal: a historical review. Int J Psychiatry 6(3):185–208, 1968

Halleck S: Forensic psychiatry after World War II, in American Psychiatry After World War II: 1944–1994. Edited by Menninger RW, Nemiah JC. Washington, DC, American Psychiatric Press, 2000, pp 517–542

Halpern AL: Reconsideration of the insanity defense and related issues in the aftermath of the Hinckley trial. Psychiatr Q 54:260–264, 1982

Hinckley wants more visits. New York Times, August 16, 2006

Hornstein GA. To Redeem One Person Is to Redeem the World: A Life of Frieda Fromm-Reichmann. New York, Free Press, 2000, pp 383–385

Janofsky JS: Lies and coercion: why psychiatrists should not participate in police and intelligence interrogations. J Am Acad Psychiatry Law 34:472–478, 2006

Klerman GL: The psychiatric patient's right to effective treatment: implications of Osheroff v Chestnut Lodge. Am J Psychiatry 147:409–418, 1990

Menninger KA: The Crime of Punishment. New York, Viking Press, 1968

Osheroff v Chestnut Lodge, 62 Md App 519 490, cert denied, Chestnut Lodge, Inc v Osheroff, 304 Md 163, 497 A2d 1163 (1985)

Perr IN: The insanity defense: a tale of two cities. Am J Psychiatry 140:873–874, 1983

Reisner R, Slobogin C, Rai A: Law and the Mental Health System: Civil and Criminal Aspects, 4th Edition. St Paul, MN, Thomson/West, 2004

Report of the U.S. Delegation to assess recent changes in Soviet psychiatry. Schizophr Bull 15 (4, suppl):1–219, 1989

Roche PQ: The Criminal Mind: A Study of Communication between the Criminal Law and Psychiatry. New York, Farrar, Straus & Cudahy, 1958

Sharfstein SS: President's column: medical ethics and the detainees at Guantanamo Bay. Psychiatr News 40(22):3, 2005

Shuchman M: Falling through the cracks: Virginia Tech and the restructuring of college mental health services. New Engl J Med 357:105–110, 2007

Simon RI, Gold LH (eds): The American Psychiatric Publishing Text-book of Forensic Psychiatry. Washington, DC, American Psychiatric Publishing, 2004

Slater D, Hans VP: Public opinion of forensic psychiatry following the Hinckley verdict. Am J Psychiatry 141:675–679, 1984

Stone AA: The right to treatment and the psychiatric establishment. Psychiatr Ann 4(9):21–42, 1974

Tarasoff v Regents of the University of California, 131 CalRptr 14, 551 P2d 334 (Cal 1976)

United States v Brawner, 471 F2d 969 (DC Cir 1972)

Zarin DA, McIntyre JS, Pincus HA, et al: Practice guidelines in psychiatry and a psychiatric practice research network, in The American Psychiatric Press Textbook of Psychiatry, 3rd Edition. Edited by Hales RE, Yudofsky SC. Washington, DC, American Psychiatric Press, 1999, pp 1655–1665

10

Evidence-Based Diagnosis and Treatment

*T*he plan for publication of DSM-III, initiated by the American Psychiatric Association (APA) in 1975, was the most important decision taken by the profession in the latter part of the twentieth century. From my perspective, it marked the end of the post-war years for psychiatry and the beginning of an evidence-based clinical practice that was much more adaptive to a new constellation of economic, social, political, professional, and scientific forces. While the selection of specific disorders for inclusion in the *Diagnostic and Statistical Manual of Mental Disorders* (DSM) and their precise description were extremely important, the most significant advance was the official adoption of a clear evidence-based system of nosology. No other country in the developed world had rejected psychiatric diagnosis as strongly as had the United States in the postwar decades (Menninger 1963). No country moved more decisively in an opposite direction after 1975. The publication of DSM-III (American Psychiatric Association 1980) and subsequently the Practice Guidelines (Zarin et al. 1999) were the key events in American psychiatry that gave a powerful new direction to the field.

As time passes, however, the understanding of the enormity of the change has begun to fade. A new generation in the mental health field is attempting to cope with a new set of problems, and what happened thirty years ago seems less relevant to them. I believe that understanding how American psychiatry changed its course is still important for problem solving in today's climate.

Some historians and psychiatrists have characterized the adoption of DSM-III as the reassertion of descriptive biological psychiatry's previous stance that had prevailed before the war; a stance that had been interrupted by what Shorter (1997) called the "hiatus" of psychoanalytic domination after World War II. Others, such as Paris in his book *The Fall of an Icon* (Paris 2005), have emphasized the leadership of a few influential nosologists, such as Robert Spitzer, who cleverly steered the APA through many hurdles. These formulations are correct, especially in acknowledging Spitzer's central role, but incomplete. Taken at face value, they characterize organized psychiatry as a beleaguered entity that responded somewhat passively and belatedly to outside pressures by adopting the old St. Louis diagnostic criteria (Feighner et al. 1972; see Blashfield 1982) as a straightforward defensive maneuver. This approach trivializes the decisive action taken by the APA leadership to change the field. One of the major purposes of this book is to demonstrate that the changes in American psychiatry reflected in the adoption of DSM-III were initiated by a profession eager to achieve a more evidence-based practice.

I acknowledge, of course, that I am not a neutral observer of these events. As a matter of fact, DSM-IV (American Psychiatric Association 1994) was dedicated to me, and understandably my perspective may be regarded by some as an effort to justify my role. Nevertheless, I believe that I ought to provide my personal perspective on the events leading to the publication of DSM-III and DSM-IV for current practitioners and also for the consideration of future historians. The failure to recognize the crucial role of the APA in changing American psychiatry is a serious, if understandable, mistake.

How could a professional organization engineer a scientific revolution that changed its core? According to conventional wisdom, organizations respond; they do not initiate. By the 1970s psychiatry in the United States had begun to undergo massive changes. The postwar glow had been replaced by the new pressures for accountability on all of medicine. Many leaders in psychiatry deplored the ideological rifts that had divided the field, and they called for a more unified, scientifically based profession. They deplored the "demedicalization" of psychiatry and its severe loss of credibility.

I was one of the young leaders who had criticized the ideological divisions within psychiatry and had been searching for ways to improve its scientific status throughout my career (see Sabshin 1977, 1990, 1999, the last two of which are reprinted in Appendix 1). The field's ideological schisms had weakened us seriously, and psychiatrists' bitter public disagreements were self-destructive (Shore 1979). To cover up these differences or to act solely because of the criticism was not in itself sufficient; psychiatry had to adopt a genuine commitment to science rather than to ideology. It needed to change the profession fundamentally if it was to become a respected part of medicine. To accede to the pressures without radical modifications of the field would not have convinced others that the profession had changed. A new strategy was essential!

Producing the DSM-III stated emphatically that psychiatry in America chose an evidence-based practice rather than ideology. In a published debate on DSM-III in 1984, Gerald Klerman, the distinguished administrator of the Alcohol, Drug Abuse, and Mental Health Administration (ADAMHA), enunciated this principle when he stated,

> In my opinion the development of *DSM-III* represents a fateful point in the history of the American psychiatric profession. In discussing the history of psychiatry, one of my premises is that professional groups, such as medical specialties, are able to determine their own destiny to a greater extent than most other occupational groups. The decision of the American Psychiatric Association first to develop the DSM-III and then to promulgate its use represents a significant reaffirmation on the part of American psychiatry of its medical identity and its commitment to scientific medicine. (Klerman 1984, p. 539)

No one has made the point better.

Ideologues tend to perceive criticisms of their ideas by outsiders as prejudiced and based on false assumptions. By the 1970s the post–World War II intentions of the American public and decision makers to give high priority to psychiatric casualties and to support the field enthusiastically had faded; psychiatrists were no longer perceived primarily in positive terms. Criticism of the field had grown, and not all of it was coming from antipsychiatry groups. It became widely recognized, especially among medical colleagues, that some psychiatrists would routinely prescribe medication, whereas others would recommend psychodynamic psychotherapy for patients with similar problems. The choice of treatment had clearly become based on the bias of the physician's ideology rather than on a reliable diagnosis and rational therapeutic guidelines. In addition to growing professional concerns about this trend, family members of mental patients were also becoming vocal in this criticism of psychiatric practice, as enunciated by, for example, the then National Alliance for the Mentally Ill (NAMI; now National Alliance on Mental Illness) and E. Fuller Torrey (1974, 1983), and began questioning the basic priorities of the field. Equally important, however, was the growing recognition by APA's leadership that it was time for a change (Brodie 1983; A. Freedman 1974; D. Freedman 1981, 1982; Pardes 1989; Tarjan 1984).

During the two decades after World War II, the costs of medical care had risen dramatically (Lazarus and Sharfstein 1998; Myers 1970).Those responsible for the fiscal management of newly developed health reimbursement programs, both private and governmental, became alarmed and sought new controls over expenditures. As attempts were made to reduce the overall costs of medical care, systems were organized to provide review and management of the choice and length of treatment that insurers were prepared to finance. Such attempts to reduce costs were inevitable in a nation that relied so heavily on work-related private insurance to pay most of the medical bills. Increasingly, insurance companies and government agencies sought to regulate physicians' choice of treatment and the fees paid to them. What evidence justified the specific therapy employed and its duration was the key question of the fiscal agencies responsible. They required physicians to provide data justifying their charges. Most often these data included responses to questions about diagnosis and plans for treatment. Accountability became the rule whenever reimbursement was sought from a "third party." When previous fiscal models proved to be ineffective in lowering costs sufficiently, insurers developed their own payment criteria and demanded compliance with them for reimbursement. Rarely in the history of medical economics has a relatively free market system been replaced so quickly by new regulatory constraints.

Psychoanalysts faced mortal danger from such external review of their practices. Despite their protestations, their field lacked clear diagnostic standards or guidelines for specific choice of therapies. There was no objective or convincing way to explain the reliability, let alone validity, of psychodynamic formulations to the regulators. Arbitrary constraints upon all forms of psychotherapy became common and grew more severe over time. These limitations on practice were criticized by psychiatrists; there was no doubt that some of the decisions were indeed based on gross misunderstanding. Nevertheless, the lack of sufficient clarity or precision about the fundamentals of psychiatric diagnosis and treatment took its toll. The failure to achieve parity of reimbursement for psychiatric treatment with other medical interventions could not be reversed solely by pleading for equal status with other medical disciplines. Such argument without adequate data was grossly insufficient.

In my judgment psychiatry had to change radically to meet the new challenges, and it needed to demonstrate that it possessed the leadership, determination, and capacity to become a respected part of medical science. In accomplishing all these purposes, the profession also needed to seek strong allies who supported the field's changing direction. Most significant was the relationship with organized medicine that had weakened in the postwar years but grew steadily closer since the 1970s and is very close today. Support by other physicians for psychiatry's new scientific status is now indispensable, as discussed in Chapter 6 ("En Route to Equity").

Psychiatry was not alone in medicine in attempting to become accountable to the increasingly restraining regulation of its fiscal practices. Its lack of a clear evidence-based diagnostic or therapeutic system, however, was a special weakness, and this deficit accounted for some of the harsh restrictions that were placed upon the field. Becoming fully aware of this fundamental deficit was a very powerful and important insight. Of course, we had to correct the deficit!

For psychoanalysis, the clash with the new systems of accountability was decisive. Coping with new policies of fiscal reimbursement was difficult for analysts (Raney 1983). For several decades they essentially resisted allegations of their weak evidential basis. Part of the problem was that many analysts believed that only those trained as psychoanalysts understood the field well enough to be capable of conducting outcome evaluation of psychoanalytical treatment. In addition, they asserted that their classical techniques of evaluating patients were superior to oversimplified quantitative methods. They believed that understanding their individual patients in-depth was much superior to applying pedestrian diagnostic labels. Some, such as Karl Menninger, raised questions about the entire value of nosological classification in solving these patterns of discrimination. In 1956 Menninger noted that "[t]he old Kraepelinian terms have largely disappeared" (Menninger 1995, p. 851). In 1963 he said, "Gone forever is the notion that the mentally ill person is an exception. It is now accepted that most people have some degree of mental illness at some time, and many of them have a degree of mental illness most of the time" (Menninger 1963). The analysts stated passionately that the plans to develop a new diagnostic system in psychiatry were unnecessary or retrogressive; the medical principle of providing specific treatments for specific disorders seemed antithetical to the conceptual framework for the general application of psychoanalytic treatment. The battle lines were drawn. Psychiatry chose to establish a new diagnostic system and accompanying practice guidelines.

Psychiatry, on the whole, had also been weak in providing convincing outcome data for the success rate of alternative methods of treatment. While there had been extensive efforts to provide such data, most of the early findings were criticized as unclear and biased. The need to proceed with reliably based outcome studies had to be widely understood and accepted, and for this there had to be a development of clear diagnostic criteria if adequate investigations of patients' improvement were to be conducted. DSM-II (American Psychiatric Association 1968) would have been grossly inadequate. A common language for such study was basic to a new beginning.

Research on diagnostic categories and specific treatments for them was also a fundamental part of a better ultimate understanding of the etiology of psychiatric disorder. Reliable nosology was a prerequisite for research on etiology. The lack of specific diagnostic and treatment guidelines was hindering the profession at many levels. Variations in treatment response would help to clarify which symptoms of which disorder were more or less effectively treated. Psychoanalysts, however, continued to believe for a long time that their own formulations explained the primary causes of most neurotic disorders. Many of them were not interested in systematic diagnostic research that sought to change our understanding of etiology. Psychiatry's decision to formulate a new nosology was interpreted by some as a direct attack on psychoanalysis. As Paris (2005) emphasizes, "Otto Kernberg was right: the DSM was indeed an attack on psychoanalysis."

During the debates about DSM-III, DSM-III-R, and DSM-IV, analysts were often critical of what they perceived as DSM's "narrow, descriptive approach." It is important to note, however, that in recent years, psychoanalysts have begun more serious efforts to develop their own diagnostic formulations, as presented in the *Psychodynamic Diagnostic Manual* (Alliance of Psychoanalytic Organizations 2006) and discussed in Chapter 8 ("Psychoanalysis"). Whatever its limitations, the PDM is a laudable effort.

For me, the old anti-nosology perspective was mostly vividly expressed by Jose Barchilon, who told me that he much preferred to describe his patients as Hamlet or Raskolnikov than in terms of the constricting, pedestrian language of the DSM. It is true that few films or engrossing novels could be based upon the six criteria for "borderline personality disorder." Psychoanalytic formulations are marvellous subjects for films and theater (Gabbard and Gabbard 1999), but another approach is necessary to justify scientific status and reimbursement. No matter how brilliant the art form, psychoanalysis did not have the accountability and predictability for medical practice. The publication of the PDM is a sign that the message has begun to be heard.

For psychiatry to develop a new diagnostic system, there were many problems to confront. Diagnostic studies that included samples of patients from diverse backgrounds were needed both for shaping policy within the United States and for carrying out studies across national boundaries. Psychiatry, like all of medicine, requires transnational and cross-cultural data to understand the role of social variables transacting with biological and psychological factors in the pathogenesis of illness. Co-operation across a variety of entities is essential in conducting such studies. The World Health Organization (WHO) had begun to advocate more precise diagnostic categories for international research and collection of data, and this led to the *International Classification of Diseases* (World Health Organization 1977; see Jakob et al. 2007). No other country had rejected serious study of nosology as much as American psychiatry had in the post-war years, and only American psychiatry could be effective in changing its own ideological morass.

Today, many psychiatric commentators seem to have forgotten (or to never have known) how much American psychiatry neglected diagnosis in the postwar years. Since that time we have moved almost in the opposite direction. Psychiatrists in the United States also needed to demonstrate that they understood the importance of epidemiology for policy decisions. I find it particularly significant that epidemiology is still rarely mentioned in the psychoanalytic literature. While analysis continues to emphasise its major interest in data about individuals rather than aggregates of people, the neglect of epidemiological data to test some of its hypotheses is, in my judgment, a revealing and important flaw. Lack of interest in prevalence and incidence of disorders weakens analysts' role in policy decisions. To be interested also in data about how many people might need to be helped by psychodynamic treatment does not necessarily reduce the importance of individual patients' needs. Lack of serious psychoanalytic interest in what is meant by "normal" behavior is also a reflection of insufficient interest in policy implications of theoretical constructs. To describe normality in Freud's words as "the capacity to love and to work" is poetic but of limited epidemiological utility.

Some current critics of psychiatric efforts in developing the DSM system have mistakenly stated that psychiatry was "inventing" many new diagnoses to increase the number of people needing its services (e.g., Shorter 1997). Such opinions fail to recognize that, on the contrary, DSM-III served a purpose opposite to the effect of implicit psychoanalytic assumptions of widespread disorder. In our books about the concept of normality, Offer and I have written extensively about how psychoanalysts and others have seemed to utilize a concept that psychopathology is almost universal (Offer and Sabshin 1966, 1984, 1991), as the quote from Menninger earlier in this chapter demonstrates; they imply that all children and adults employ pathological defensive measures at times and that these defenses become basic elements in the structure of disorders. Few of us adapt without some deficit in our mental structure. Many analysts today would deny the validity of this criticism; they would state that they never advocated a system of universal psychopathology. An emphatic denial made much earlier, along with an understanding of the need to collect reliable epidemiological data, would have been helpful. Not doing so was a powerful denial that psychoanalyisis was a medical discipline. Physicians rely on epidemiological studies as well as on case reports, but psychoanalysts do not.

DSM-III challenged the "universality of psychopathology" concept by its formulation of specific criteria for the various disorders and developed clear principles for including and excluding parts of the population. It paved the way for more reliable epidemiological studies that would be useful in policy formulations of health expenditures. No other field in medicine had employed a model that implied the universality of pathology so passionately. Such models became a centerpiece of the public perception of psychiatry's adoption of a nonmedical stance. Open discussion by psychoanalysts upon the policy implications of their concepts might have been helpful in clarifying some of the misunderstandings. A conference focusing on these policy implications, if held in the 1970s, could have been a positive contribution. It still could be useful today.

By the early 1970s psychiatry in the United States had undergone a massive "demedicalization" (Sabshin 1990; see Appendix 1A). Despite occasional lip service to agreement with Freud's "Project" and the importance of brain functions (Freud 1895[1950]), there was little everyday practical interest by most psychoanalysts in modern neuroscience, and at that time they did not pay much attention to the advances in neurochemistry and psychopharmacology. To quote Freud's project today without acknowledging its lack of widespread understanding by analysts is misleading. Interest in neuroanalysis by psychoanalysts is a recent phenomenon. I recall the efforts of some of my psychoanalytic supervisors to curb "medical zealousness" and their semihumorous questions about wearing white coats. In their judgment, the authoritarian physician identity had serious drawbacks when psychoanalysts were dealing with patients. Medical models were also frequently criticized. The great debate by psychoanalysts in 1927 about their medical identity (Schröter 2004) was most significant, including, as it did, Freud's fundamental doubts about the need for analysts to be physicians. My own view paralleled the points made in 1927 by Ernest Jones about the importance of medical qualifications for making reliable diagnoses and to develop rational treatment options (International Psycho-analytic Association 1927). For a variety of reasons, however, the American Psychoanalytic Association ultimately changed its admission criteria in 1991 and opened the door for nonmedical groups to be fully accepted in the association as qualified practitioners. Psychiatry had split itself off from psychoanalysis by adopting DSM-III, and, in effect, the analysts confirmed the split by changing their own membership requirements.

By the 1970s the demedicalization of American psychiatry had weakened not only our ties to medicine but also our pleas for "parity" with other medical fields in reimbursement plans. A commitment to nosology was a basic step in the long road toward achieving parity, and an empirically derived basis for choice of treatment was also a practical necessity. Psychiatry's adoption of DSM—and, later, the new Practice Guidelines—was an adaptive step that changed its public image, because the work represented in these publications was decisive in changing the profession's core approach to training, research, and practice. Such adaptation was quite different from the purely defensive maneuvers depicted by Shorter (1997).

Professional organizations are rarely praised for taking courageous or progressive steps. It is widely assumed that motivations for policy changes are only self-protective. Almost all descriptions by historians of the DSM process assume that the APA was forced to change. It is assumed that without the severe social and economic pressures, the profession would have staunchly resisted changes. Pavlov would heartily agree with this reflexive explanation! That a significant number of leaders within the APA wished to see an end to ideological dominance and wanted to bring about a paradigm shift that encouraged evidence-based practice seems to have been misunderstood. The DSM itself is more important than the array of motives that induced its acceptance. It is also important, however, to note that psychiatry chose to change its basic foundations in diagnosis and treatment.

In Shorter's book *A History of Psychiatry* there is a one-paragraph description of his understanding of my role in the development of the DSM-III (Shorter 1997, p. 301):

> Meanwhile the American Psychiatric Association was under pressure to revise the DSM II. Gay groups were unhappy that homosexuality had been included as a disorder. Insurance companies wanted more precise diagnoses if they were going to pay for long term psychotherapy. Many clinicians were becoming disaffected from psychoanalysis wanted diagnoses based on symptoms rather than on dubious theories about underlying causes. Early in 1973, Walter Barton, initiated a task force "to revive DSM II and to prepare DSM III within the next two years." Melvin Sabshin, a Young Turk, then succeeded Barton as Medical Director. Sabshin realized that if the group who had designed DSM II were to take on the revision DSM III would become a 'minor variant' of its predecessor. What was needed was something completely different. In April, 1974, Sabshin summoned Spitzer and Theodore Millon, another Young Turk who was a Ph.D. psychologist at the Neuropsychiatric Institute of the Uni-

versity of Illinois Medical Center in Chicago[,] for an all day conference. Out of this conference came the leadership that would drive forward DSM III published in 1980.

Professor Shorter, of course, had every right to publish that paragraph without talking to me about it. From my standpoint, however, it might have been useful for me to explain why I wanted something "completely different." Of course, Shorter was right in describing the pressures that had been placed on the APA. A response was needed, and I came to the APA to help in addressing the issues raised by these pressures. I also came to the APA because I wanted psychiatry to behave like a medical science, and my appointment assured me that that there was powerful support for this position. That the APA strongly wished to change American psychiatry radically does not seem to have been one of Shorter's explanatory options.

To some extent Joel Paris also takes a similar position to Shorter's when he discusses "The DSM Revolution." In his book *The Fall of an Icon* (Paris 2005, p. 86), he praises Robert Spitzer quite deservedly for his superb leadership role. But his language does not imply that the APA itself preferred the "Revolution" on scientific grounds as well as on the basis of economic necessities. It is difficult for some to perceive that a professional organization can act primarily on a rational scientific basis. In this case the adoption of a new scientific stance was also useful, but utility was not the only motive.

Janet Williams has provided an excellent summary of the basic processes involved in the formulation of DSM-III (Williams 1999). Williams, who, along with Robert Spitzer, deserves special credit for that edition of DSM, captures the nuances of specific inclusion and exclusion of disorders, the emergence of the multiaxial systems, the extensive research behind the choice of criteria, the reliability and limited construct validity of the diagnoses, the transcultural implications of the findings and attempts to cope with comorbidity. These were the core scientific issues that were involved in producing a new diagnostic system. In this chapter I do not wish to attempt to reproduce the detail of DSM-III approach. My emphasis is upon the process of changing the field. As a matter of fact, even though DSM-IV (American Psychiatric Association 1994) was dedicated to me, I am not a nosological expert. What I contributed to the process of preparing DSM-III and DSM-IV was an emphasis on policy implications; its key authors respected my part and dealt with these considerations. I was particularly impressed by the chair of the DSM-IV Task Force, Allen Frances. He understood the full implications of the changes in American psychiatry and the continuing efforts to update the system.

Of course, Spitzer and others had played a decisive role in the policy debates. Paris is right when he points out, for example, how Spitzer's notion to include some of the old categories in parentheses after the new ones permitted a useful temporary compromise. One of my most important roles was to attempt to anticipate the full panoply of policy arguments against the DSM and to seek to emphasize why we needed to approve its basic principles. I spoke at many APA District Branch meetings and area councils. In addition I had several opportunities at special conferences to support the adoption of the DSM. In every medical director's report to the Board and Assembly I reinforced the relationship between new science and new economics. When the crucial debates took place, I was encouraged to give my opinion. Given that the medical director was not chief executive officer of the APA at that time, I needed to be judicious about the use of power. Every leader of the APA, however, knew that I was exerting considerable influence in the DSM process, and the passage of time, allowing me to reflect on what really happened, allows me to acknowledge that role more frankly.

As I write this chapter in 2007, the APA's nosological system is once again being revised and DSM-V is under development, to appear by 2012. This continuing process of review and correction is precisely what was anticipated when the DSM was created. Research and clinical practice would investigate the reliability and the utility of the nosology, and then the DSM would be modified accordingly. The multiaxial system of placing the diagnoses in a variety of contexts (e.g., the presence of other medical conditions) has not been employed by clinicians as widely and vigorously as anticipated and will need to be reexamined carefully. There is also a significant need to reconsider how social and cultural variables will be integrated better in DSM-V. The entire review process is a remarkable illustration of how clinical research has become a central feature of today's psychiatry. We look forward to the time when laboratory diagnosis begins to provide reliable complementary data supporting clinical diagnostic methodology.

Most importantly, the development of the DSM has made it possible to create evidence-based Practice Guidelines for treatment of specific disorders. Such guidelines, in turn, permit outcome studies that will help in ongoing revision of the nosological system. Empirical research on clinical practice outcomes will become a major basis for the next stage of revision. There will be a continuing interaction between the review process and the modifications in diagnoses and therapeutics. This effort must be a vital part of clinical psychiatry in the next several decades.

The international acceptance of DSM-III and DSM-IV has been remarkable. It became obvious that there was a great need for such a classification. The DSM is continuing to be employed in many countries across the world. Its overall acceptance and adoption, including its enormous employment in forensics, has been much more widespread than expected. Of course, some lawyers have tried to interpret the classifications and guidelines as absolute standards; others have raised many questions about their reliability. Just recently, my stepson, a senior British lawyer, drew my attention to an interesting case in which there was an appeal against a verdict of murder. The question at issue was whether the mental status of the accused fitted the classification of a disorder that could have been responsible for the crime. It also raised the question of the employment of subthreshold diagnoses—those in which the symptoms do not fully meet the criteria for the disorder but are suggestive of it. The frequent use of the DSM in forensic work is an important indicator of its worldwide employment.

While more needs to be done in further improvement of diagnostic reliability, the acceptance of the DSM has been phenomenal, and the original expectations, including what it has meant for the scientific image of the field, have been exceeded. Once a new, rational nosological system was developed it became essential to follow it up with an increase in the scientific precision of psychiatric therapeutics. Clarification of diagnostic categories has led to the development of a much more empirically based system of practice guidelines. Currently such guidelines have been completed for many disorders, and ultimately they will be compiled for most, if not all, of the categories of disorder. (The very use of the word "guidelines" rather than "standards" or "options" reflected intense discussion of the reliability of the current empirical evidence.)

Use of these guidelines in outcome research will increase the reliability of comparing international therapeutic trials. It will also lead to a better understanding of the nosological variables themselves and help in their subsequent refinement. This wide acceptance and use of the DSM and the practice guidelines places the entire field of psychiatry at a higher scientific level. The process of investigation has brought together research and clinical communities in a manner not previously achieved in psychiatry. I recognize that there is a danger in being so enthusiastic about the implications of nosology and guidelines in that insufficient attention might be given to the need for further changes. I have also been concerned that the many practical issues in fiscal accountability experienced by American psychiatrists today will obscure the importance of the establishment of scientific rigor in the field. This chapter, and the book as a whole, are intended to reinforce that rigor.

Three individuals have played crucial roles in the development of the practice guidelines. The deputy director of the Office of Psychiatric Research, Deborah Zarin, was the lead investigator of the project from the beginning and contributed greatly to the thoroughness and precision of the guideline preparation. Her imaginative approaches to the details of evidence criteria for levels of therapeutic confidence, of sequential components of guideline development, and the formation of a clinical research network were particularly important (Zarin at al. 1999). Her capacity to conceptualize and organize the project as a whole has been extraordinary.

The leadership by the director of the Office of Research, Harold Pincus, was also decisive. With the vital leadership of Allen Frances, Chair of the DSM IV Task Force, Pincus was one of the chief architects of DSM-IV, and very few investigators conceptualized the research implications of the bridge from nosology to practice as well as he did. In Chapter 11 ("Psychiatric Research") I discuss Dr. Pincus's overall leadership role in psychiatric research in greater detail, but no area was more important than the nosological–therapeutic linkage.

John McIntyre has been one of the APA's most important overall leaders in the latter part of the twentieth century. He was very effective as speaker of the Assembly (1988–89) and also as president of the APA (1993–94). His grasp of the full implications of Practice Guidelines for psychiatric clinicians has been unrivalled. The first sentence of the superb article he coauthored with Zarin, Pincus, and Siegel conveys his belief that "[o]ver the past two decades, the field of psychiatry has moved systematically toward the goal of evidence-based clinical practice" (Zarin et al. 1999. p. 1655). McIntyre's leadership made the guidelines much more easily grasped by Assembly and Board of Trustees members. While a few critics expressed concern about the guidelines as "cookbook medicine" or "inhibitory to novel therapeutic approaches," McIntyre argued forcibly about their flexibility and the inclusion of many opinions in producing the various drafts of the documents. He also emphasized the series of careful reviews to make sure that the guidelines would be periodically revised. The approval process for the guidelines has been somewhat easier than was the approval of DSM-III. Clearly there was broad understanding that American psychiatry had changed dramatically.

Much of the continuing work on the practice guidelines has been conducted since my departure from the APA. Both Jay Scully, Medical Director, and Darrel Regier, Director of the Office of Research, are devoted to the full implementation of the project. Dr. McIntyre also continues his work on integrating the APA's Practice Guidelines with those produced by other medical specialties and accomplishes this coordination with other leaders in the American Medical Association and other medical leadership.

The APA began a vigorous process of fundamental change in 1975 when it undertook development of DSM-III. Work has expanded tremendously for over 30 years with a continuing cycle of evidence-based modifications in diagnosis and treatment guidelines. The transactions of new nosology and new therapeutics are the best indicator of how much psychiatry has changed and will continue to change. A genuine scientific pathway has been constructed for the field's continuing progress.

REFERENCES

Alliance of Psychoanalytic Organizations, PDM Task Force: Psychodynamic Diagnostic Manual. Silver Spring, MD, Alliance of Psychoanalytic Organizations, 2006

American Psychiatric Association: Diagnostic and Statistical Manual of Mental Disorders, 2nd Edition. Washington, DC, American Psychiatric Association, 1968

American Psychiatric Association: Diagnostic and Statistical Manual of Mental Disorders, 3rd Edition. Washington, DC, American Psychiatric Association, 1980

American Psychiatric Association: Diagnostic and Statistical Manual of Mental Disorders, 4th Edition. Washington, DC, American Psychiatric Association, 1994

Blashfield RK: Feighner et al., invisible colleges, and the Matthew effect. Schizophr Bull 8(1):1–12, 1982

Bourne PG: The psychiatrist's responsibility and the public trust. Am J Psychiatry 135(2):174–177, 1978

Brodie HK: Presidential Address: psychiatry—its locus and its future. Am J Psychiatry 140:965–968, 1983

Feighner JP, Robins E, Guze SB, et al: Diagnostic criteria for use in psychiatric research. Arch Gen Psychiatry 26:57–63, 1972

Freedman AM: Presidential Address: creating the future. Am J Psychiatry 131:749–754, 1974

Freedman DX: Response to the Presidential Address. Am J Psychiatry 138:1017–1020, 1981

Freedman DX: Presidential Address: science in the service of the ill. Am J Psychiatry 139:1087–1095, 1982

Freud S: Project for a scientific psychology (1895[1950]), in Standard Edition of the Complete Psychological Works of Sigmund Freud, Vol 1. Translated and edited by Strachey J. London, Hogarth Press, 1966, pp 281–397

Gabbard GO, Gabbard K: Psychiatry and the Cinema, 2nd Edition. Washington, DC, American Psychiatric Press, 1999

Galatzer-Levy IR, Galatzer-Levy RM: The revolution in psychiatric diagnosis: problems at the foundations. Perspect Biol Med 50(2):161–180, 2007

Hall BH (ed.): A Psychiatrist's World: Selected Papers. New York, Viking Press, 1959

Ingham J: The public image of psychiatry. Soc Psychiatry 20(3):107–108, 1985

International Psycho-analytic Association, Sub-committee on Lay Analysis: Abbreviated report of the Sub-committee on Lay Analysis. Bulletin of the International Psycho-analytical Association 8:559–560, 1927

Jakob, R, Ustün, B, Madden, R, et al: The WHO Family of International Classifications. Bundesgesundheitsblatt Gesundheitsforschung Gesundheitsschutz 50:924–931, (2007)

Klerman GL, Vaillant GE, Spitzer RL, et al: A debate on DSM-III. Am J Psychiatry 141:539–553, 1984

Lazarus JA, Sharfstein SS: New Roles for Psychiatrists in Organized Systems of Care. Washington, DC, American Psychiatric Press, 1998

Menninger KA: The Vital Balance: The Life Process in Mental Health and Illness. New York, Viking, 1963

Menninger KA: The Selected Correspondence of Karl A Menninger, 1946–1965. Columbia, University of Missouri Press, 1995

Mollica RF: From asylum to community. The threatened disintegration of public psychiatry. N Engl J Med 308(7):367–373, 1983

Myers ES: Insurance coverage for mental illness: present status and future prospects. Am J Publ Health 60:1921–1930, 1970

Offer D, Sabshin M (eds): Normality: Theoretical and Clinical Concepts of Mental Health. New York, Basic Books, 1966

Offer D, Sabshin M (eds): Normality and the Life Cycle: A Critical Integration. New York, Basic Books, 1984

Offer D, Sabshin M (eds): Diversity of Normal Behavior: Further Contributions to Normatology. New York, Basic Books, 1991

Pardes H: Response to the Presidential Address: the research alliance: road to clinical excellence. Am J Psychiatry 146:1105–1111, 1989

Paris J: Fall of an Icon: Psychoanalysis and Academic Psychiatry. Toronto, University of Toronto Press, 2005

Raney JO: The payment of fees for psychotherapy. Int J Psychoanal Psychother 9:147–181, 1982–1983

Sabshin M: On remedicalization and holism in psychiatry. Psychosomatics 18(4):7–8, 1977

Sabshin M: Turning points in twentieth-century American psychiatry. Am J Psychiatry 147:1267–1274, 1990

Sabshin M: The future of psychiatry, in The American Psychiatric Press Textbook of Psychiatry, 3rd Edition. Edited by Hales RE, Yudofsky SC, Talbott JA. Washington, American Psychiatric Press, 1999, pp 1693–1701

Schröter M: The early history of lay analysis, especially in Vienna, Berlin and London: aspects of an unfolding controversy (1906–24). Int J Psychoanal 85(pt 1):159–177, 2004

Shore MF: Public psychiatry: the public's view. Hosp Community Psychiatry 30(11):768–771, 1979

Shorter E: A History of Psychiatry: From the Era of the Asylum to the Age of Prozac. New York, Wiley, 1997

Tarjan G: Presidential Address: American psychiatry: a dynamic mosaic. Am J Psychiatry 141:923–930, 1984

Torrey EF: The Death of Psychiatry. Radnor, PA, Chilton Book Co., 1974

Torrey EF: The Mind Game: Witchdoctors and Psychiatrists. New York, J. Aronson, 1983

Williams JBW: Psychiatric classification, in The American Psychiatric Press Textbook of Psychiatry, 3rd Edition. Edited by Hales RE, Yudofsky SC, Talbott JA. Washington, American Psychiatric Press, 1999, pp 227–252

World Health Organization: International Classification of Diseases, 9th Revision. Geneva, World Health Organization, 1977

Zarin DA, McIntyre JS, Pincus HA, et al: Practice guidelines in psychiatry and a psychiatric practice research network, in The American Psychiatric Press Textbook of Psychiatry, 3rd Edition. Edited by Hales RE, Yudofsky SC. Washington, DC, American Psychiatric Press, 1999, pp 1655–1665

11

Psychiatric Research

*T*he *Diagnostic and Statistical Manual of Mental Disorders* (DSM) and the Practice Guidelines project (Zarin et al. 1999) were the centerpieces in the structure of a changing American psychiatry (see Chapter 10, "Evidence-Based Diagnosis and Treatment"). While these developments were bitterly opposed by many psychoanalysts, the overwhelming majority of psychiatrists supported the field's adoption of an evidence-based position. To achieve their enormous impact, however, several accompanying contextual changes were absolutely vital. In Chapter 6 ("En Route to Equity"), I have described how the effectiveness of the American Psychiatric Association in government affairs, economic issues, and public relations cleared the pathway for an acceptance of a new psychiatry. Jay Cutler's understanding and appreciation of the centrality of psychiatric research to our government affairs activities was indispensable. Equally important was the development of a strong APA Office of Research, headed first by Harold Pincus and then, subsequent to my retirement, by Darrel Regier. The promotion of an evidence-based psychiatry has dramatically changed clinical practice and the image of the field among colleagues and the public.

In this chapter I wish to describe how the commitment to psychiatric research that had begun intensively in the 1970s contributed to the structure, the reinforcement, and the concepts of a new psychiatry. It is difficult for the current generation of psychiatrists to begin to realize the extent of psychiatry's research weakness during the three post-war decades. The field has changed so radically since that time that the old practices are difficult to discern. Even some of America's most distinguished psychiatric research policy makers do not seem to grasp how much clinical psychiatry has changed since the 1970s. I believe that failure to understand the basis and extent of these changes may weaken our efforts to cope with current problems. In this chapter and throughout the book, I wish to emphasize how strongly the scientific developments we achieved have already changed the clinical practice of psychiatry and have moved the profession toward increasingly precise diagnosis and therapeutics.

By 1970 medical colleagues, policy makers and most of the general public had begun to believe that psychiatry was more like a collection of diverse cults rather than a medical science. The problems were compounded by the psychiatric ideologues themselves when they poured scorn on other psychiatric practitioners. At Michael Reese Hospital, as discussed in Chapter 3 ("Implicit Preparations for a Leadership Role in Psychiatry"), I noted much public caricaturizing of the biologically oriented psychiatrists by the psychoanalysts, who in turn were mocked by their ideological opponents. Self-criticism was rare. By the middle 1970s, however, the number of external critics of psychiatry from a wide variety of backgrounds was growing quickly. There were many psychiatrists who genuinely advocated scientific principles and research, but their voices were not generally accepted at first as examples of rationality. Rather they were heard by the general public as more noise in a controversial system. Changing psychiatry was vital, but it was going to be difficult. That the profession changed itself so radically is important for the present generation to understand. Recognition of the importance of an evidence-based core was the key to changing the basic direction of the field even before managed care exerted its powerful impact.

The growth and development of the National Institute of Mental Health (NIMH) into a research colossus was a crucial step in achieving the ascendancy of a psychiatric science, but it was a long time before it became primarily a research-based institute (Kolb et al. 2000). In the beginning NIMH emphasized training, and then it focused heavily on improving mental health service systems, followed by a combination of services and research. Several structural reorganizations led to separate administrative systems for drug abuse and alcoholism. Mental health service agencies were organized and separated from research functions. Funding for training was significantly reduced, especially when convincing evidence was presented that psychiatry should no longer be designated as a shortage specialty. By the middle 1980s research had become the primary function of the institute. The 1990s were designated the "decade of the brain," and NIMH became the premier funding body in the world for psychiatric research. The change was truly astonishing.

When the NIMH was first formed in 1946, it was not yet a powerful research agency. By the start of the new century it was the second highest research funding institute in the National Institutes of Health. The APA's Office of Government Affairs, with much help from our Office of Research, contributed significantly to growing dominance of research activities. The APA was particularly effective in seeking political support for the funding. Determined psychiatric leadership was very important in obtaining advocacy for the mental health field by executive and legislative governmental agencies. Alliances with citizens' groups and other health organizations were vital. Jay Cutler and his staff played a key role in the metamorphosis of mental health agencies toward an extraordinarily strong research base. Major supporters in the U.S. Senate included Sen. Pete V. Domenici (R-N.M.), Sen. Jacob K. Javitz (R-N.Y.), Sen. Edward M. Kennedy (D-Mass.), Sen. Arlen Specter (R-Pa.), Sen. Paul Wellstone (D-Minn.), Sen. Ron Wyden (D-Ore.), and Sen. Barbara A. Mikulski (D-Md.). In the U.S. House Of Representatives the chief champions for budgetary increases for research included Rep. John E. Porter (R-Ill.), Rep. James Ramstad (R-Minn.), Rep. Thomas J. Downey (D-N.Y.), Rep. Howard Berman (D-Calif.), Rep. Gerald E. Sikorski (D-Minn.), Rep. Steny H. Hoyer (D-Md.), Rep. Pete Stark (D-Calif.), Rep. Rosa DeLauro (D-Conn.), Rep. Vic Fazio (D-Calif.), Rep. Jim McDermott (D-Wash.), Rep. Gus Bilirakis (R-Fla.), Rep. Constance A. Morella (R-Md.), Rep. Edward J. Markey (D-Mass.), and Rep. James Bacchus (D-Fla.).

During my time at the APA several mental health administrators of the NIMH and Alcohol, Drug Abuse and Mental Health Administration (ADMHA) provided extraordinary leadership. I was particularly close to NIMH Directors Drs. Herbert Pardes, Lewis Judd, Shervert Frazier; ADMHA Administrators Drs. Gerald Klerman and William Mayer; ADAMH Acting Administrator Robert Trachtenberg; and National Institute on Drug Abuse (NIDA) Director Dr. Alan Leshner. My contacts were useful, but APA's main impact for over two decades was accomplished by Jay Cutler and his staff, along with Dr. Pincus and his colleagues. During her tenure as senior deputy medical director of the APA, Carolyn Robinowitz was particularly effective in a variety of liaison functions with NIMH. She continued with that activity after she left the APA, in her role as a Dean at the Georgetown School of Medicine. She has also increased her work with federal agencies since she became president-elect of the APA in 2006. The APA was a major driving force in the advance of psychiatric research, and it is important that the current generation—practitioners and researchers—understand the significance of what our association has accomplished. Failure to recognize our early determination to change could weaken our adaptation to future problems. Research support of evidence-based practice has been the catalyst that has changed the public image of psychiatry.

I wanted a strong APA research capacity when I became medical director in 1974, but we did not have the resources to accomplish this at that time. The Board had agreed to establish a small administrative research office to work with the DSM-III project. I recognized, however, that it would be important to develop a much stronger research office headed by a leader who could assume a national coordinating role in achieving the primacy of research. Fortunately, the success of DSM-III (American Psychiatric Association 1980) and the anticipation of DSM-IV (American Psychiatric Association 1994) and beyond provided us with the resources to build up an organization and to search for a founding director.

Not surprisingly, we found our new director at the NIMH. From 1979 to 1984, Dr. Harold Pincus served as special assistant to the director of the Department of Health and Human Resources at NIMH. Interested in federal systems involving mental health research policies early in his career, Pincus served as a legislative intern during medical school. As a psychiatry resident at George Washington University, he was appointed clinical scholar in the Robert Wood Johnson program, which helped prepare him for a future as a research policy leader. In 1978 and 1979, Dr. Pincus served as a Fellow for The President's Commission on Mental Health, which played an important role in transforming the field of psychiatry at the time. Established by President Jimmy Carter soon after he took office in 1977, the Commission was eventually chaired by First Lady Rosalynn Carter, who had actively campaigned in Georgia for the creation of community mental health services. Rosalynn Carter's intelligence, determination, and compassion helped revitalize the mental health system.

Dr. Pincus has had a most distinguished career in psychiatric research policy and in academic psychiatry. When he left the APA in 1999 he was appointed professor and vice chair of the Department of Psychiatry at the University of Pittsburgh School of Medicine. This was followed by his appointment as vice chair of the Department of Psychiatry at Columbia University's College of Medicine. Pittsburgh and Columbia are two of the most prestigious medical research centers in the country, and Dr. Pincus's academic leadership reflects his high national status in research policy.

The APA was fortunate to have the services of Dr. Pincus as a deputy medical director and founding director of the Office of Research for 14 pivotal years (1985–1999). Those were crucial years during which psychiatric research rapidly became a powerful force in reshaping American psychiatry.

During the 1980s and 1990s research replaced education as the top priority in academic psychiatry (Weissman et al. 1999). About 20% of the departments became research behemoths as defined by their higher success in obtaining research grants; almost all of the remaining departments were also involved in seeking funds for investigations. As psychiatry rejoined the rest of the medical community, an extraordinary change occurred in the selection of departmental chairs in psychiatry. As a reflection of the shifting priorities in academic psychiatry, search committees no longer considered psychoanalyst educators as their top candidates for these positions. Departments deeply rooted in psychoanalytic theory and practice now sought potential leaders with a track record of directing large research projects and obtaining grants. As in internal medicine and other large clinical departments, research prowess became the currency by which top faculty members were recruited and educational funding obtained. Ironically, only two decades earlier, research in psychiatry had relied on whatever monies could be spared from its overall educational funds. Since the clinical segments of academic psychiatry were much less profitable than, for example, the lucrative high therapeutic technology of the surgical departments, they generated little in the way of funding for research.

Our Office of Research often provided help to search committees in identifying suitable candidates for departmental chairmanships. Dr. Pincus and his staff were also a practical source of help to academic departments seeking new faculty with high research credentials. The Office compiled and published directories of psychiatric research programs. It put together the extraordinarily popular "Psychiatric Research Reports," which have been utilized across the world as a major source of information. Along with our Office of Education, our research staff had close ties with the Association of American Medical Colleges (AAMC), and psychiatry's image with medical colleagues improved dramatically. Deans of medical schools perceived psychiatry in a new light, and, as a matter of fact, an impressive number of psychiatrists became deans. Our Office of Research was seen as very helpful in promoting the new scientific psychiatry at every level, and it has continued these functions until the present time.

Most important for the current stage of American psychiatry is the dominance of neuroscientific, biological, and pharmacological research. There are many reasons for these priorities, including the great success of the "decade of the brain" and the exponential growth in evidence-based diagnosis and treatment (Weissman et al. 1999). The biological advances have vastly outpaced the psychosocial aspects of the field. Exceptions can be found, but the trend toward the hegemony of biological psychiatry cannot be denied.

At the APA Annual Meeting, as described in Chapter 14 ("Annual Meetings"), the industry-sponsored symposia have become dominant and tremendously popular. Almost all of the presentations feature a neuroscientific topic. One can still find some high-quality programs in psychotherapy and social psychiatry at our mammoth meeting, but the prominence of pharmacology is apparent in our exhibit halls and our symposia. APA President Steven Sharfstein sounded a warning with which many would agree when, in his president-elect address in 2005, he bemoaned the "bio-bio-bio model" becoming so dominant as compared to a bio-psycho-social model (Sharfstein 2005).

Research has brought psychiatry out of its ideological morass, but the results include significant imbalances in areas of investigation and clinical practice. It is somewhat unlikely that the pharmaceutical industry would support research in psychosocial psychiatry unless there were strong evidence that combined biological and psychotherapeutic treatment does indeed augment pharmacotherapy (Lazar and Gabbard 1997).

In the United States we will need to rely heavily on the willingness of federal agencies and private foundations to become more interested in stimulating high quality research in the psychosocial sphere. The long history of ideological dominance in the mental health field has rendered federal agencies, political leaders, family groups, and much of the general public somewhat wary of psychosocial explanations of mental illness. I believe that the growing strength of evidence-based employment of psychological and social variables will lead to an increase in their level of support. Restoring a more balanced research portfolio should be one of our goals. Many colleagues do not agree with this position.

At least some discernible difference of opinion exists among the most advanced neuroscientific researchers about the future course of our profession. Some advocate a union between psychiatry and neurology into a joint neuroscientific specialty that will focus upon neuron signaling, neurotransmitters, neuropeptides (especially the endorphins), and co-localization. Neuroanatomy and neurophysiology, including molecular neurobiology, would be central areas of investigation and would ultimately become a base for a new nosology and a new generation of even more effective medications. Understanding specific genomic influence will become enormously important. Some see this exciting area as the center of a new research era in psychiatry. Those advocating a merged neuroscientific specialty believe that emphasis upon such variables will help us in the development of a new understanding of the etiology of mental illness and provide a base for superior pharmacological treatments. Many believe that present-day psychiatry is still too engaged in psychosocial issues that do not have major research potential; they do not envisage psychosocial psychiatry as a central part of the future of our profession.

One example of this point of view can be seen in the following quotation from Thomas Insel, the current NIMH Director:

> While research in psychiatry has begun to embrace the power of molecular, cellular, and systems neuroscience, the scientific excitement has not yet influenced clinical practice by refining diagnosis and informing treatment. Furthermore, these advances have been conspicuously ignored by training programs. Most psychiatric residency programs remain focused on psychodynamic psychiatry or applied psychopharmacology with little exposure to the revolution in neurobiology or cognitive science. While many of America's best colleges have developed departments or majors in neuroscience, medical schools continue to divide the mind from the brain, forcing students to choose between psychiatry and neurology. Judged from recent recruiting statistics, both psychiatry and neurology are stalled, in spite of the enormous interest in neuroscience from students entering medical school. The intellectual framework [Eric] Kandel foresees for psychiatry may ultimately require that both psychiatry and neurology are reframed in clinical neuroscience disciplines. (Insel 2005, pp. 29–30)

Insel represents an extremely important perspective on the prospect of a new scientific revolution for psychiatry. He is eager to support neuroscientific research that will lead to a new paradigm for the field. In my judgment, however, he minimizes the clinical changes that have occurred during the last 25 years.

I believe that what has already occurred in research and clinical practice during the last quarter of a century paves the way for further development. Psychoanalytic teaching in residency training programs has been greatly reduced and indeed its dominance has been questioned by most faculties. As Altshuler (1990) notes, "More than 60% of the psychiatrists now in training may complete their training without ever seeing a patient in twice-a-week or more intensive psychotherapy." I recognize that Insel and others are dissatisfied with the amount of neuroscientific education filling the newly available time, but qualitative change has begun.

To Insel and some of his colleagues, the DSM and the Practice Guidelines may not be perceived as major advances. Ironically, in this opinion, they agree with many psychoanalytic critics, but of course for contrasting reasons. To me and to many of my contemporaries, new diagnostic and new therapeutics have brought about a qualitative change in clinical practice. To ignore the development of an evidence-based system in the passion for an even more radical alteration of the field is, in my judgment, incorrect. At the very least the subject requires very careful discussion. I believe that such discussion and debate could be very helpful in resolving or at least defining the differences. In addition, I believe that psychiatry's problems in recruiting residents are not likely to be solved by an integration with neurology. That merger would not attract potential candidates who still are interested in psychosocial aspects of the field. Perhaps Dr. Insel would not wish to attract such candidates. Did the peak recruitment for psychiatric residency in the 1960s and 1970s during a time of psychoanalytic dominance argue against changing its ideological base? The causes for high and low recruitment are more complex than Insel implies. Psychiatry, like the rest of medicine, is under siege today largely because of managed care. The field also seems less attractive to some students, for whom it lacks a strong enough psychosocial emphasis. Insel and I disagree on the solutions to the present problems faced by psychiatry. He favors a new neuroscientific specialty, whereas I favor support for an evidence-based psychosocial renaissance for the field coordinated with neuroscience and embedded in a new and more rational health system.

Other research leaders advocate varying degrees of support for psychosocial aspects of psychiatry. After a superb review of neuroscience developments in psychiatry and a reiteration of how the field must continue to incorporate neuroscience, Coyle and Hyman (1999), in their textbook chapter "The Neuroscientific Foundations of Psychiatry," conclude:

> Psychiatry, as the medical specialty primarily involved in the diagnosis and management of behavioral disorders, must by necessity incorporate neuroscience into its scientific foundation. Based on the breathtaking growth of neuroscience research over the last decade, advances in the understanding of the structure, organization, and function of the brain promise to offer powerful new methods for diagnosing psychiatric disorders, clarifying their pathophysiology, and developing more specific and effective therapies.
>
> Fears that these advances will undermine the humanistic tradition of psychiatry and negate the important relationship between physician and patient are unfounded. First, even when genetically based techniques become feasible for identifying certain of the hereditary major mental disorders, the clinical method for developing provisional diagnosis that is used at present will still be necessary to determine which individuals warrant testing. Second, diagnoses should be neither offered nor accepted in a mechanical fashion; making a definitive diagnosis requires ongoing humane psychological management. Third, clinical research on psychopharmacological treatments for several psychiatric disorders is now demonstrating that pharmacotherapy alone is insufficient for the complete and effective management of many patients. To the contrary, evidence is growing that specific behavioral, psychological, and psychosocial strategies must often be coupled with pharmacotherapy to achieve optimal outcome in the management of psychiatric disorders. Fourth, the methods for rigorously establishing the efficacy of somatic therapies will have to be applied to behavioral and psychological therapies to determine the most effective inter-

ventions for particular disorders. Thus, clinicians will be able to tailor the treatments, be they somatic or psychological, with increasing confidence about their efficacy and specificity. (p. 32)

I agree with the implication in this formulation and would emphasize that more research on the coupling of psychological and biological variables is vital. Ultimately such research should bring about increased support for exploring new psychosocial hypotheses and also perhaps some very old ones.

The current APA Office of Research under Darrel Regier is very much involved in all of the questions raised in this chapter and, with the support of Drs. Scully and Robinowitz, is active in the policy implications. Dr. Regier came to the APA after my departure, but I knew him during many of his leadership roles at the NIMH. His large-scale epidemiological studies, interest in social psychiatry research, and international policy leadership have been very important. The creation by the APA of the American Psychiatric Institute for Research and Education (APIRE), which Dr. Regier directs, affords a new system to support all of the research activities.

It is now widely appreciated that research is a vital element for psychiatry's goal of parity and equity. APA's current president, Carolyn Robinowitz, and its medical director, Jay Scully, understand the importance of research for the future of psychiatry. I believe that this message must be reiterated frequently; it can easily be overwhelmed by the pressure of current economic problems. Most of our members are absorbed with the encroachments of managed care and could easily overlook the underlying vital role of research for the scientific image and basic support of psychiatry, yet their continuing support will be crucial for our profession's progress. I know that our current leadership will emphasize the importance of new data and an evidence-based practice. I also hope that American psychiatry will play a significant role in a reorganization of our national health system so that a new scientifically balanced biopsychosocial psychiatry can be genuinely supported.

REFERENCES

Altshuler KZ: Whatever happened to intensive psychotherapy? Am J Psychiatry 147:430, 1990

American Psychiatric Association: Diagnostic and Statistical Manual of Mental Disorders, 3rd Edition. Washington, DC, American Psychiatric Association, 1980

American Psychiatric Association: Diagnostic and Statistical Manual of Mental Disorders, 4th Edition. Washington, DC, American Psychiatric Association, 1994

Coyle JT, Hyman SE: The neuroscientific foundations of psychiatry, in The American Psychiatric Press Textbook of Psychiatry, 3rd Edition. Edited by Hales RE, Yudofsky SC, Talbott JA. Washington, DC, American Psychiatric Press, 1999, pp 3–33

Insel TR: Commentary: "A new intellectual framework for psychiatry," in Kandel ER:Psychiatry, Psychoanalysis, and the New Biology of Mind. Washington, DC, American Psychiatric Publishing, 2005, pp 27–31

Ivanov I: Common problems in psychotherapy training for psychiatry residents. J Psychiatr Pract 13(3):184–189, 2007

Kolb LC, Frazier SH, Sirovatka P: The National Institute of Mental Health: its influence on psychiatry and the nation's mental health in American Psychiatry After World War II: 1944–1994. Edited by Menninger RW, Nemiah JC. Washington, DC, American Psychiatric Press, 2000, pp 207–231

Lazar SG, Gabbard GO: The cost-effectiveness of psychotherapy. J Psychother Pract Res 6:307–314, 1997

Sharfstein SS: Response to the Presidential Address: advocacy for our patients and our profession. Am J Psychiatry 162:2045–2047, 2005

Weissman S, Sabshin M, Eist H (eds): Psychiatry in the New Millennium. Washington, DC, American Psychiatric Press, 1999

Zarin DA, McIntyre JS, Pincus HA, et al: Practice guidelines in psychiatry and a psychiatric practice research network, in The American Psychiatric Press Textbook of Psychiatry, 3rd Edition. Edited by Hales RE, Yudofsky SC. Washington, DC, American Psychiatric Press, 1999, pp 1655–1665

12

Psychiatric Education

*T*he field of psychiatric education is massive, complex, and a splendid indicator of changing professional goals. Discussion of its full scope would fill several large volumes and would indeed give an important insight into psychiatric history. I have been particularly impressed by the excellent summation of the field by Scully, Robinowitz, and Shore (Scully et al. 2000). They reviewed all levels of psychiatric education, decade by decade, since World War II, and their conclusions have very much influenced this chapter. Consonant with the basic objectives of this book, I am emphasizing *how* changes in American psychiatric education have been influenced by the replacement of ideology by scientific principles. The interaction of new science and the new economics of health care is also discussed, as are potential educational alternative directions for the field. I start with medical school education, concentrating on how it affects specialty choice and then discuss postgraduate training and lifelong learning. In each case I have emphasized the context of the education at least as much as the content.

MEDICAL STUDENT EDUCATION IN PSYCHIATRY

Even during these days of powerful genetic and biological formulations about the causes of mental disorders and, indeed, much of human behavior, medical students' selection of a specialty is still primarily understood on psychological, social, and economic grounds. Of course, during the time of psychoanalytic domination of American psychiatry (see Chapter 8, "Psychoanalysis"), one could have argued that genetic tendencies to be "psychologically minded" might have influenced the choice of specialty. Today, even with the neuroscientific domination of the field, it would be still hard to develop a biological hypothesis to distinguish the choice of psychiatry as compared with neurology or even internal medicine. Some specialties, such as orthopedics and general surgery, continue to attract fewer women, and this has been the topic of intense scrutiny in the literature (Sanfey et al. 2006).

Most medical educators agree that, whatever the predilections before medical school, the experiences during training heavily influence the final choice. In this section, I consider several aspects of that decision, recognizing that the primary goal of psychiatric education for medical students is to help their future work in whatever specialty they enter. I also explore recruitment into psychiatry and discuss postgraduate psychiatric education, including subspecialty careers.

As time passes, the realities of psychiatric education during the postwar years are becoming increasingly hazy in the minds of many of today's psychiatrists. They know from teachers, books, and articles that the field has changed enormously, but it would be hard for most of them to comprehend the full extent of the differences. The most radical changes have taken place in the residency training area, but teaching in the medical student program has also undergone massive revision (Scully at al. 2000).

During the postwar years, a revolution took place in the content, style, and the amount of time devoted to psychiatric education for all medical students. From a pre-war limited exposure to a few "insane" individuals, the medical student educational field burgeoned by 1970 to be one of the five clinical departments in medical schools with the most curriculum time. (The four others were surgery, internal medicine, pediatrics, and obstetrics-gynecology.) In addition to clinical clerkships in psychiatry during the last 2 years of medical school, most psychiatric departments were allocated time in both the first and second years to teach Principles of Behavioral Science, Introduction to Clinical Examination, and Basic Psychopathology. Psychiatric departments at that time were more invested in education than they were in research, and they tended to believe that they possessed a special ability to communicate well with most people, including medical students. Some psychiatric educators were gifted teachers, with humor and a flair for being interesting and persuasive. Few, however, were truly empathetic with the basic attitudes, experiences, and academic concerns of medical students. They were quick to diagnose "resistance" to learning about psychodynamics but slow in perceiving the problems in their own teaching. Psychoanalytic principles often seemed extraneous to students deeply involved in the study of gross anatomy and physiology during their first year, or the complexity of pathology in their second year. Their future depended on their comprehension of the basic subjects; psychodynamic principles were at the periphery and, besides, somewhat controversial. The sexual content was particularly difficult for some students at that time. The scientific validity of what was being taught seemed questionable to many students when compared with the clarity of histology, pathology, and internal medicine.

Despite what I consider to have been an overall negative reaction to the teaching of psychiatry to medical students during the postwar period, a fascinating paradox occurred. The proportion of American medical graduates (AMGs) choosing psychiatry surged from 3%–5% to 6%–7% during the immediate postwar period up through 1969 (Sierles and Taylor 1995). AMGs choosing psychiatry dropped to 4%–5% during the next twenty years. This figure dropped further to about 3% during the 1990s. In 1980, an all-time nadir of 2.6% alarmed academic psychiatrists, triggering a careful analysis of factors that may have led to the drop (Weissman and Bashook 1991). By default, the decrease in available AMGs has led to more international medical graduates (IMGs) filling these slots, but because of many variables, the number of IMGs applying to the field may also be insufficient (Rao 2003). Recruitment into psychiatry varies among medical schools, but workforce trends in psychiatry continue to concern psychiatry educators (Sierles et al. 2003). It should be noted, however, that in the postwar years more students entered medical school with an interest in psychiatry than did graduates of the school; there was either a fall-off of interest or a greater attraction to other career possibilities, or both. A survey of new medical students in three Southwestern U.S. medical schools found that although strongly valuing actual traits about the field psychiatry (close interpersonal contact, attractive lifestyle, challenging), 35.3% of students considered it unlikely that they would pursue psychiatry, and 27.1% had already ruled it out (Feifel et al. 1999). Fortunately, subsequent studies have found that favorable experiences during the psychiatry clerkship may impact students' eventual choice of psychiatry as a specialty (Clardy and Thrush 2000).

By 1980 psychiatric research had replaced education as the highest priority for most academic departments of psychiatry. This was not universally true, and some academic centers continued their special interest in education. The American Psychiatric Association (APA) took over publication of the *Journal of Psychiatric Education* in 1989 when it was realized that the *American Journal of Psychiatry* had reduced its educational content so as to include a much higher percentage of research articles. (The *Journal of Psychiatric Education* was renamed *Academic Psychiatry* in 1989.) By this time, however, the *Journal of Psychiatric Education* revealed less psychodynamic content than existed in the pedagogy of the 1960s. It would be interesting to classify academic departments of psychiatry into high and low commitment to the educational aspects of psychiatry and to compare recruitment into psychiatry in both samples.

By the early 1990s, the recruitment of American students to psychiatry had reached a low point; since that time, the number entering psychiatry has slightly increased but is not up to the peak of the earlier period.

During the last two decades, the teaching of psychiatry to medical students has become much less ideologically dominated than it had been previously. Today, the emphasis is upon clinical examination, nosology, and psychopathology. Some psychiatrists assert that the changes have not been significant enough (Insel 2005), but I believe that this opinion comes from leaders who would prefer a full merger of psychiatry with neurology into a clinical neuroscience program. For them, that is the proper future direction of psychiatry. From my perspective, however, there is now a much better scientific base in both preclinical and clinical teaching of psychiatry to medical students (Scully et al. 2000). Derision of psychiatric education has reduced considerably among medical students and the overall medical faculty. The difference in current psychiatric education is noticed by both groups. The psychiatric subspecialties have provided excellent scholarly education for medical students in child psychiatry, gerontology, and psychosomatics. These educators are much more knowledgeable and practical than their clinical predecessors, and they are particularly helpful for those contemplating a career in pediatrics, internal medicine, and geriatrics. The general improvement in psychiatric education for medical students, however, has not brought psychiatry back to its peak level of recruitment. Among a number of possible factors for this, I wish to concentrate on a few that seem particularly relevant.

During the three decades after World War II, psychiatry was officially designated a "shortage" field. There was strong government support to increase the number of medical students entering the field. In addition, higher-than-usual resident stipends were provided for physicians in other medical specialties or in general practice to switch fields and take up psychiatric residencies. The "shortage definition" no longer applies to psychiatry; some even perceive an oversupply of psychiatrists. Furthermore, although earnings of physicians and surgeons are among

TABLE 1. **MEDIAN TOTAL COMPENSATION OF PHYSICIANS BY SPECIALTY, 2004**

	Less than two years in specialty	Over one year in specialty
Anesthesiology	$259,948	$321,686
Surgery: general	228,839	282,504
Obstetrics/Gynecology: general	203,270	247,348
Psychiatry: general	173,922	180,000
Internal medicine: general	141,912	166,420
Pediatrics: general	132,953	161,331
Family practice (without obstetrics)	137,119	156,010

Note. Total compensation for physicians reflects the amount reported as direct compensation for tax purposes, plus all voluntary salary reductions. Salary, bonus, and/or incentive payments, research stipends, honoraria, and distribution of profits were included in the total compensation.
Source. Medical Group Management Association Physician Compensation and Production Report, 2005. Cited in Bureau of Labor Statistics 2007.

the highest of any occupation, the income of psychiatrists when compared with other medical specialists has been relatively low (see Table 1). Income prospects obviously play a role in selecting a specialty; many students are heavily in debt when they graduate from medical school, and the opportunity to repay that debt in as short a time as possible affects their career choice. Surgical specialties have been especially attractive for those seeking higher incomes. More recent trends in specialty choice suggest that medical students highly prioritize "controllable" lifestyle factors such as number of work hours, lifestyle, income, and years of training more so than their predecessors (Dorsey et al. 2003). Considered a "controllable lifestyle" specialty, psychiatry may become the beneficiary of medical students' preference for a "balance" between their personal and professional lives.

The percentage of female medical students has grown rapidly in recent decades, and a higher proportion of them are now entering psychiatry than men, as discussed in Chapter 13 ("A Changing Membership"). But the opportunities for women to be accepted by all medical specialties has grown, including in some fields, such as orthopedics and general surgery, that previously discouraged their entry. This success story has meant that while more women are entering psychiatry, the proportion is not larger. The proportion of male graduates choosing psychiatry has declined to less than 3%.

In addition to the demographics just described, I would like to suggest the presence of other variables that might affect specialty choice but are not often mentioned. If psychiatry, as some propose (Cowan and Kandel 2001), merges with neurology in some not-too-distant future, why not choose neurology rather than psychiatry? Why not choose internal medicine, which overlaps with the subspecialty of liaison psychiatry (now called psychosomatic medicine)? Some previously important reasons to choose psychiatry have been reduced in the real world of comprehending distinctions among the specialties.

Another variable relates to the impact of the current decline of interest in the psychological and social aspects of psychiatry. Those subjects may have been attractive to some students in the past, but their present lack of emphasis (Wallerstein 2006) may now be discouraging to a group previously attracted to the psychodynamic concentration.

Discouragement about third-party payors and its impact on patient care is common in the medical profession. Lack of reimbursement parity with other medical disciplines may further be eroding psychiatrists' professional morale. For primary care and specialist physicians, declining income appears to be less important in determining career satisfaction than systemic factors such as threats to physician autonomy and the decreased ability to manage daily patient interactions (Landon et al. 2003). The negative mood of many psychiatrists is communicated to students and does indeed affect today's specialty choices. For many medical students, the field seems less pleasurable, less rewarding, and less intellectually exciting than other fields. Of course, all of medicine is facing difficulty with managed care, and concerns about the future of medicine affect the choice of a medical career.

I believe that a revitalization of a scholarly psychosocial psychiatry genuinely integrated into a biopsychosocial model would spark an interest among some students who are turned off today by a field that seems insufficiently interested or unable to find time to systematically explore the relevance of psychological experience to the etiology of illness or to treat patients with psychotherapy. A broader clinical practice in psychiatry needs exploration on several grounds, including its potential attractiveness for some talented young medical students. To be successful in these efforts, the determination to change in this direction will need to match the motivation that led us to develop DSM-III (American Psychiatric Association 1980).

POSTGRADUATE EDUCATION IN PSYCHIATRY

Postgraduate training in American psychiatry has not yet found a calm equilibrium after a dramatic half century of change. The therapeutic ideologies (Strauss et al. 1964) that dominated the field's clinical practice and educational priorities after World War II have been pushed into the background. Psychiatry is now a more respected medical specialty. It has ended a period during which its basic identity as a part of medicine was challenged and it could have become one member of a group of "mental health disciplines." It chose a different course. With its new scientific agenda and the many economic questions facing all of American medicine, new decisions about psychiatry's basic future priorities will be required, and these decisions will have a major impact on residency training.

In order to determine psychiatry's best future course, I believe that two somewhat competing models would need to be explored in depth. The very names of the two approaches have already stirred controversy; in part the debate depends considerably on how the terms are defined. The first approach is the "biopsychosocial" model, which was originally formulated by Meyer (1952; see Lidz 1966) and elaborated by Engel (see Engel 1982) The second model is aptly described as the "clinical neuroscience model," and its explicit and implicit advocates include distinguished researchers and educators (Andreasen 1997; Kandel 1998). My presentation of this debate throughout much of this book will not be an impartial balanced discussion of both sides; I am very much in favor of the first position and concerned about the consequences of the second. Much depends on the details included within the two points of view.

I favor a biopsychosocial system that includes efforts to examine all three levels (biological, psychological, and social) hierarchically transactional over time (Grinker 1967). The final common pathway of causality for psychopathology always involves neural pathways. All three levels are involved, however, in the etiology of mental disorders, but to varying degrees and through varying mechanisms in different illnesses. Treatment also affects all the levels, but most psychiatrists' interest in changes at the social level will be limited to those variables that have a demonstrable direct impact on the mental illnesses. Cognition, executive competence, mood state, and rational behavior are key levels for evaluating outcome of treatment. Effects of biological and psychological therapies on the central nervous system are vital for understanding therapeutic outcome, but I hope that clinical psychiatrists will continue to pay attention to the psychological responses. "Biopsychosocial" psychiatry is not meant to imply equivalent interest and confidence in all three hierarchical levels. It does imply paying attention to the levels that are relevant to etiology, to treatment, and, ultimately, to prevention (Engel 1980). It is the interest in the transaction of these variables over time that will differentiate the psychiatrist, on the one hand, from the neurologist and the clinical psychologist, on the other hand. The neurologist will focus primarily on the "bio" side, whereas the clinical psychologist will focus primarily upon the psychological; the psychiatrist's unique role will be to understand the relevance of both to etiology and treatment.

The clinical neuroscience model for psychiatry primarily differs from the biopsychosocial model in its reduction of the salience of psychological and social variables as central to understanding the etiology and treatment of mental illnesses. From this point of view, understanding the central nervous system is the key to the etiology of mental illness and its treatment. Psychological and social variables are not central. The basic central nervous system "hardware" is what is important, not the psychosocial "software." If the advocate of the clinical neuroscience model asserts a serious commitment to psychological or social importance in etiology and treatment, she or he has implicitly accepted a biopsychosocial stance.

Psychoanalytic interest in neural image changes accompanying psychoanalytic therapy (Insel 2005) is primarily intent on demonstrating a correlation. It appears to be less interested in studying how these structural changes could be involved as a decisive pathogenetic factor in causing a disorder like "character neurosis." The clinical neuroscientist will, on the other hand, be interested in the neural mechanisms that are vital in the etiology of schizophrenia and personality disorders. In all likelihood, the psychosocial variables will be handled by a mental health professional in the same manner that neurologists ask other mental health specialists to deal with the behavioral consequences of multiple sclerosis or myasthenia gravis.

Adoption of a neuroscience model would indeed require a major change in postgraduate education in psychiatry. The biopsychosocial model would require somewhat less of a change, with the assumption that psychological and social aspects of the training would not decline below the current required levels. The emphasis would be on evidence-based factors that appear important in etiology and treatment. Special emphasis should be placed on empirically based combined employment of psychotherapy and pharmacotherapy by the psychiatrist. It is to be hoped that over time, however, research on what type of psychotherapy to combine with what particular medication will provide helpful information on the nuances of specific methodology. The choice of psychotherapies has broadened considerably in recent years, as has the availability of alternative medications, with the number of such medications growing almost geometrically. We are still at an early stage in the rationale for combined treatment, but many advances are occurring.

Looking back to the postwar years and postgraduate psychiatric education helps us to understand the more recent trends (Whitehorn and Mitchell 1953). By the 1960s, residency training in psychiatry had altered markedly from the pre-war years. Adolf Meyer had stimulated some modification, but prewar psychiatry had been hospital based, and there was not great optimism in learning to work with very sick patients. My residency at Tulane, as I described in Chapter 2 ("A Pathway to Psychiatry"), involved some of the pre-war employment of insulin, malaria, and electric shock, but that program was steadily overtaken by the new psychodynamic psychotherapy. While maintaining broad standards to meet accreditation requirements and preparing residents for board certification, the education in psychodynamic psychotherapy became the centerpiece and the crown jewel of the program. A few residency programs resisted the trend, but the overall image was overwhelming. At some centers, the new emphasis was so strong that residency was like a "prep school" before the "real work" at the psychoanalytic institute. Scientific education in training programs that emphasized biological or social psychiatry (Strauss et al. 1964) were usually not better in presenting scientific data as the base of their clinical judgment. Opinions rather than research highlighted the educational programs. As in Psychoanalytic Institutes, where clinical supervision was the most important way to evaluate psychoanalytic candidates, clinical supervision for psychotherapy became central to successful completion of residency programs. Supervisory styles varied, but relatively few of these clinical teachers emphasized the research background for their teaching. Instruction in biological and social psychiatry occurred mostly in case conferences or classrooms. The intimacy and the power of individual supervision had major personal impact; the decision to be analyzed also often affected psychiatric residents' subsequent career choice as well as their personal development. Positive growth during their analysis tended to reinforce the choice of an analytic career.

In Chapter 3 ("Implicit Preparations for a Leadership Role in Psychiatry"), I described the charismatic effect of several psychodynamic educators during my psychiatric training. Such powerful teaching is found in all fields; in scientific education the availability of data can enhance the personal magnetism of the teacher; if the data are weak, other persuasive talents are at work in student indoctrination into an ideology. Wallerstein (2006) has pointed out how much emphasis was placed on psychodynamic psychiatry at its peak in the post war years. The data also reveals a significant fall after that time (Lipsitt 2000).

A remarkable event in 1969 marked the nadir of the demedicalization of American psychiatry. Prior to that time, before entering a psychiatric residency, future psychiatrists were required to complete an "internship" year that involved a special commitment to working as a physician. It was practical learning, and for many of us it was a powerful personal experience that symbolized and reinforced the physician identity. The decision to terminate internship requirement was made in the context of other changes in medical training in general, but it sent a shock wave through most of psychiatry. John Romano, one of the most distinguished psychiatric educators of his time, noted that

> the psychiatrist, as physician, brings to the field his ancient heritage of the physician and broad experience in biology and clinical medicine, as well as in psychology and the social sciences. To reduce the dimensions of the role of psychiatrist as physician would seriously impair his contributions as practitioner, teacher, scholar, and investigator. It is a degradation of quality. (Romano 1970, p. 1575)

The impact of this decision was a catalyst for many psychiatrists who finally recognized that the demedicalization of psychiatry had gone too far. The reaction was powerful, and when its implications were widely recognized, the decision was reversed in 1973 with the establishment of an additional first year of psychiatric residency that primarily involved work in other medical departments. Psychiatric residency became a four-year program.

The explosive reaction to the termination of the internship requirement was connected by many psychiatrists to the nosological weakness of the field. The remedicalization of psychiatry received a powerful impetus in the development of the DSM-III (see Chapter 10, "Evidence-Based Diagnosis and Treatment"). The alienation of psychiatrists from other physicians had become disturbing. The power of those who wanted psychiatry to be brought back into medicine became dominant at the APA and in the field as a whole. The reversal of the internship decision was a powerful indicator that the tide had changed.

DSM-III, DSM-III-R (American Psychiatric Association 1987), and DSM-IV (American Psychiatric Association 1994) have had great success across the world, including producing a powerful impact on psychiatric educational programs. Practice Guidelines also became influential in a similar fashion. Although not intended, the combination of DSM and the guidelines became the de facto textbook for psychiatric residents.

Another shock wave was widely experienced when psychologists began to seek prescription privileges after they had become leading investigators and practitioners of psychotherapy (Lavoie and Barone 2006). The validity of the entire medical training system for the learning of pharmacotherapy was under attack. The increasing complexity for pharmacotherapy, however, and its prominence in psychiatric residency training by the 1990s strengthened key differences between psychiatrits and clinical psychologists. For a psychologist to learn how to prescribe adequately, the training would, in effect, require a medical education. The prescription debate sharpened the psychiatrists' motivation to emphasize the full medical educational foundations of the profession. The decision by psychoanalysts to include nonphysicians as fully qualified clinical candidates was also a powerful stimulus to clarify that psychiatric training was not the grammar school leading to a later higher stage of learning. By 2007 the number of psychiatric residents subsequently seeking psychoanalytic training had declined, while the number of other candidates, such as psychologists and social workers, had increased.

Psychoanalysis is not likely now to develop into a psychiatric subspecialty in the United States as it is in the United Kingdom, but five other areas have been approved as subspecialties. Child psychiatry was approved in the mid–twentieth century; geriatric psychiatry, addiction psychiatry, forensic psychiatry, and psychosomatic medicine (consultation-liaison psychiatry) have received formal accreditation as subspecialties in more recent times. To be approved by the accreditation agencies, each of these areas had to pass steep hurdles demonstrating their special core of knowledge and research, their fundamental ties to medicine, the public need for the new subspecialties, and the plans for specific education and board certification. The American Board of Medical Specialties has the authority to approve new subspecialties. The American Board of Psychiatry and Neurology (ABPN) develops the criteria for assessing candidates who seek certification in subspecialties.

Child psychiatry has changed rapidly since the postwar years. It has paralleled adult psychiatry in its being influenced heavily by psychoanalysis in the 1950s and 1960s. Child psychiatry has altered its course thoroughly, and its scientific accomplishments have been models for all of psychiatry. The *Journal of the American Academy of Child and Adolescent Psychiatry* has been first rate in its commitment to broad-based scientific models for many years and published articles that emphasize psychological and social data. While genetics, neurochemistry, immunology, psychopharmacology, and neural pathways for learning are a high priority, the psychological development of children and their vulnerabilities cannot be ignored, as I believe has tended to occur in some areas of adult psychiatry. Hypotheses about children's psychological development are clearly vital areas for the future of child psychiatry.

Adolescence has been a very special and occasionally controversial cohort of child psychiatry. Along with my colleague Daniel Offer, I have been interested in the field for many years (Offer and Sabshin 1974, 1984, 1991; Offer et al. 2004). In my judgment, the psychoanalysts' formulation about the teenage period poses several theoretical as well as practical concerns. In effect, they conceive of adolescence as a period of universal psychopathology. Of course, it is true that adolescence can be a tumultuous period with many substantial problems to solve. The presentations of these difficulties by analysts in the postwar years were hard to distinguish from a concept of the "universality of psychopathology" (Erikson 1968). Studies of "normal" populations were rare; interest in adolescents who were quite resilient and coped especially well during those years and subsequently were also infrequent. A more balanced view of adolescence is beginning; this approach still seeks to assist the teenagers who experience problems, but it also emphasizes that adolescent resilience, sexual adaptation, enduring healthy friendships, educational progress, and preparation for adulthood should also be a central theoretical and clinical part of the field.

The biopsychosocial model is central in working with adolescents. The "clinical neuroscientist" who genuinely dismisses or underemphasizes psychological and social variables will have special problems with adolescent psychiatry. Obviously, however, biological variables are highly relevant for recognizing adolescent problems. One cannot understand teenagers without paying attention to the biological stresses, but neither can the psychological and social causes be ignored. The biopsychosocial changes may indeed be stressful for many adolescents and may contribute to unhealthy adaptations, but frequently they may be handled quite effectively in the course of healthy maturation.

The future relationships of all components of child and adolescent psychiatry to pediatrics will vary to some extent depending on what models of psychiatry are chosen during the next quarter century. I believe the biopsychosocial model will continue to recruit more trainees into child psychiatry than the clinical neuroscientists who have not so far shown any great interest in the field. As of this writing, there is a shortage of child psychiatrists (Thomas and Holzer 2006), but the subspecialty is becoming more popular.

Geriatric psychiatry, like child psychiatry, is growing rapidly. The lengthening of the average life span in the United States is a reflection of improved medical care and of better welfare facilities; the problems of

American medicine are enormous, but the progress deserves acknowledgment. Both geriatric psychiatrists and geriatricians are currently in great demand. Increased training for general psychiatrists to work with older populations is needed, but subspecialists dealing with the full biological and psychological effects of aging are now needed more than ever before. Psychodynamic psychiatry made a few inroads into geriatrics, but the effect was limited. The major impact of analysts had been upon earlier stages of life. The aging population was less interesting to psychoanalysts for a long time. The *Journal of Geriatric Psychiatry*, in my judgment, has revealed a very balanced perspective. Education in geriatric psychiatry has needed less restructuring than other aspects of the field. Future changes will involve quantitative accretions of knowledge at all levels including the transaction of the variables for an ever extending time.

The subspecialty of addiction psychiatry is a reflection of the marked increase of addictive behavior in America during the latter part of the twentieth century and up to the present. It relates closely to addiction medicine, and the two have overlapping involvement in diagnosis and treatment. Today abuse of drugs is seen frequently in all parts of medical and surgical practice. The prevalence of drug abuse among young people is a major national tragedy. Today's psychiatrist must be mindful of diagnosing the disorders and the toxicity induced by drug abuse. He or she must also note its impact on the signs and symptoms of other psychiatric disorders. Addicted individuals constitute a significant part of a population seen in today's emergency rooms of general hospitals by psychiatric residents. Education in this subject is much more intense today than it was during my residency training. The excellent evidence-based work of the National Institute on Drug Abuse (NIDA) has contributed greatly to our ability to cope with this major problem.

The genetic factors involved in vulnerability to substance abuse are very important, but the recognition that psychosocial factors, such as restlessness and ennui in youths and deployment of military personnel far from home, transact with the biological predilection that undoubtedly exists is also important. This relationship must be understood by the general psychiatrist as well as the addiction specialist. It is very difficult to work with patients with addictions, and psychiatry has needed a group dedicated enough and wise enough to deal with the problems. Once again, I believe that when the genetic factors predisposing people to addiction are further clarified, there will still be a need to integrate the education and the practice in biopsychosocial terms. The higher prevalence of substance abuse in certain groups cannot be explained by genetics alone.

Forensic psychiatry is a relatively new formal subspecialty, but it has had a long history in American psychiatry. Chapter 9 ("Forensic Psychiatry") is devoted to this subject and includes those aspects of forensic psychiatry that accompanied the very formation of the APA in 1844. A plethora of legal constraints affects current practice. Education in this subject is now important for all psychiatrists (Simon and Gold 2004). Also required are subspecialists who have been prepared to deal with the full range of subtle legal interpretations, precedents, and opinions concerning mental competency, disability, patient rights, and insanity.

Education in forensic psychiatry is a profound reminder that psychiatric practice can flourish only in a democratic society. Without the full protection and regulation by a democratic justice system, psychiatry and psychiatric patients would be constantly abused.

Subspecialty work in consultation-liaison psychiatry has replaced the older psychosomatic medicine of the 1950s and 1960s. My own education in psychosomatic medicine was influenced by two conflicting streams. The specificity theories (Alexander [Alexander and Visotsky 1955] and French [1941]) of the unconscious conflicts causing hypertension, peptic ulcers, asthma, and other illnesses were strongly endorsed by the Chicago Institute for Psychoanalysis and cited positively in several psychiatric textbooks. These formulations, however, were based primarily on limited populations, usually derived from patients already in psychoanalysis; few long-term empirical studies with sufficient samples were available. Psychiatrists employing these formulations when seeing patients in consultation would render a psychodynamic formulation rather than a diagnosis. Often the consultation did not lead to practical suggestions for management. To suggest that the patient might need to be psychoanalyzed was not always received positively. The older specificity theories of psychoanalysis are a glaring illustration of the weaknesses of its research formulations and methodology. They are rarely cited today.

My other introduction to psychosomatic work, as described in Chapter 3 ("Implicit Preparations for a Leadership Role in Psychiatry"), was at the Psychosomatic and Psychiatric Institute (PPI) in Chicago under the direction of Roy Grinker (Grinker and Robbins 1959). His research studied the impact of multiple emotional states, such as anxiety, depression, and anger, that were rated quantitatively in volunteers and then correlated with a large number of biochemical and physiological measures. This research was not, and is not yet, clearly relevant for current clinical practice, but it was a good opportunity for me to note the differences between a scientific and an ideological stance. Grinker employed a biopsychosocial model well before this was a widely accepted practice.

Today's consultation-liaison psychiatry is much superior to the earlier version. The psychiatrists working in these fields understand a great deal about the experiences of those whom they serve as consultants. They have accumulated a great deal of experience in learning about the psychiatric disorders that often accompany particular medical conditions. Even if the psychiatric disorder is subclinical the symptom can be appraised and helped by both cognitive therapies and medication. This subspecialty of psychiatry is an excellent symbol of the remedicalization of the field. It also requires special experience in understanding how psychosocial variables interact with the biological factors in the illness. This special psychosocial knowledge differentiates the liaison consultant from those she or he is attempting to advise.

Liaison psychiatry epitomizes the best of modern practice. It was weak when it relied on psychoanalysis to understand people with overlapping medical and psychiatric disorders. It would weaken again if psychiatry were to merge with neurology into a narrowly defined clinical neuroscience. Psychosocial knowledge and the current nosology, coupled with experience in clinical medicine, enable consultants to be helpful and evidence-based in their recommendations to medical colleagues.

Psychiatric education does indeed have a life after residency training. Mandatory continued education is now in force (Scully et al. 2000), and failure to comply may now result in the loss of one's medical licence. This language is harsh, but the goal is laudable. Fifty years ago, continuing education was not conceived to be very important for psychiatrists. At that time, one's education was expected to remain relevant indefinitely. Scientific information changes constantly; ideology has a permanent quality. The same implications for maintaining life-time competence applies to the development of a recertification system for psychiatric practitioners. During the 1970s fewer psychiatrists were board certified compared with other medical specialists (Greenblatt et al. 1977; Levit and Holden 1978). If psychiatry was merely a preparatory experience on the way to later psychoanalytic work, the "real" certification was conducted by the Psychoanalytic Institute, not by the ABPN. After the 1970s the number of board-certified psychiatrists increased markedly. Recertification is now required. A changing field must enforce continuing education; practice in a democracy requires legislation that protects patients. Certification, recertification, and continuing education are testaments to a changing American psychiatry. The ABPN plays a much more central role in psychiatry than ever before and the assessment of candidates' learning is much more precise.

Psychiatric education has had a profound effect on American psychiatry; it has also been radically changed by theoretical and scientific constructs. New economic conditions and new science have produced a complex lifelong educational system in psychiatry. A new confidence in basic research and in the achievement of reimbursement parity should help to broaden the capability of psychiatry to educate and to recruit even more successfully.

REFERENCES

Alexander F, Visotsky H: Psychosomatic study of a case of asthma. Psychosom Med 17:470–472, 1955

American Psychiatric Association: Psychiatry and Medical Education; Report (Conference on Psychiatric Education, Cornell University, 1951), Washington, DC, American Psychiatric Association, 1952

American Psychiatric Association: Diagnostic and Statistical Manual of Mental Disorders, 3rd Edition. Washington, DC, American Psychiatric Association, 1980

American Psychiatric Association: Diagnostic and Statistical Manual of Mental Disorders, 3rd Edition, Revised. Washington, DC, American Psychiatric Association, 1987

American Psychiatric Association: Diagnostic and Statistical Manual of Mental Disorders, 4th Edition. Washington, DC, American Psychiatric Association, 1994

Andreasen NC: Linking mind and brain in the study of mental illnesses: a project for a scientific psychopathology. Science 275:1586–1590, 1997

Beutel ME, Stern E, Silbersweig DA: The emerging dialogue between psychoanalysis and neuroscience: neuroimaging perspectives. J Am Psychoanal Assoc 51:773–801, 2003

Bureau of Labor Statistics, Office of Occupational Statistics and Employment Projections: Occupational Outlook Handbook, 2006–07 Edition: Physicians and Surgeons. Washington, DC, U.S. Department of Labor, 2007. Available at: http://www.bls.gov/oco/ocos074.htm. Accessed August 28, 2007.

Cherpitel CJ: Trends in alcohol- and drug-related ER and primary care visits, 1995–2000: are Healthy People 2000 objectives met? Am J Addict 14:281–290, 2005

Clardy JA, Thrush CR: The junior-year psychiatric clerkship and medical students' interest in psychiatry. Acad Psychiatry 24:35–40, 2000

Cowan WM, Kandel ER. Prospects for neurology and psychiatry. JAMA 285:594–600, 2001

Dorsey ER, Jarjoura D, Rutecki GW: Influence of controllable lifestyle on recent trends in specialty choice by US medical students. JAMA 200:1173–1178, 2003

Earley LW, et al.: Teaching Psychiatry in Medical School: The Working Papers (Conference on Psychiatry and Medical under the auspices of the American Psychiatric Association and the Association of American Medical Colleges Education, Atlanta, 1967). Washington, DC, American Psychiatric Association, 1969

Engel GL: The need for a new medical model: a challenge for biomedicine. Science 196:129–136, 1977

Engel GL: The clinical application of the biopsychosocial model. Am J Psychiatry 137:535–544, 1980

Engel GL: Sounding board: The biopsychosocial model and medical education. Who are to be the teachers? New Engl J Med 306:802–805, 1982

Erikson EH: Identity, Youth, and Crisis. New York, WW Norton, 1968

Feifel D, Yu Moutier C, Swerdlow NR: Attitudes toward psychiatry as a prospective career among students entering medical school. Am J Psychiatry 156:1397–1402, 1999

French T: Physiology of behavior and choice of neurosis. Psychoanal Q 10:561–1941

Greenblatt M, Carew J, Pierce CM: Success rates in psychiatry and neurology certification examinations. Am J Psychiatry 134:1259–1261, 1977

Grinker RR (ed): Towards a Unified Theory of Hunan Behavior: An Introduction to General Systems, 2nd Edition. New York, Basic Books, 1967

Grinker RR, Robbins FP: Psychosomatic Case Book. New York, Blakiston, 1954

Hales DJ, Rapaport MH: From the Editors: an introduction to FOCUS. Focus 1:5–6, 2003

Hammersley DW (ed): Training the Psychiatrist to Meet Changing Needs: Report of the Conference on Graduate Psychiatric Education, Washington, DC, December 2–6, 1962, with the co-sponsorship of the Canadian Psychiatric Association). Washington, DC, American Psychiatric Association, 1963

Horwath E, Johnson J, Klerman GL, et al: What are the public health implications of subclinical depressive symptoms? Psychiatr Q 65:323–337, 1994

Insel TR: Commentary: "A new intellectual framework for psychiatry," in Kandel ER: Psychiatry, Psychoanalysis, and the New Biology of Mind. Washington, DC, American Psychiatric Publishing, 2005, pp 27–31

Kandel ER: A new intellectual framework for psychiatry. Am J Psychiatry 155:457–469, 1998

Kay J: The essentials of psychodynamic psychotherapy. Focus 4:167–172, 2006

Landon BE, Reschovsky J, Blumenthal D: Changes in career satisfaction among primary care and specialist physicians, 1997–2001. JAMA 289:442–449, 2003

Lavoie KL, Barone S: Prescription privileges for psychologists: a comprehensive review and critical analysis of current issues and controversies. CNS Drugs 20:51–66, 2006

Levit EJ, Holden WD: Specialty board certification rates: a longitudinal tracking study of US medical school graduates. JAMA 239:407–412, 1978

Lidz T: Adolf Meyer and the development of American psychiatry. Am J Psychiatry 123(3):320–332, 1966

Lipsitt DR: Psyche and soma: struggles to close the gap, in American Psychiatry After World War II: 1944–1994. Edited by Menninger RW, Nemiah JC. Washington, DC, American Psychiatric Press, 2000, pp 152–186

Meyer A: Twenty-fourth anniversary of the Henry Phipps Psychiatric Clinic, in Collected Papers, Vol 2. Edited by Winters EE. Baltimore, MD, Johns Hopkins University Press, 1952

Offer D, Sabshin M: Normality: Theoretical and Clinical Concepts of Mental Health, Revised Edition. New York, Basic Books, 1974

Offer D, Sabshin M (eds): Normality and the Life Cycle: A Critical Integration. New York, Basic Books, 1984

Offer D, Sabshin M (eds): The Diversity of Normal Behavior: Further Contributions to Normatology. New York, Basic Books, 1991

Offer D, Offer MK, Ostrov E: Regular Guys: 34 Years Beyond Adolescence. New York, Kluwer Academic/Plenum, 2004

Rao NR: Recent trends in psychiatry residency workforce with special reference to International Medical Graduates. Acad Psychiatry 27:269–276, 2003

Romano J: The elimination of the internship—an action of regression. Am J Psychiatry 126:1565–1576, 1970

Romano J: On the teaching of psychiatry to medical students: does it have to get worse before it gets better? Psychosom Med 42(1, suppl):103–311, 1980

Sanfey HA, Sallwachter-Shulman AR, Nyhof-Young JM, et al: Influences on medical student career choice. Arch Surg 141:1086–1094, 2006

Scully JH, Robinowitz CB, Shore JH: Psychiatric education after World War II, in American Psychiatry After World War II: 1944–1994. Edited by Menninger RW, Nemiah JC. Washington, DC, American Psychiatric Press, 2000, pp 124–151

Sierles FS, Taylor MA: Decline of US medical student career choice of psychiatry and what to do about it. Am J Psychiatry 152:1416–1426, 1995

Sierles FS, Yager J, Weissman SH: Recruitment of US medical graduates into psychiatry: reasons for optimism, sources of concern. Acad Psychiatry 27:252–259, 2003

Simon RI, Gold LH (eds): The American Psychiatric Publishing Textbook of Forensic Psychiatry. Washington, DC, American Psychiatric Publishing, 2004

Strauss A, Schatzman L, Bucher R, et al: Psychiatric Ideologies and Institutions. New York, Free Press, 1964

Sussex JN, et al: The Working Papers of the 1975 Conference on Education of Psychiatrists, as prepared by members of the Preparatory Commissions for the Conference (Lake of the Ozarks, Mo), Washington, DC, American Psychiatric Association, 1976

Thomas CR, Holzer CE 3rd: The continuing shortage of child and adolescent psychiatrists. J Am Acad Child Adolesc Psychiatry 45:1023–1031, 2006

Wallerstein RS: Psychoanalytic therapy research: its history, present status, and projected future, in Psychodynamic Diagnostic Manual (PDM). Silver Spring, MD, Alliance of Psychoanalytic Organizations, 2006

Weissman SH, Bashook PG: Forty year trends in selecting a psychiatric career. Psychiatr Q 62(2):81–93, 1991

Whitehorn JC, Mitchell J McK (eds): The Psychiatrist: His Training and Development. Report from the Conference on Psychiatric Education, Cornell University, 1952. Washington, DC, American Psychiatric Association, 1953

13

A Changing Membership

Both the typical and the symbolic American psychiatrist have changed radically since the formation of the APA in 1844. For the first 100 years the most typical psychiatrist was male, Protestant, and salaried and worked in a state hospital. He was deeply interested in clinical description and forensic questions. During the next quarter century after World War II, the most popular stereotype of the profession was the consultant analyst portrayed in the Hitchcock's 1945 film *Spellbound*. White bearded, avuncular, wise, and probably Jewish, he was somewhat admired early on, but his image became tarnished and even moderately threatening by the 1980s. Today the typical American Psychiatric Association member has no predominant image; she[1] may work in a clinic as a salaried employee, seeing many patients and adjusting their medication dosages; she may participate in a research project on the treatment of bipolar disorder; she may work in a private child psychiatric practice dealing with several patients with attention-deficit/hyperactivity disorder and their families. Younger versions of Barbra Streisand or Jane Fonda would probably get the film role today rather than the regal Ingrid Bergman of 60 years ago.

---

[1]I describe the psychiatrist as "she" and provide several examples to highlight the increased number of women entering psychiatry as well as to emphasize that there is no simple stereotype for the current generation of American psychiatrists, whether male or female. Our membership is quite diverse, but we are no longer an organization composed of competing ideologues.

The choice of psychiatry as a career is determined by many motives; I have discussed some of these in Chapter 12 ("Psychiatric Education"). The highest percentage of medical students entering psychiatry in the United States occurred during the period of psychoanalytic dominance of academic departments and training centers (see Table 1). Might the number have been even higher if that period had also included a substantial amount of high-quality biopsychosocial research? Would fewer students have selected psychiatric careers if the field had been neuroscientifically oriented? We do not know the answer to these questions nor can we be sure about what is most attractive or unattractive in today's recruiting efforts—an intriguing question and one that I think about very often. One of the physicians succeeding in keeping me well enough to finish this book is a distinguished academic nephrologist. He told me that he would choose a career in psychiatry today because of the current quality and challenges of neuroscientific research. I told him how proud I was of psychiatry being able to interest such an eminent medical leader, but I also expressed some of my concerns about losing the psychiatrist's psychological and social skills if the field were to become totally integrated with neurology. I am not sure that I convinced him.

In Chapter 12, I discussed the predominant patterns of entry into American psychiatry. Membership increased rapidly from 4,010 in 1946, just after World War II, to a peak of almost 41,000 members in 1997 (see Appendix 5). Since that time there has been some decline in total APA membership, although the most recent decade shows a slight increase.

Psychiatry is one of the medical specialties that has recruited a substantial number of foreign medical graduates to fill its allotted residency openings and also to work in some less attractive caretaker positions. While the total number of APA members has remained around 39,000, there has been both a significant loss of and a gain in psychiatrist membership since the late 1980s. Some members of the APA believed that the organization was not helping them enough in coping with managed care and resigned. Several were quite bitter as well as pessimistic about the future of the profession. The overwhelming majority of our members, however, understood that the fight for parity and equity by the APA was important for them, and they retained their membership during these challenging times. Some psychoanalysts resigned after DSM-III (American Psychiatric Association 1980) and DSM-IV (American Psychiatric Association 1994) were published. They found the new direction disturbing. Others left the APA when, in 1991, the American Psychoanalytic Association changed its policy about accepting nonphysician candidates for training. That so many psychoanalysts chose to remain in the APA was noteworthy. I have also been pleased to note that the development

TABLE 1. PERCENTAGE OF MEDICAL SCHOOL GRADUATES ENTERING A SPECIALTY, 1900–1993

	1900–1924 (%)	1925–1939 (%)	1940–1954 (%)	1955–1964 (%)	1990–1993 (%)
General practice	47.09	35.18	24.14	18.94	10.9[a]
Internal medicine	8.46	16.43	18.51	16.32	14.8
General surgery	8.41	11.03	11.89	9.23	7.6
Psychiatry	2.80	4.63	6.60	5.97	4.3

[a]Family practice.
Source. Reprinted from Scully JH, Robinowitz CB, Shore JH: "Psychiatric Education After World War II," in *American Psychiatry After World War II: 1944–1994.* Edited by Menninger RW, Nemiah JC. Washington, DC, American Psychiatric Press, 2000, pp. 124–151; p. 133. Used with permission.

of several psychiatric subspecialties has not caused a significant decline in APA membership. The professional identity of these subgroups still includes general psychiatry.

In this chapter I discuss some of the major constituencies that make up the APA's membership. Almost all of these members belong to an additional formal group that signifies their primary interest, but despite the heterogeneity of today's psychiatrists there is much less ideological divisiveness now than existed in the postwar years. How these groups evaluate APA policies will be very important for overall future membership trends.

We are on the verge of achieving a majority female membership of the APA. While the overall percentage of women members is still less that 50%, the majority of psychiatric residents are women. With the number of female medical students continuing to rise (Lambert and Holmboe 2005), there is every reason to assume that the female majority of the APA will continue to grow.

Some parts of the "glass ceiling" for women have been pierced, whereas others remain difficult to penetrate (Dickstein and Nadelson 1986). Carol Nadelson became the first woman president of the APA in 1986. Since that time there have been six other women elected as president. They have served with powerful administrative leadership, strong policy orientation, and academic prominence. Several have been extremely active in educational and editorial roles. They have been particularly good models for medical students considering a career in psychiatry. The APA Assembly has been somewhat slower in achieving leadership by women, having elected its first female speaker, Donna Norris, in 1998, followed, in 2002, by Nada Stotland. Other candidates are now on the pathway.

The glass ceiling is still powerful in the selection of academic chairs of psychiatry, with less than a handful of women ever having served in that role. Another example of barriers in women's psychiatric careers can be found in the relatively small number of senior women researchers in the field. Many exceptional leaders have contributed enormously but to develop a distinguished research career often requires a long apprenticeship with strong support and flexibility. If a woman chooses to have a family as well as to become a well published, internationally renowned researcher, she will require enormous strength to get past many hurdles.

While many women are quintessential practitioners of today's psychiatry, a large number of those now selecting a career in this field are still extraordinarily gifted in psychological mindedness. This is a personal opinion, based, no doubt, upon my experience of women teachers and supervisors, many colleagues, my wife Edith, and my two granddaughters, who have become psychiatrists. Today young psychiatrists face the fact that economic pressures limit the amount of time that can be spent on psychotherapeutic work. I do hope, however, that the future majority of women psychiatrists will play an important role in supporting a psychological renaissance in the field. APA Past-Presidents Michelle Riba and Marcia Goin's advocacy of combined psychotherapy and pharmacotherapy are good examples of this kind of leadership. Presenting evidence that psychotherapy is a significant part of the therapeutic combination can facilitate its scientific and economic resurgence.

While visiting outside the United States, I have noted in some countries that women psychiatrists constitute an overwhelming majority of the working caretakers in the large mental hospitals; the men hold the administrative leadership positions and the chief academic posts. This was most apparent in the old Soviet Union and will require strong attention to avert this type of discrimination in the United States. Psychiatric leadership by women in the APA and elsewhere will be important in producing a balanced scientific profession

In Chapter 11 ("Psychiatric Research"), I expressed concern about current research-oriented chairpersons of academic departments of psychiatry becoming somewhat less interested in assuming organizational leadership in the APA itself. Other opportunities have become more attractive especially in neuroscientific areas. As more women researchers become psychiatric leaders and departmental chairs, from my perspective it would be particularly important to ensure their substantial participation in the major psychiatric policy decisions of the next decade. I hope that they will tend to encourage a psychiatry that includes a serious research oriented involvement in the psychological and social variables. Such support would be decisive.

The story of American psychiatrists whose medical school training and/or postgraduate experience took place in another country is a very important part of understanding psychiatry in the United States. Not surprisingly, some of the best practitioners, teachers, and researchers come from abroad. What they succeeded in accomplishing has been vital for America, but we must face the fact that our gain may be a loss for their home countries. Any discussion of this policy brings to mind the current great debate in the United States about overall immigration practices. Our International Medical Graduates (IMGs) are indeed here legally, but the economic incentives that bring them here require careful consideration and most likely some changes of policy. I do not possess any simple solution, but I believe that the problems relate fundamentally to the basic economics of health practice in the United States. We do not produce enough motivated, home-grown psychiatrists to deal with the poorest, underserved psychiatric populations. Reconfiguration of our health care system must include modification of our training programs and career patterns. Negotiations should take place with countries that educate large numbers of physicians but do not have enough work for all of them. We benefit at all levels from international psychiatrists, but our dependence on them and our exploitation deserve serious attention.

Those IMGs already in the United States should continue to be our colleagues, our teachers, and our students. We cannot and should not attempt to discourage immigration by practicing less favorable treatment of our international colleagues. But while treating them fairly is vital for our basic professional principles, we need policies that regulate their entry built in tandem with our reform of United States health care. The recent decline of psychotherapy in the United States facilitates the recruitment of some IMGs whose weakness in English language and their cultural experience may hinder their development of psychotherapeutic skills. Paradoxically, psychoanalytic psychotherapy came to the United States from Europe and was taught to us by people who somehow learned English, even if heavily accented. While exceptions are quite visible, many of today's foreign-born physicians do not seem to possess the language skill or the strong motivation to practice psychotherapy. Complex "medication adjustments" can be learned by the bright foreign trained psychiatrist and that capacity may be become an attraction to bring more of them to this country.

The APA has welcomed IMGs and "international" members with special programs. Able APA leaders with foreign training have served as chairs of committees and as APA elected officers. Several foreign-born presidents and speakers of the APA—Jack Weinberg, George Tarjan, Pedro Ruiz, Prakash Desai—have been particularly close personal colleagues of mine and have been extremely active in innovative leadership roles in the organization and the profession. I recognize that I am attempting a delicate balance in being so pleased with our international colleagues but also seeking to limit their exploitation.

It is important to note that some of the foreign-trained U.S. psychiatrists are U.S. citizens who went abroad for their medical school experience, being unable to find a place at home, and came back to the United States for residency work. There are also many foreign-born psychiatrists whose medical training took place entirely in the United States. Every variety of foreign experience is well represented in American psychiatry. With the leadership of Ellen Mercer, as described in Chapter 7 ("International Affairs"), a category of international membership was established. Our Office of International Affairs paid special attention to the welfare of these members, and this support needs to be reestablished.

Throughout my life I have had the good fortune to learn a great deal from people who were born or educated abroad. The diversity of their psychological and cultural experience has always intrigued me. My foreign-born mother and father, cross-cultural expertise in my training, close contact with internationalists like Norman Sartorius and J. Jose Lopez-Ibor, the support for my work from internationalists of all backgrounds—all have been very important for my career. I have attempted to support international cooperation throughout my working life, and I have regretted the economic, social, and political pressures that exploit rather than encourage such a relationship.

I have also been a consistent advocate of APA efforts to recruit psychiatrists from diverse minority groups. This has been true since early in my career, when I learned a great deal about psychiatric racism in the context of providing services in African American communities (Kellam et al. 1975). At one point at the University of Illinois, we were fortunate to have in our program several African American psychiatric residents who were particularly active in pointing out how racism remained an important issue even when some of us thought that the problems had been solved. Part of my interest in this subject included the belief that minority psychiatrists might be more inclined to use their special cultural knowledge as a buffer against biological reductionism. The excellent contribution on cross-cultural psychiatry by Ezra Griffiths and colleagues includes many good examples of intellectual leadership principles in this area that I hope will become even more widely incorporated into our nosological and therapeutic guidelines (Griffiths et al. 1999).

I have been fortunate to have been close to African American colleagues throughout my career. Charles Pinderhughes, Charles Wilkinson, Hiawatha Harris, Chester Pierce, and Robert Phillips were special friends, as was Jeanne Spurlock, who worked with me at the University of Illinois as well as at the APA. Dr. Spurlock was a widely respected and powerful spokesperson for minority psychiatrists who spearheaded our child psychiatry activities. She organized fellowships for minority trainees, arranged conferences on special problems for minorities, and fought against discrimination in services for patients wherever it was found (Spurlock 1999). I worked with her to establish an Office of Minority Affairs at the APA and was particularly pleased to note how she paid special attention to psychiatrists from all minority groups. African American leadership was present in our Board and Assembly, but the APA has not yet elected a African American president. As I write this, I am aware of past African American leaders who might well have been considered for presidency and should have been nominated many years ago. Recently, I have been told that several African American leaders, including Donna Norris, are well on their way to be considered as presidential candidates. I am also hopeful that their candidacy will include support for special psychosocial interests.

Efforts to recruit African American physicians into many medical specialties is more apparent today than ever before, and the competition to attract them to our field is now substantial. At times, during "blue" periods I find myself needing to be reassured that our field is worthy to recruit minorities to our profession. I do not want us to recruit minorities to a field still rampant with discrimination. Our new scientific status and our new image have raised our standing and reduced my anxiety.

Spanish-speaking psychiatrists have become much more active in the APA leadership during the past two decades. The high concentration of Spanish-speaking populations in Florida, California, and Texas has played an important role in calling attention to the special health needs of this group. Hispanic and Latino psychiatrists in these regions, as well as in many other population centers, also serve as a special bridge to psychiatry in Mexico, Latin America, the Caribbean, and all of South America. The different Spanish-speaking groups experience culturally specific problems and possess unique talents in many areas. Ties to Spain have also been established, especially during the brilliant leadership of Jose Lopez-Ibor when he was president of the World Psychiatric Association. He has been one of the most visible figures in global psychiatry in America.

The two Hispanic psychiatrists who have been elected as presidents of the APA, Rodrigo Muñoz (1998–99) and Pedro Ruiz (2006–7), have been distinguished leaders for many years; their differences in professional work also demonstrate that stereotyping of Spanish-speaking leadership or membership is incorrect. While both Muñoz and Ruiz have been interested in improving the care of Hispanic patients, their own research has involved separate areas of the field (Muñoz 2006; Muñoz and Amado 1986; Ruiz 1998; see also Mezzich et al. 1999).

The impact of race and cultural variables on all therapies is an important area that deserves increased scientific attention. The proposition that pharmacotherapy might have more predictable effects across diverse cultural groups than psychotherapy requires careful investigation; both types of treatment can be affected by cultural, familial, and economic circumstances.

New minority groups of psychiatrists and patients are becoming more visible in the United States. With the influx of Vietnamese into the country during the last three decades, they have begun to receive specific attention, so that a new generation of Asian and East Asian American psychiatrists has become increasingly prominent. Psychiatrists of

Chinese, Japanese, Central Asian, Indian, Pakistani, and Bangladeshi descent have become increasingly active in the APA. Psychiatrists of Middle Eastern descent have organized to deal with culturally significant clinical questions. Given that special attention is being paid to that part of the world today, social psychiatric studies of that population may be particularly important. Psychiatry needs to pay special attention to the recruitment from diverse minority groups for multiple reasons, including the need to understand subcultural variations in behavior during a time of biological hegemony in American psychiatry.

Questions about homosexuality have had a profound impact on the APA and its membership for many years. Before World War II most Americans agreed with popular prejudices that homosexuals were sexual deviants. After the War, the dominance of psychoanalysis inculcated a new pathological theory that homosexuals were fixated at an early stage of psychosexual development and thus suffered from a pathological condition. The formulation was prevalent throughout the world of psychoanalysis, and homosexuality was accepted as a disorder in the APA's early diagnostic publications such as DSM–II (American Psychiatric Association 1968). Ronald Bayer has provided a detailed and accurate picture of the APA's policies on homosexuality (Bayer 1987). Larry Hartmann, the only acknowledged gay APA President, gave the John Fryer Award Lecture, entitled "Homosexuality and Ignorance," at the APA 2007 Annual Meeting. For most of the postwar period, homosexual groups, including members of the APA, were highly critical of the organization's stance on homosexuality. The protests increased in scope and intensity, and by the opening session of the APA's Annual Meeting in San Francisco in 1973, the discontent had become highly visible. There was a demonstration at the session by hundreds of gay activists, who demanded a change in policy.

Around the world, psychiatrists and psychoanalysts were perceived by homosexuals as obdurate villains and theoretical leaders of the antigay movement. In addition to demonstrations, the gay groups tried to reason with members at various APA meetings; one incident including a masked figure providing testimony at an APA committee deliberation. The act was theatrical but made its point vividly. (Later, the masked man was revealed to be Dr. John Fryer, whose work for the abolition of discrimination against homosexuals has now been recognized by the institution of an annual award lecture delivered at the Annual Meeting.) Finally all these efforts led to a reconsideration of the evidence that brought about a dramatic change in much of the world's attitudes about homosexuality. A large part of the credit for the changing policy should go to progressive leadership by several APA presidents, such as Judd Marmor and Larry Hartmann, who has made many presentations and is a leading authority on the subject (Drescher 2006; Hartmann et al. 1996). Marmor was one of the country's leading psychoanalysts and, against bitter criticism from many of his colleagues, argued for a more flexible theoretical and practical approach, including the acceptance of alternative normal sexual pathways (Marmor 1972; Stoller et al. 1973). Members of the Task Force on DSM-III (see Chapter 10, "Evidence-Based Diagnosis and Treatment" and Appendix 12, "DSM Task Forces and Working Groups"), led by Robert Spitzer, were key players in the removal of homosexuality from the disorders manual. The Task Force on DSM-IV, chaired by Allen Frances, completed the elimination of homosexuality from the classification of disorders. These actions, like the considerations of DSM-III's model overall, were bitterly debated. Several psychoanalytic groups and many other APA members struggled vociferously at many levels against the changes (Socarides and Volkan 1981). Some politically conservative members quoted religious sources and continued to fight a long-term rearguard battle over homosexuality. The conflict rocked the APA and included lengthy arguments and ultimately a referendum. Homosexuality was removed as a disorder category, and this decision was supported by the majority of the membership. A final effort to reaffirm that homosexuality was a mental disorder was also defeated in 1974.

This decision was strongly supported by the homosexual membership of the APA, many of whom had had to hide their sexual orientation. International gay organizations had been bitter about the APA's previous stance and were delighted with the change. The homosexual membership of the APA is now an open group that encompasses gay, lesbian, bisexual, and transgender members; has an excellent newsletter; carries out broad professional activities; and, as the Association of Gay and Lesbian Psychiatrists, is proud to be accepted by and supportive of the APA.

The APA action was important for homosexual groups in many countries. It took several decades for most of the world to accept the American decision fully. Several European psychiatric and psychoanalytic groups at first attacked the APA decision, and in some of their textbooks, such as those in Finland, continued to describe homosexuality as a disorder until recently. Psychoanalysts ultimately, but in a few cases reluctantly, altered their developmental models that insisted on the pathogenetic definition of homosexuality. Many at last admitted openly gay analysts to membership of their association.

Not all of America has accepted the APA judgment, and homosexuality is still perceived as an unnatural sexual disorder by many conservative political spokespersons. It remains as a divisive issue for Republican presidential candidates in the 2008 race. Some religious leaders also continue to argue that homosexuality must be pathological, but the number of extreme critics seems to be declining. The U.S. Department of Defense is accepting more gays as members of the armed forces, but they still do not permit gay service people to be open about their sexual orientation. Of course, in some parts of the world, homosexuals are still the victims of discrimination.

The decision to remove homosexuality from DSM-III was recommended by Spitzer and his task force after careful evaluation of the scientific evidence. The task force did not accept the earlier psychoanalytic formulation of psychosexual fixation and its lifetime consequences. The DSM directly challenged psychoanalytic concepts about the formulations of psychosexual fixation and regression. It attempted to establish empirically based definitions of psychopathology and adopted a more traditional medical model of normality and illness. Illness ordinarily involves a minority of the population rather than being a widespread phenomenon, except during epidemics. Therefore, the implication of DSM's decision went beyond the issue of homosexuality itself; it struck at the base of much psychoanalytic pathogenesis that included a very wide theoretically based formulation of disorder without strong epidemiological or other empirical evidence. It was a time for clear action. The decision was of course vital for therapists who are homosexual as well as for other gay people who did not perceive their behavior as mentally ill. The pattern of modifying psychoanalytic assumptions of the universality of psychopathology became an important part of the APA's modern stance. For many psychoanalysts the decision to exclude homosexuality, combined with a major overall nosological revision, was a bitter defeat (Socarides et al. 1981). As of 2007, however, alternative psychosexual pathways have become much more acceptable to psychoanalysts, and most of the battle about homosexuality is over. It is interesting to note that the American Psychoanalytic Association and colleagues do not use the term "homosexual" in their recent *Psychodynamic Diagnostic Manual* (Alliance of Psychoanalytic Organizations 2006). Homosexual therapists are now active members in both psychiatry and psychoanalysis.

Another major change in APA membership policy relates to the inclusion of psychiatric residents as full members of the APA. The decision to move in this direction was also somewhat controversial. Previously, many psychiatrists wanted to maintain membership of the organization as an honorific category that reflected completion of training. In the Royal College of Psychiatrists of the United Kingdom and in other national psychiatric associations, candidates, after completing training successfully, have to pass an examination before being permitted to join the national society as full members.

The APA continues to have several membership categories and, as it should, maintains ceremonies to honor its older members. Nevertheless, the organization, somewhat belatedly in my judgment, recognizes that young psychiatrists have an important part to play in the decision making and reconfiguration of the field. Residents are not only full members; some of them are also elected to the Board and to the Assembly, where they contribute a great deal to new policy formulations.

Psychiatric residents are also an important presence at our national meetings, and special programs are planned by them and for them. The current active role of residents is a major sign of the profession's continuing change. An association that is fully committed to maintaining its traditional stances tends to treat its inductees as apprentices who need to learn the field as it has been practiced. While psychiatry requires a great deal of such learning, the young members must also help to shape the next stages of policy deliberations and growth. From my point of view, the decision about residents has been helpful in several ways. Residents have contributed many new ideas in policy discussions; in addition, they have been particularly helpful as teachers of medical students, providing an excellent portrait of modern psychiatry. Resident participation has invigorated the APA.

The APA's Office of Research has been a major advocate for the profession's scientific image and has assisted in shaping the consequences of that dramatic change, as discussed in Chapter 11 ("Psychiatric Research"). It encourages research careers, promotes the research knowledge of all psychiatrists, and is a vital part of the profession's transformation from ideology to science. For some researchers, however, the field has still not changed enough, as shown in Insel's commentary on Eric Kandel's paper "A New Intellectual Framework for Psychiatry," discussed in Chapter 11 (Insel 2005). The majority of researchers, however, feel more positively about the APA now, even though the association is not viewed by many of them as an organization at the frontier of neuroscience. The APA needs research members and leaders, and this topic needs careful attention in the policy decisions of the next few decades. The scientific image of psychiatry is vital for continued public acceptance of the profession, and a vigorous role assumed by research members facilitates that image. Psychiatric researchers should not lose sight of how the profession has placed research in a much more important role.

From my perspective, the APA is the organization most likely to support a resurgence of a research emphasis in psychological and social aspects of psychiatry. We need more members who have a major interest and capacity in this particular area. How to accomplish this task without alienating neuroscientific researchers will take special understanding and leadership. Biopsychosocial investigations that study the interaction of multiple variables should help in increasing the popularity of this approach. The high quality of broad-based science in the preparation of the DSM-V and the new practice guidelines will help in supporting the APA's pivotal role in promoting a more inclusive attitude to research, as discussed in Chapter 11. The importance of this issue for the general membership of the APA requires reiteration and continued leadership. The scientific advances in the field have opened the pathway for parity and equity.

The current importance of subspecialty psychiatry has been discussed in several chapters and is also critical to the future membership of the APA, as discussed in Chapter 12 ("Psychiatric Education") and Chapter 9 ("Forensic Psychiatry"). In Chapter 9, I discussed how the subspecialty of forensic psychiatry emphasizes its need to keep up with changes in general psychiatry; each of the other subspecialties requires similar understanding of the current changing models of the field as a whole. I have been most impressed with the superb leadership of Medical Director Jay Scully in promoting close educational and research ties with all the psychiatric subspecialties. Assembly liaison activities have also been helpful in supporting the efforts of subspecialties to achieve equity in the new health care system.

Regional differences in membership continue to be visible especially in the deliberations of our Assembly of District Branches. While there have been few studies of political and social values of psychiatrists in different parts of the country, the South and the Mountain West seem more conservative in political and social orientation than the Northeast and Pacific Coast. Our three District Branches in Canada have been particularly active in teaching us about the advantages and disadvantages of an alternative health system.

In recent years, psychiatrists have tended to become more cautious about taking stances on general social issues. Such stances in the postwar years caused considerable confusion about the boundaries of psychiatrists' competence. The more conservative members have been particularly strong on separating professionally related questions from more generic social issues. Occasionally there is a flare up of disagreement about where the professional boundary lies in these discussions. I am not certain how regional membership perspectives will affect APA's decision on national health policies. It is a very important topic, but I have had too little contact with the Area Councils in the past decade to have a clear opinion about how regional membership differences will shape the discussion.

The APA membership as a whole has undergone massive changes and has been buffeted by enormous economic, political, social, and scientific upheavals during the last half century. The association is the primary organization that can pay close attention to the totality of current heterogeneous American psychiatry. It can also best understand the perspectives of the various subgroups of psychiatrists in the context of policies that fit the needs of the overall membership and their patients. Preparing the membership as a whole for determining the next major changes in American psychiatry on the pathway to equity will be the most important task for the APA during the next decades. Accomplishing this will require the best possible unification of a diverse membership.

REFERENCES

Alliance of Psychoanalytic Organizations: Psychodynamic Diagnostic Manual. Silver Spring, MD, Alliance of Psychoanalytic Organizations, 2006

American Psychiatric Association: Diagnostic and Statistical Manual of Mental Disorders, 2nd Edition. Washington, DC, American Psychiatric Association, 1968

American Psychiatric Association: Diagnostic and Statistical Manual of Mental Disorders, 3rd Edition. Washington, DC, American Psychiatric Association, 1980

American Psychiatric Association: Diagnostic and Statistical Manual of Mental Disorders, 4th Edition. Washington, DC, American Psychiatric Association, 1994

Bayer R: Homosexuality and American Psychiatry: The Politics of Diagnosis. Princeton, NJ, Princeton University Press, 1987

Dickstein LJ, Nadelson CC (eds): Women Physicians in Leadership Roles. Washington, DC, American Psychiatric Association, 1986

Drescher J: An interview with Lawrence Hartmann, MD. Journal of Gay and Lesbian Psychotherapy 10(1):123–137, 2006

Griffiths EEH, Gonzalez CA, Blue HC: The basics of cultural psychiatry, in The American Psychiatric Press Textbook of Psychiatry, 3rd Edition. Edited by Hales RE, Yudofsky SC, Talbott JA. Washington, DC, American Psychiatric Press, 1999, pp 1463–1492

Hartmann L, Hanson G: Latency development in prehomosexual boys, in Textbook of Homosexuality and Mental Health. Edited by Cabaj RP, Stein TS. Washington, DC, American Psychiatric Press, 1996, pp 253–266

Insel TR: Commentary: A new intellectual framework for psychiatry, in Kandel ER: Psychiatry, Psychoanalysis, and the New Biology of Mind. Washington, DC, American Psychiatric Publishing, 2005, pp 27–31

Kellam SG, Branch JD, Agrawal KC, et al: Mental Health and Going to School: The Woodlawn Program of Assessment, Early Intervention, and Evaluation. Chicago, IL, University of Chicago Press, 1975

Lambert EM, Holmboe ES: The relationship between specialty choice and gender of U.S. medical students, 1990–2003. Acad Med 80:797–802, 2005

Mezzich JE, Ruiz P, Muñoz RA: Mental health care for Hispanic Americans: a current perspective. Cultur Divers Ethnic Minor Psychol 5(2):91–102, 1999

Marmor J: Homosexuality—mental illness or moral dilemma? Int J Psychiatry 10(1):114–117, 1972

Muñoz RA: Life in Color: Culture in American Psychiatry. Chicago, IL, Hilton Publishing, 2006

Muñoz RA, Amado H: Anorexia nervosa: an affective disorder. New Dir Ment Health Serv 31:13–19, 1986

Ruiz P: The role of culture in psychiatric care. Am J Psychiatry 155:1763–1765, 1998

Scully JH, Robinowitz CB, Shore JH: Psychiatric education after World War II, in American Psychiatry After World War II: 1944–1994. Edited by Menninger RW, Nemiah JC. Washington, DC, American Psychiatric Press, 2000, pp 124–151

Socarides CW, Volkan VD: Challenging the diagnostic status of homosexuality. Am J Psychiatry 138:1256–1257, 1981

Spurlock J: Black Psychiatrists and American Psychiatry. Washington, DC, American Psychiatric Association, 1999

Stoller RJ, Marmor J, Bieber I, et al: A symposium: should homosexuality be in the APA nomenclature? Am J Psychiatry 130:1207–1216, 1973

14

Annual Meetings

The American Psychiatric Association convenes two large annual scientific meetings, and they are markedly different from each other. When examined carefully, their history and their contrasting content reveal a great deal about changes in the substance and direction of American psychiatry. One of the meetings is an extraordinarily massive convention, with up to 23,000 registrants, that attempts to encompass today's full range of American psychiatry; the other meeting concentrates on such matters as hospital psychiatry, social and community psychiatry, treatment of the most vulnerable patients, managed care, and regulatory issues affecting practice. There are many other national psychiatric and mental health meetings each year; it would be hard to find a week in the United States without one such meeting. The field has grown enormously, and each area of interest has adherents who gather annually. A large number of psychiatric groups meet in the same city as the APA just before its Annual Meetings. Several organizations that used to meet in conjunction with the APA now meet at a different time of the year in another city. The American Society of Biological Psychiatry, for example, now holds a very large, separate annual meeting that includes major presentations at the frontiers of biological research in psychiatry.

The American Psychoanalytic Association recently decided to hold both its yearly meetings at a different site from the APA's meeting. One of the American Psychoanalytic Association's meetings takes place each year at the Waldorf Hotel in New York in December, but its spring meeting has been held in tandem in the city in which the APA holds its convention. The American Psychoanalytic Association will begin to meet separately starting in Spring 2008. The decision for this change was explained by both groups as being based primarily on logistic grounds, but perhaps the more significant factor was that the two organizations had drifted apart sufficiently to weaken any effective protest. I regret that decision.

It would be useful to have a catalogue describing the full range of annual mental health meetings in the United States. This thick volume would illustrate the permeable boundaries and contours of an enormous field. Even a catalogue limited to psychiatric annual meetings would be large and would demonstrate a diverse range of interests.

In this chapter, in order to clarify recent changes in psychiatry most sharply, I have chosen to focus on the APA's two annual meetings. They both have a rich history, with several alterations in their titles over the years and varying functions and changes in their relationship with each other over time. For example, the current Institute on Psychiatric Services was the Institute of Hospital and Community Psychiatry until 1995.

The APA Annual Meeting began in 1844 as a small group of superintendents of mental hospitals who gathered to discuss the management of their facilities. The APA started an additional annual meeting in 1949 to focus on issues of psychiatric service delivery. Now called Institute on Psychiatric Services, these gatherings ensure the centrality of mental hospitals and community facilities to the APA as it faces many competing priorities such as new education and research.

The APA Annual Meeting has grown in spurts to become our "big tent." After World War II, the meeting grew rapidly in size. From the 1940s through the 1960s, the average attendance was about 5,000. During the 1980s, attendance grew to more than 17,000. The Institute on Psychiatric Services, by contrast, has been smaller in size but has carried out several vital functions. Its current title reflects the increased scope of the meeting, especially in the many services affected by the dominating role of managed care. In this sense, the Institute is no longer maintaining an old tradition but is now in the vanguard of rapid systemic changes in psychiatric services.

With an emphasis on mental health hospitals, pre-war Annual Meetings were relatively small in terms of attendance and size of venue and had less breadth and depth of topics. With only 5,000 attendees, procuring large convention halls was not essential. However, the postwar dominance of psychodynamic psychiatry and psychoanalysis dramatically changed the mood and content of the APA Annual Meetings. In addition to psychoanalysis and psychodynamic psychiatry, academic psychiatry rose in prominence because of the dominance of education in academic departments of psychiatry. Presentations on research topics were relatively few in number.

Neglected during World War II, American psychiatric hospitals, especially state-run facilities, were underfinanced and understaffed. Reform-oriented citizens and professionals raised questions about "grim warehouses" of patients that were depicted in books such as *The Shame of the States* by Albert Deutsch (1948). With a public shocked by the inhumane conditions of some institutions, advocates' pleas to overhaul mental health care gained momentum (Grob 1991). Presenting grim pictures of hospitalized mental patients, Deutsch described the plight of "hundreds of patients sleeping in damp, bug-ridden basements. Noisy and violent patients made life intolerable in barn-like day rooms because there weren't seclusion rooms where they might be isolated until they had calmed down."

The APA, responding to several simultaneous challenges and new opportunities, decided to organize new central headquarters in Washington, D.C., and appointed its first medical director, Daniel Blain, in 1948. Blain, the only medical director later to become the APA's president, had extensive relevant leadership experiences as chief of neuropsychiatry in the Veterans Administration. That role brought him in touch with critically important changes that were taking place in American psychiatry and prepared him to become a national leader of a newly energized and dynamic profession. He made a point of visiting almost every state in America and paid particular attention to their mental institutions, criticizing several of them but also reporting on some effective treatment models (Blain 1951). He led a reform movement on several fronts by strengthening the mental health services of the APA and organizing the Mental Hospital Institute. The first meeting, in 1949, involved a cathartic series of plenary sessions with a registration of almost 200. Most appropriately it was held at the Institute of the Pennsylvania Hospital in Philadelphia, the place where the APA had started in 1844.

The Annual Meeting in May has continued to include some sessions on mental hospitals, but the decision to hold a separate meeting on these and other psychiatric services was an effort to maintain strong interest in the topics that previously had dominated American psychiatry. For some the content of the Institute is the "real" matter of psychiatry. For example, the distinguished scholar of psychiatric history Gerald Grob focuses on psychiatry's public systems in his important contribution "Mental Health Policy in Late Twentieth-Century America" (Grob 2000). Recently, the APA has once again become much more involved in coping with these policy questions, and the APA's current strong alliance with the National Alliance on Mental Illness (NAMI) particularly reflects that trend ("NAMI Wants Stronger Partnership" 2006; see also Bender 2007). At the 2007 Annual Meeting, NAMI's president, Suzanne Vogel-Scibilia, accepted an award from APA President Pedro Ruiz.

Several APA presidents have also strongly focused their attention on overall mental health policy (Robinowitz 2007). President Sharfstein, in 2006, took as his theme "From Science to Public Policy: Advocacy for Patients and the Professions." He also wrote about such issues in his president's column in *Psychiatric News* (Sharfstein 2005b, 2006). A list of APA presidential themes for 1984 through 2008 is given in Appendix 3. Back in 1949 Daniel Blain wanted to ensure that such policy issues would not be neglected in the face of a new psychiatric agenda and a radically changing field. The APA Annual Meeting in the 1950s and 1960s attempted to straddle the new post-war interests with the old hospitalpsychiatry. Later, a surge of developments in biological psychiatry made this expanding subject the most prominent feature of the Annual Meetings.

I was appointed chairman of the APA's Program Committee in 1972 and continued in that role for two years. In addition to the basic task of selecting the Annual Meeting content, the role served as an excellent learning experience for me. After assuming the post of medical director of the APA in 1974, I became even more interested in new possibilities for the Annual Meeting and assumed leadership in its restructuring. Through the years, the changes have been so dramatic that the overall experience of attending the meeting is qualitatively different for the new generation of psychiatrists, for instance, the regular use of enormous new convention halls. Not all the changes have been positive. As with psychiatry as a whole, some of the effects, such as the complexity and coordination of programs, were not fully anticipated and have produced problems for some members. Other changes were planned, but the "success" of the plans brought about new problems. The sheer size of the Annual Meetings poses difficulties, especially for older members. I often heard the comment "Our Annual Meeting is too big for me. I like smaller meetings." The gigantic conference centers, with many simultaneous sessions, are sometimes difficult to navigate. The utilization of many hotels for additional parts of the program adds to the coping problems. Furthermore, if a registrant wishes to attend sessions at one of the other conventions held in conjunction with the APA, the management of scheduling is not simple. The APA tries very hard to be helpful with buses, signs, and easily available staff assistance. Above and beyond the physical magnitude of the coping, the tendency for some people to feel nostalgic about the simpler old times adds to the mood. I played a key role in adding to the complexity of the Annual Meeting, but I definitely have to deal with nostalgia as well as sore feet. I also envy the energy of younger colleagues walking past me quickly in the long corridors.

The enormous exhibits area at the modern convention center also serves as a colorful image of the entire Annual Meeting. A new "city" has been quickly constructed in the exhibit hall—one that is dominated by pharmaceutical companies. New psychiatric medications are featured, but old "favorites" continue to get some attention. Audiovisual presentations are provided, and helpful employees are eager to assist attendees in employing their products. The exhibits area also features many institutional and hospital programs. It has a special publishers' section. When American Psychiatric Press (APPI) began to occupy the best and largest space in the exhibits area, there were concerns that other publishers might be offended. In actuality, it appears that APPI has helped to draw a larger crowd to the entire publications area. Important for the APA, the exhibit area provides booths for different APA offices to feature their efforts. There is also a large area where members who are considering or seeking new employment may be helped to get in contact with prospective employers. In the age of managed care, the Annual Meeting has become particularly important for learning about employment and practice opportunities.

The new complexity of the Annual Meeting has not changed the fact that the primary attraction for most members and guests is still the scientific program itself. This program, which is selected and organized by a committee months before the meeting, except where the recency of new data is very important, has become quite different from that of the earlier postwar years. The changes in American psychiatry in the late part of the twentieth century are clearly demonstrated by comparing the content, style of presentation, degree of popularity of the various topics, and demographics of the attendees. Neuroscientific psychiatry has dramatically emerged as the favorite subject of an overwhelming majority, and research topics are very popular, in contrast with the early postwar years. All-day courses on pharmacological treatments of major psychiatric disorders are heavily subscribed. The Annual Meeting has a vast continuing education function. Papers, symposia, and workshops on new pharmaceutical agents are popular. Lectures by some of the major contributors to the neurosciences, neurochemistry and psychopharmacological systems are often attended by audiences of several thousand people. Occasionally, a lecture at the Annual Meeting has had tremendous influence on the field. In 1894 S. Weir Mitchell's lecture on the significance of scientific psychiatry had a great impact (Mitchell 1894), as did the 1956 lecture by Percival Bailey when he raised questions about the dominance of psychoanalytic theory and practice at a time when psychoanalysis was powerful in American psychiatry (Bailey 1956). By an interesting coincidence, at the same Chicago meeting where Bailey spoke, Ernest Jones, the great biographer and follower of Freud, lectured on psychoanalysis on the occasion of the 100th anniversary of Freud's birth (Jones 1956).

Starting in 1983, a change was made in the program that has had a powerful effect on the Annual Meeting as a whole. Up to that time most contributors to the program had volunteered to be accepted by sending to the program committee an abstract of what they might present. There was an exception to this for "named" lecturers, that is, those invited to speak by the APA. A decision was made to permit "industry"-sponsored programs in which organizations like pharmaceutical companies could submit a proposed presentation by a panel of experts who could be paid by the company for participating. If the industry-sponsored program was accepted, the company also paid a fee to the APA. The first such industry symposia were presented at the 1983 Annual Meeting, which was held in New York, for which ten symposia were selected. By the turn of the century, more than fifty had been held at the Annual Meeting every year. The number has grown significantly in this first decade of the new century. Many are in the evening, and the company serves dinner for the attendees. Some are early-morning sessions and breakfast is provided.

These symposia are meticulously prepared with rehearsals before the meeting, and they have excellent audio-visual content. They employ modern educational principles with clear learning objectives and make pertinent written summaries available to the audience. The industry-sponsored programs are very popular with the registrants, but, of course, such sponsorship raises important questions about fairness and objectivity of the presentation. The Program Committee has carefully monitored the sessions to ensure balanced presentations. For the pharmaceutical companies, these rules still permit discussion of their products with a large audience. For work in the psychological and social aspects of psychiatry, there are very few, if any, "industries" or "companies" that would be motivated to provide such a symposium. Psychotherapy and social aspects of psychiatry receive attention at the industry symposia only when a comparison is made among various types of therapies or when combined treatment is employed. But undoubtedly the major attention is given to biological psychiatry per se—a focus that reflects and reinforces current American psychiatric practice. In later chapters, I express the hope of a revitalization of psychotherapy and social psychiatry in American psychiatry that might increase their visibility at the Annual Meeting and Institute.

Despite the decision of the American Psychoanalytic Association to meet separately, interest by the attendees in analytic topics continues, and indeed a new generation of psychodynamic leaders is now very popular at the APA meetings. When Glen Gabbard lectures, he draws a very large audience. His lectures are presented superbly and include discussion of the relationship between neuroscience and psychoanalysis, as, for example, when he gave the 2004 Adolf Meyer Award Lecture entitled "Mind, Brain, and Personality Disorders" (Gabbard 2005). Nevertheless such presentations are the exception; the content and the superb organization of the industrial symposia dominate the meeting.

There are also relatively few papers on social and community psychiatry at the Annual Meeting. This paucity is in part a result of the Institute on Psychiatric Services's becoming the primary place for such presentations. It also reflects some decline in attention currently given to "social psychiatry." In the postwar years, the broad definition of social psychiatry included social questions issues such as poverty, racial discrimination, and the Vietnam war. More recently the social issues included for discussion at the Annual Meeting are those that directly affect psychopathology and its treatment.

Poster materials are selected for prominent display each year. The hundreds of such posters accepted by the Program Committee cover varying topics, but the majority involve somatic research. "Academic" biological psychiatrists would now probably prefer to present their most exciting new findings at a neuroscience meeting. There is still good motivation to present at the APA Annual Meeting, but communicating the most important *new* findings is best done in more specialized settings.

During the last two decades there has been a surge in international registrants at the Annual Meeting. The number of registrants from outside the United States is nearly equal to the number of American registrants. The international registrants are often the majority of attendees at certain popular lectures. They enjoy the courses and the industry-sponsored symposia, and they frequently purchase books in the publishers' exhibition. Many factors have contributed to this surge. American psychiatry is now quite popular across the world; DSM-III (American Psychiatric Association 1980) and DSM-IV (American Psychiatric Association 1994) have had international success, and American psychopharmacological developments have had a major impact worldwide.

Pharmaceutical companies often pay for the travel of foreign psychiatrists to the APA Annual Meeting and Institute on Psychiatric Services. The rate of growth in the number of psychiatrists in some countries has significantly increased, and information about the APA now reaches a large segment of this group. The current reduced value of the dollar compared with other currencies makes travel cheaper, and popular tourist sites, such as New York and San Francisco, add to the attraction of the meeting for many foreign attendees. Equally important in stimulating the surge were the efforts of the APA's Office of International Affairs. Foreign attendees were given personal attention, with a large hotel area made available for their collective use, and APA staff available there, under the management of Ellen Mercer, to assist them. This genuine hospitality made the visitors feel most welcome, and many have told me how important it was for their attendance at the meeting. As I have indicated in Chapter 7 ("International Affairs"), the closing of that office after my departure from the APA was most disappointing to me, and I was concerned with the long-term effects of the weakened communication and hospitality. I am pleased that the current APA leadership is in process of restoring this office. Some of the APA membership wanted to focus our spending on the many economic problems affecting the profession, and they perceived international affairs as a luxury. I am a strong advocate of international activity, even during hard times. International attendance at Annual Meetings is cost effective in that it brings in delegate fees and increases the sale of publications. Perhaps more important, it is a useful source of scientific information; an internationally sensitive American psychiatry has many positive ramifications enhancing cooperation at multiple levels. Insensitivity to international attendees at our Annual Meetings is not wise.

Large numbers of psychiatric residents now attend the Annual Meeting. Efforts to make it more attractive to these trainees have included development of special targeted learning sessions and social events. The fact that residents have become elected voting members of APA governing bodies and are much better organized than before in communicating with one another heightens the popularity of the Annual Meeting. In addition, more medical students attend; contacts are made with medical schools with representatives at the meeting to enable their students to attend without fee. The trainees who attend seem to adapt much more efficiently to the complexity and the magnitude of the program. Study of the sessions popular with the residents and medical students indicates future as well as current trends in the profession.

The sheer size and complexity of the Annual Meeting has limited the number of American and Canadian cities where it can be held. Only Atlanta, Atlantic City, Boston, Chicago, Dallas, Detroit, Los Angeles, Miami, New Orleans, New York, Philadelphia, San Diego, San Francisco, Toronto, and Washington, D.C. now have adequate venues with a spacious conference center and nearby large hotels. Many cities that previously hosted the Annual Meeting quite successfully cannot do so any more. That is unfortunate, because holding the Annual Meeting in a city helps to improve the local public image of psychiatry.

For me, nostalgia about conventions held many years ago is still very strong. The first APA Meeting I attended was in 1953 in Cincinnati. I had a marvellous time and thoroughly enjoyed the town, including the hospitality of the faculty and students at the University of Cincinnati. Today Cincinnati is a big city but is not quite large enough in its facilities for a "mega" convention.

The Canadian Psychiatric Association has made a point of meeting in many of its provinces, but logistics and economic factors will at some point affect the choice of meeting sites as they do in the United States. I have been a devotee of the Canadian Psychiatric Association's Annual Meeting. During my tenure at the APA I did not miss a single one.

The largest number of registrants consistently appear at APA meetings in New York and San Francisco. This has made it advisable for the organization to plan more of its meetings in those two cities. Decisions about meeting sites must be made several years in advance, and the APA meetings are coveted by officials in America's largest cities, even though facilities in some of these cities are currently booked for many years in advance.

Surprisingly, the selection of one Annual Meeting site became one of the most controversial issues during my time as medical director. In the late 1970s we had selected New Orleans as the site for our 1981 meeting. During the intervening years, states across the United States were considering an amendment to the U.S. Constitution on full support of equal rights for women. The State of Louisiana failed to ratify the amendment, and by 1980 many of our members had begun to support a proposal that we should not be meeting in states opposed to equal rights for women. The argument was intense and involved two referenda of our members and much Board and Assembly debate. One of our past presidents stated that the cancellation of our Annual Meeting was vital to our integrity, even if it meant that the APA might be sued and brought close to bankruptcy. The likelihood of successful suits against the APA if we cancelled our New Orleans contract was pointed out to us by our attorneys. Therefore, as much as I supported women's rights, I felt that my first duty was to ensure the continuation of the APA. I was active in the dispute and alienated several APA leaders by my support of a referendum to go ahead with the New Orleans meeting. A majority of the membership voted to sustain the decision, and we did not cancel the meeting. A number of APA leaders have still not forgiven me. Had the membership voted differently, I doubt that I would now be writing this book.

Many allied psychiatric and mental health groups continue to meet in association with the APA. They are featured in the APA program, and their liaison with our membership can be facilitated by joint sessions.

For example, the American Association of Chairs of Departments of Psychiatry has consistently held one of their meetings during the APA Annual Meeting. As discussed elsewhere, the new generation of chairs is composed of people with career backgrounds different from those of the post–World War II chairs. Today, in marked contrast to 1970, few psychoanalysts are department chairs. Many are biological research–oriented psychiatrists, and relatively few of them, as compared with their predecessors, now seek leadership positions in the APA. Nevertheless there are good relationships between the chairs and the APA. Dr. Scully, the present APA medical director, was a chair before he came to the APA, and he has facilitated very close ties between the APA and academic leadership. His high standing among academic psychiatrists is important for the APA.

The Annual Meeting affords the APA an opportunity to publicize psychiatry's scientific status, and its actions on policy issues. Today, more reporters attend the Annual Meeting than ever before, and the APA staff host them in a professional manner. Occasionally national and international coverage develops from scientific sessions or even business meetings; for example, APA's statement that homosexuality was not a psychiatric illness drew wide attention in the national and international press. Most often the coverage is by local newspapers, television, or radio. Understandably, the reporters' conception of what is interesting is not always that of the membership. Sometimes a presentation with a catchy title on an unusual subject becomes the story, despite the APA leadership's wish for press coverage on, for example, excellent treatment results employing conjoint psychotherapy and medication. Despite the dubious newsworthiness of covering the predictable annual demonstration at the Annual Meeting by antipsychiatry demonstrators, such as the Scientologists, some local press will capture images of these modest demonstrations of trained protestors carrying signs with provocative messages such as "Psychiatry Kills!" By and large this annual protest, with about 150 demonstrators, is contained well by APA security and local police. Our members have become disciplined and do not overreact to deliberate provocations, which sometimes include personal taunts. Once, at a meeting in Miami, the Scientologists hired a small plane with a streamer saying "Psychiatry Kills," primarily referring to the death of patients for whom "dangerous" psychopharmacological treatments had been employed but implying something even more sinister.

As often as possible, there is an attempt by APA leaders to meet with editorial boards of newspapers; such discussions during the Annual Meeting are particularly useful. During Steve Sharfstein's presidency, his visits with editorial boards about the mistreatment of detainees at

Guantanamo Bay Prison by U.S. military personnel received significant attention (Sharfstein 2005a). Other presidents—for example, Mary Jane England, Joseph English, Jack McIntyre, George Tarjan, and Jack Weinberg—have been particularly successful in meeting with the press.

APA's business meetings for its internal divisions use the meeting site with great advantage. The Assembly of District Branches, as discussed in the chapter on governance, holds one of its two annual sessions just before the Annual Meeting. The Board holds two short meetings in sequence, primarily to change from the jurisdiction of the retiring Board to the newly elected one. There is an Annual Membership Meeting, which any members may attend and seek the floor to raise questions to APA officers about the association's actions or nonactions. Thirty-five years ago some of these meetings attracted well over a thousand members, with homosexuality and the war in Vietnam being particularly passionate topics. Today these meetings are much less stormy and sparsely attended.

The American Psychiatric Foundation, which was created by the APA in 1991 as an independent organization to pursue philanthropic endeavors that would improve the treatment of mental illness, has grown to be a significant dispenser of research funds and holds a large social gathering, as well as its business meetings, during the convention. It has become a powerful force in supporting and advocating psychiatric research. Many other groups utilize the Annual Meetings as an opportunity to hold receptions which serve as a reunion for previous students and staff. That such social gatherings occur enhances the value of the meeting for many attendees.

By contrast, the Institute on Psychiatric Services has less than one-tenth the attendance of the Annual Meeting, but it nevertheless has unique special objectives. These are well expressed in the APA's mission statement for the Institute:

> The Mission of the Institute on Psychiatric Services is to train and support psychiatrists to supply quality care and leadership through the study of the array of clinical innovations and services necessary to meet the needs of individuals who suffer from serious mental illness, substance abuse, or other assaults to their mental health due to trauma or adverse social circumstances, in order to assure optimal care and hope of recovery.

"To fulfil its mission," the mission statement elaborates in a subsequent section, "the IPS [Institute on Psychiatric Services] holds an annual meeting each fall that focuses on clinical and service programs, especially those that provide a complex array of services and innovations to meet the needs of the more difficult to serve patients." It is further noted that "[t]he Mission of the IPS is of particular significance for an important subset of APA members who are its prime constituents." Undoubtedly that is true, and the APA is wise to value this relationship.

Careful study of the wording of the mission statement is most revealing about many aspects of changing American psychiatry. Before World War II it was clear that American psychiatry focused on those with "serious mental illness" as written in the mission statement. During the three postwar decades, the focus changed, and, especially with the new emphasis on psychodynamic psychotherapy conducted primarily with ambulatory patients, the scope of psychiatry's activities enlarged. By the 1980s some critics were asserting that American psychiatry was paying too much attention to the "worried well." The National Alliance for the Mentally Ill (now National Alliance on Mental Illness, or NAMI) grew very rapidly during the last quarter of the twentieth century, and it concentrated on what was defined as those who were "severely mentally ill." Fuller Torrey's articulate writing, such as in his book *The Death of Psychiatry* (Torrey 1974), helped to stimulate NAMI's growth and also had an important impact on the APA. APA's mission statement for the Institute is in essential agreement with the policies of NAMI, and the two organizations are now close allies. Nevertheless, the APA's Institute mission statement, which acknowledges the etiological role of "other assaults to their mental health due to trauma or adverse social circumstances," leaves more flexibility in hypotheses about the etiology of mental disorders than those whose emphasis is almost exclusively on genetic/biological causality.

Social psychiatry still has an important place in the current Institute on Psychiatric Services, although its focus is much more upon those factors that can de directly related to the prevalence and the treatment of psychiatric disorders. Epidemiological research is particularly important and is a central topic at the Institute. While a number of psychiatrists still carry out distinguished research in epidemiology and social psychiatry (Lehman et al. 1984; Regier et al. 1988), it would be helpful for the field, in my judgment, if there were a resurgence of interest in the subject by psychiatrists. The growth of biological psychiatry has tended to diminish attention to social variables, though many would still agree with Sharfstein's preference for the "bio-psycho-social" model rather than the bio-bio-bio model.

As stated in its mission statement on the Institute on Psychiatric Services, the APA has a "subset" of members who are the prime constituents of the Institute meeting. Many are salaried physicians who work in state facilities. Others, salaried in private psychiatric hospitals or managed care systems, have interests in both macro- and micro-economic determinants of therapeutic care. While these salaried psychiatrists have somewhat different interests from those of the pre-war generation who tended to work in large state hospitals, they represent an important new constituency of the Institute. Also, mental health practitioners of all disciplines who work in hospital systems have been particularly welcomed at the Institute.

While several academic Departments of Psychiatry have had good relationships with state psychiatric systems (Scully et al. 2000), the attendance of academic psychiatrists at the Institute on Psychiatric Services is significantly lower than at the APA Annual Meeting.

The continuation of two annual meetings by the APA has several purposes. Daniel Blain's original vision of maintaining hospital psychiatry's prominence in the APA has been affected by deinstitutionalization, community psychiatry, judicial decisions, state funding, and federal policy decisions. Nevertheless, the current definition of "psychiatric services" still focuses attention on the needs of the sickest and most vulnerable patients. The hope is that such needs will be able to be better met when all American medicine deals more effectively to help those who are currently without insurance. Until that day the struggle for parity of care for the mentally ill remains APA's highest priority.

The APA's two yearly meetings reflect the changing of American psychiatry very well. As psychiatry began to change rapidly in the post–World War II years, the Mental Hospital Institute was established to emphasize our interest in the hospital systems. During that same period the Annual Meeting grew in size and began to feature psychodynamic psychotherapy, the education of psychiatrists and a broadly defined social psychiatry. After the tumultuous upheaval in the 1970s with the *Diagnostic and Statistical Manual of Mental Disorders* (DSM), the Practice Guideline program, and evidence-based psychiatry replacing ideology, the Annual Meeting once again grew much larger and became increasingly involved in psychopharmacology, nosology, and neurosciences and less involved in psychoanalytic and social topics. The Institute changed its name to the Institute on Psychiatric Services and now concentrates on the full array of services for "seriously disturbed patients." Perhaps at some point in the twenty-first century, with continued research and a more rational U.S. health system, the objectives of the two APA annual meetings will merge to form even clearer, uniform goals.

REFERENCES

American Medical Association: Physician characteristics and distribution in the U.S. Chicago, IL, American Medical Association, 2007

American Psychiatric Association: Diagnostic and Statistical Manual of Mental Disorders, 3rd Edition. Washington, DC, American Psychiatric Association, 1980

American Psychiatric Association: Diagnostic and Statistical Manual of Mental Disorders, 4th Edition. Washington, DC, American Psychiatric Association, 1994

Bailey P: The Academic Lecture: the great psychiatric revolution. Am J Psychiatry 113:387–406, 1956

Bender E: APA, NAMI collaborate on common goals. Psychiatr News 42(2):13, 2007

Blain D: The modern psychiatric hospital. Hawaii Med J 10(3):177–180, 1951

Deutsch A: The Shame of the States. New York, Harcourt, Brace, 1948

Gabbard GO: Mind, brain, and personality disorders. Am J Psychiatry 162:648–655, 2005

Grob GN: From Asylum to Community: Mental Health Policy in Modern America. Princeton, NJ, Princeton University Press, 1991

Grob GN: Mental health policy in late twentieth-century America, in American Psychiatry After World War II: 1944–1994. Edited by Menninger RW, Nemiah JC. Washington, DC, American Psychiatric Press, 2000, pp 232–258

Jones E: Psychiatry before and after Freud. Paper presented at the 112th annual meeting of the American Psychiatric Association, Chicago, IL, April 30, 1956

Lehman AF, Babigian HM, Reed SK: The epidemiology of treatment for chronic and non-chronic mental disorders. J Nerv Ment Disease 172:658–666, 1984

Mitchell SW: Address before the 50th annual meeting of the American Medico-Psychological Association, held in Philadelphia, May 16th, 1894. J Nerv Ment Dis 21:413–437, 1894

NAMI wants stronger partnership. Psychiatr News 41(16):12, 2006

Regier DA, Boyd JH, Burke JD Jr, et al: One-month prevalence of mental disorders in the United States: based on five Epidemiologic Catchment Area sites. Arch Gen Psychiatry 45:977–986, 1988

Robinowitz C: From the President: the art of the possible for parity. Psychiatr News 42(14):3, 2007

Scully JH, Robinowitz CB, Shore JH: Psychiatric education after World War II, in American Psychiatry After World War II: 1944–1994. Edited by Menninger RW, Nemiah JC. Washington, DC, American Psychiatric Press, 2000, pp 124–151

Sharfstein SS: President's Column: medical ethics and the detainees at Guantanamo Bay. Psychiatr News 40(22):3, 2005a

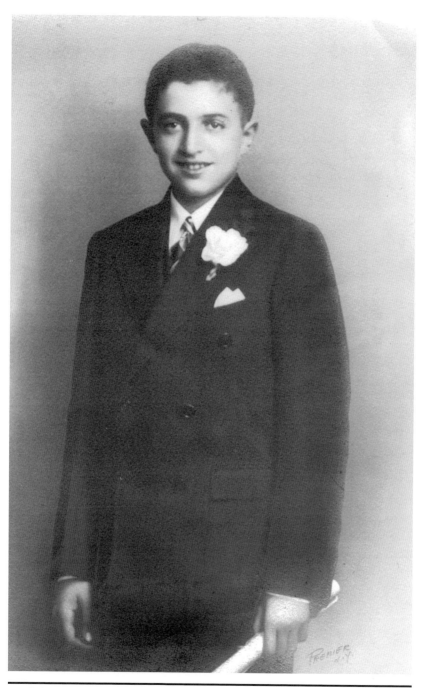

Melvin Sabshin, Townsend Harris High School, New York, 1937.

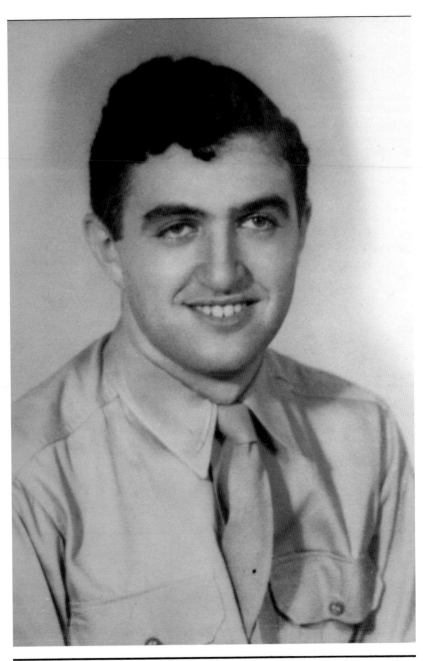

Private Melvin Sabshin, U.S. Army, 1944.

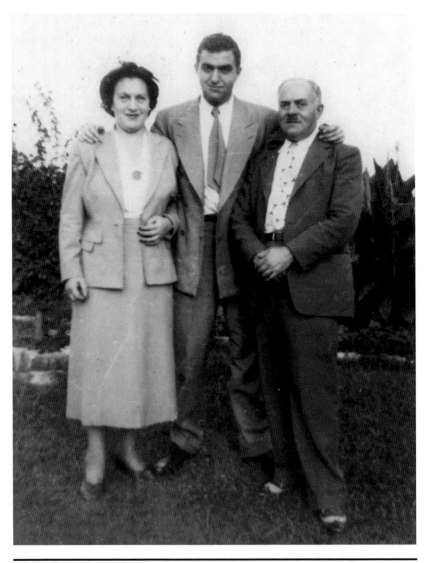

Melvin Sabshin with parents, Sonia and Dr. Zalman Sabshin.

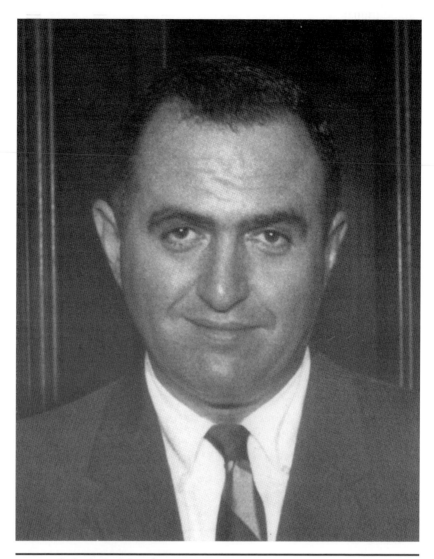

**Dr. Melvin Sabshin, Chairman, Department of Psychiatry,
University of Illinois Medical School, Chicago, 1961.**

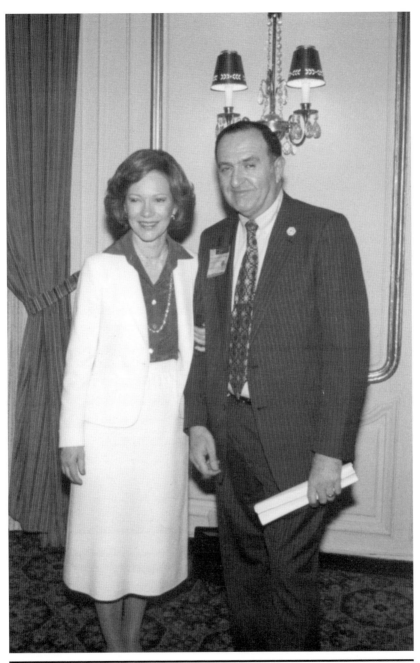

Dr. Melvin Sabshin with Mrs. Rosalynn Carter at the 132nd Annual Meeting of the American Psychiatric Association.

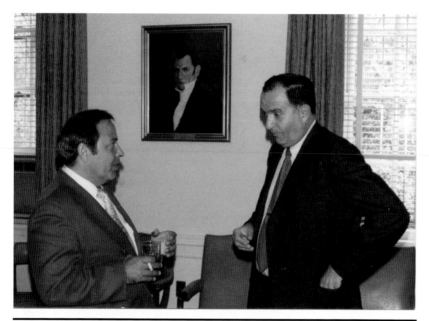

Dr. Melvin Sabshin with Jay Cutler, Director of Office of Government Affairs, at APA Main Office at 1700 18th Street, 1981.

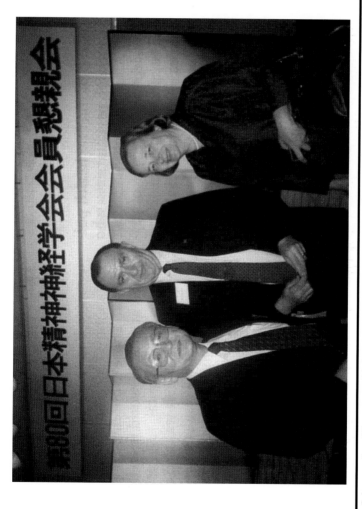

Dr. Melvin Sabshin and wife Dr. Edith Sabshin with Professor Masahisa Nishizono at the 80th Annual Meeting of the Japanese Society of Psychiatry and Neurology.

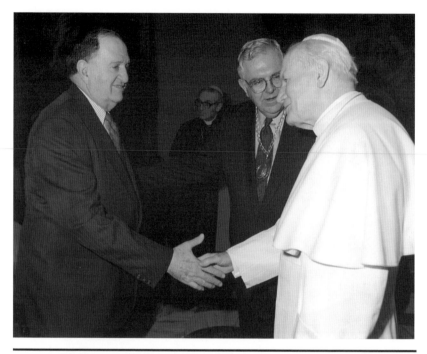

Dr. Melvin Sabshin with Joseph T. English, APA President, meeting with Pope John Paul II in Rome, 1992.

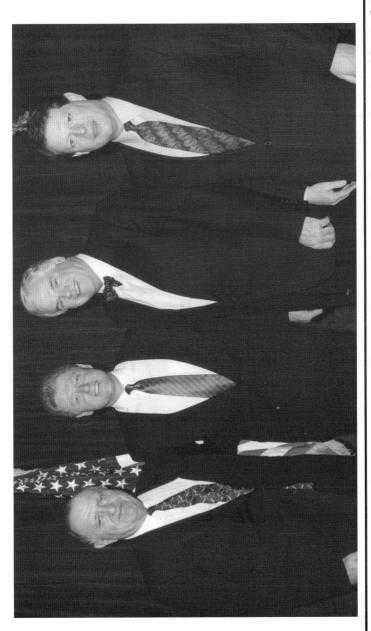

Dr. Melvin Sabshin with President William Jefferson Clinton, Dr. Jay Scully, and Vice President Al Gore, 1996.

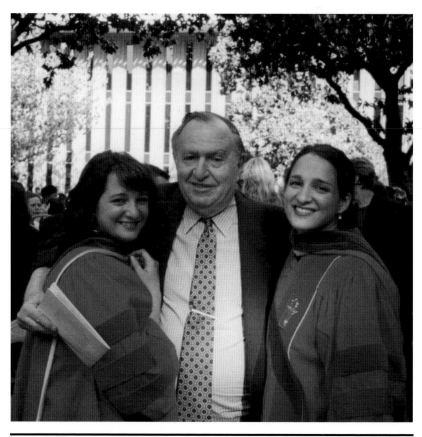

Dr. Melvin Sabshin with granddaughters Alisa Sabshin and Renée Sabshin at their graduation from medical school, June 2000.

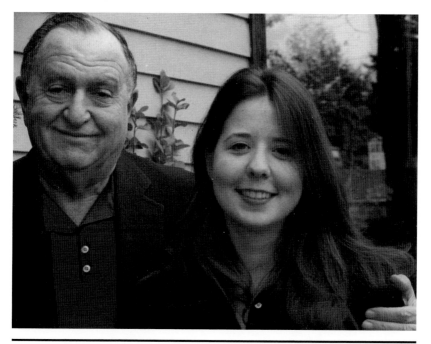
Dr. Melvin Sabshin with granddaughter Drea Sabshin.

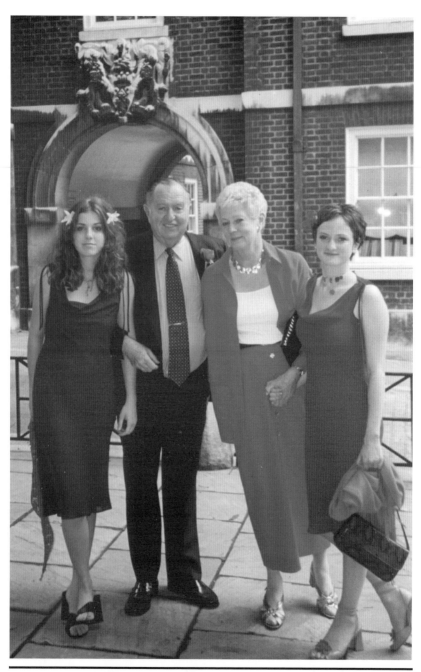

**Dr. Melvin Sabshin at his marriage to Marion Bennathan
with granddaughters Brigitte Sabshin and Ella Bennathan,
September 2000.**

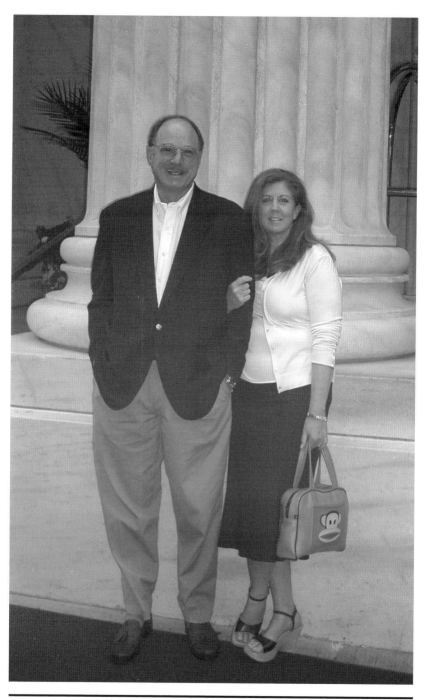

Dr. James Sabshin and wife, Mary.

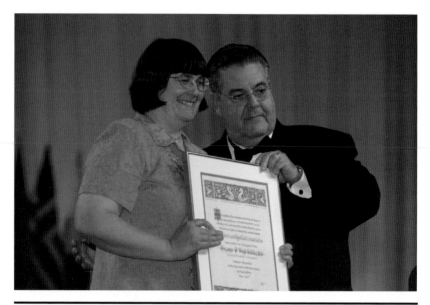

Dr. Pedro Ruiz with NAMI President, Suzanne Vogel-Scibilia, M.D., at 2007 APA Annual Meeting.

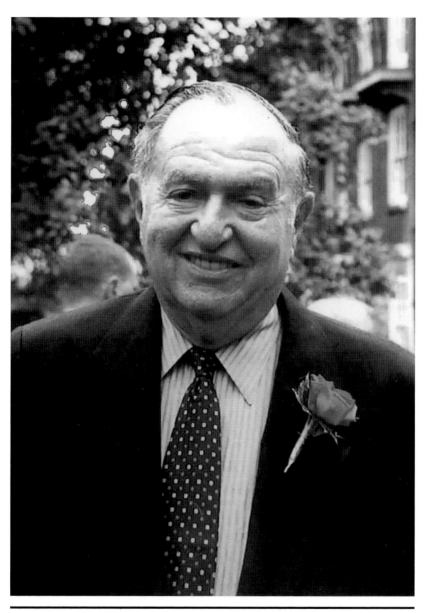

Dr. Melvin Sabshin, September 16, 2000.

Sharfstein SS: Response to the Presidential Address: advocacy for our patients and our profession. Am J Psychiatry 162:2045–2047, 2005b

Sharfstein SS: Presidential Address: Advocacy as leadership. Am J Psychiatry 163:1711–1715, 2006

Torrey EF: The Death of Psychiatry. Radnor, PA, Chilton, 1974

15

Publications

By the end of World War II, the American Psychiatric Association (APA) was publishing one dignified but somewhat staid-looking journal and a few newsletters. A half century later the APA, having fully learned the importance of the written word, has become the largest psychiatric publisher in the world, with many attractive journals, a newspaper, and a major book publishing program. Its publications have become the organization's largest source of income; they are reaching an enormous number of readers across the world and keeping our members educated and informed. I am old fashioned enough to be shocked when I find an 800-page textbook "compressed" onto one small disk or available online with fully searchable text. The American Psychiatric Publishing, Inc. (APPI) is ready for the new information technology age, even if I am not.

The *American Journal of Psychiatry* (AJP) has had the longest life span of all the APA publications. Over the years, it has changed its title, its content, and its cover several times, demonstrating dramatic alterations in the profession.

In this past decade there has been discussion about changing the name of the APA itself to reflect more clearly that psychiatrists are physicians; new names such as the "Association of Psychiatric Physicians" have been suggested. If a new name is adopted, similar changes in the title of AJP would probably follow. So far no new title for the journal has been accepted, but the current content and format of the journal clearly reflect the new American psychiatry. In this chapter I intend to highlight the general tenor of the changes to AJP and also to point out some possible future directions for the journal as well as all of the APA's publications.

The journal *Psychiatric Services* evolved from changes initiated in the middle of the twentieth century by Daniel Blain, then medical director of the APA. During a period of substantial organizational reform at the APA, he created the Department of Psychiatric Services with its publication *A.P.A. Mental Hospital Service Bulletin*. The journal that came out of this publication, whose title has changed over the years from *Mental Hospitals, Hospital & Community Psychiatry,* to the current *Psychiatric Services,* has become a leading collection of articles on the care of severely disturbed mental patients and the full range of systems required for providing that care. It publishes fewer articles on biological research than AJP and did not undergo a period of psychodynamic emphasis as did many other components of the APA. Interestingly, the APA began publishing *Academic Psychiatry* in 1989 to keep organizational and professional attention on education when biological research papers began to dominate AJP and there were fewer educational articles. Two separate journals have evolved from AJP—*Psychiatric Services* (formerly *Mental Hospitals* and *Hospital & Community Psychiatry*) and, more recently, *Academic Psychiatry* (formerly *Journal of Psychiatric Education*). Both were begun to ensure continuity of attention to their subject matter in a rapidly changing field.

The APA developed the capacity to publish several additional journals under the auspices of its then new press, American Psychiatric Press, Inc. *Psychosomatics* and the *Journal of Neuropsychiatry and Clinical Neurosciences* are examples of this trend. The formal approval of several psychiatric subspecialities (see Chapter 12, "Psychiatric Education") has led to a group of independently published journals that are extremely important in representing the scientific and professional changes brought about by those newly approved subspecialties toward the end of the century. A comparison of the full range of psychiatric journals today and 50 years ago would be useful for demonstrating various stages of American psychiatry.

I have chosen, however, to focus primarily on two journals in this chapter: *American Journal of Psychiatry* and *Psychiatric Services.* Before considering these two scholarly journals, however, I will first comment on *Psychiatric News* and then on APPI. The first is a bimonthly newspaper that is distributed to all APA members. It contains timely articles on a variety of topics affecting the practice of psychiatry as well as its public image. For example, *Psychiatric News* recently published a review about an award-winning film, "Canvas," which uncharacteristically presents psychiatrists and their patients in a realistic, more positive light (Gabbard 2007b). Pummelled by the film industry for decades, APA members need to hear that the tide of public opinion may be changing, especially from a respected psychiatry educator such as Glen Gabbard, who also co-authored the book *Psychiatry and the Cinema* (Gabbard and Gabbard 1999). *Psychiatric News* also includes regular columns by the president of the APA and by its medical director. It is full of information about APA meetings, with special coverage, for example, before and after the Annual Meeting in the Spring. *Psychiatric News* has employment columns, many advertisements, updates on a wide variety of APA activities, and detailed reports on APA elections. It also provides the best coverage of the APA's reimbursement and current legislative efforts.

As with most newspapers, *Psychiatric News* is subject to constant and occasionally rational criticism of its format and content. From my experience psychiatrists are neither shy nor passive in their reaction to news coverage, and intra-organizational debates on many stories are quite lively. For many years, the APA staff, under the direction of a managing director, selected the contents of *Psychiatric News*. This changed in 1985, when Dr. Robert Campbell was appointed editor. As a past Speaker of the Assembly, he understood very well many of the concerns about what appeared or did not appear in the *Psychiatric News*. Before he was appointed, Campbell had been editor of the newsletter of APA Area 2 (New York State). In addition, he had much writing experience and great skills in language. Campbell's appointment, like the appointment of the editors of the APA journals, involved the establishment of an administrative structure in which the staff of the publications were accountable both to the editor and to the medical director. The editor managed the choice of articles and the style of writing, while the medical director was responsible for the overall basic administration of the office. Ultimately, the Board of Trustees governed the entire process with a minimum of explicit controls.

This system could have been problematic but worked well during my tenure. My relations with the editors and managing editors involved frequent contacts and reasonable consensus. I was particularly close to the managing editor of *Psychiatric News,* Herbert Gant, and our friendly working arrangement was very helpful.

At the District Branch and Area Council organizational level of the APA, described in the next chapter (see Chapter 16, "Governance and Leadership"), the state and regional publications reflected the heart and soul of the local membership. Some of these newspapers were influential in both local and national legislative efforts. Over the years, many received special awards from the Assembly.

One of the most fateful decisions I made during my time at the APA involved my seeking and gaining approval for the creation of APPI under overall APA auspices. There were several important factors leading to this decision. The precipitating issue involved the publication of DSM-III in 1980 along with its numerous accompanying volumes. When it became apparent that DSM-III was an instant bestseller, we realized that the APA was not organized or staffed to handle such an amazing intellectual property. With my strong support, the APA Resource Development Committee, chaired by Charles Wilkinson, recommended exploring the establishment of a separate publications corporation. On March 7th 1981, American Psychiatric Press (APPI) was officially incorporated in the District of Columbia as a corporation solely owned by the APA.

The composition of the first APPI Board of Directors reflected the APA's desire to have appropriate control of the new press. The medical director served as chair and president of the board, and Jack White, the APA's Business Director, served as treasurer. The first directors were Daniel Freedman, APA President; Lawrence Hartmann, Speaker of the Assembly; and Harold Visotsky, Secretary of the APA. For me, the establishment of this structure afforded a special opportunity for a new phase of APA publications. The succes of the newly formed corporation was far beyond our most ambitious hopes.

During this development, the leadership of Dr. Shervert Frazier and his assistant, Evelyn Stone, was crucial for the founding of the press. Their practical experience in publishing was vital for the development of the new enterprise. Along with the formation of the corporation's Board, the appointment of Ron McMillen as the general manager of APPI was central to its long-term success. He continues most effectively in this role up to the present time and is now one of the leading and most experienced managers of psychiatric publishing programs in the world. Frazier was appointed as the initial editor-in-chief and served until his appointment as director of the National Institute of Mental Health.

The history of APPI has been a splendid success story for the APA. While DSM-III, DSM-III-R, and DSM-IV have been the "jewels in the crown" of the APPI publication program, the corporation has published more than 1,100 books that cover the full range of psychiatric topics, with an average of about 40 new titles each year. Psychodynamic psychiatry continues to be quite prominent, with, for example, the four editions of *Treatments of Psychiatric Disorders* (now *Gabbard's Treatments of Psychiatric Disorders*; Gabbard 2007a) and Glen Gabbard's *Psychodynamic Psychiatry in Clinical Practice* (now in its fourth edition; Gabbard 2005), being bestsellers. While the market for books on diagnosis and psychopharmacology rank highest in publication sales, APPI continues to publish many popular books on psychotherapy and psychodynamics (e.g., Person et al. 2005), indicating the continued interest of our members and many others in these subjects. This is another sign that reports of the death of psychoanalysis may be premature.

In its quarter-century history, publishing revenue has become a major source of APA income, producing 50% of overall revenue to date. Yet, when the APA Board and Assembly discussed the proposal to establish the press, there was vigorous opposition. One regional publication of the APA carried a column by its editor predicting that the press would be a dismal failure. During the debate about the new corporation, some feared that the wrath of other, competing publishers would be very hurtful to the APA membership. Fortunately, these objections did not prevail. APA's publishing over the years has magnificently proved those pessimistic forecasts wrong.

In addition to the pioneering work of Frazier and McMillen, two editors-in-chief, Carol Nadelson (1988–2001) and Robert Hales (2001–present), have worked most effectively to achieve this success. As an influential past president of the APA, Nadelson steered the press through its critical first decade. She was responsible for it rapid maturation. Hales was chosen as her successor because of his special experiences as one of the authors of a major psychiatric textbook, his chairmanship of the APA Program Committee, and his role in chairing an academic department of psychiatry. He understands the full range of important psychiatric interests and also comprehends the world of publication. He has led the press to its current unrivalled position.

APPI has become popular across the world, in part because of the extraordinary interest in the volumes of the *Diagnostic and Statistical Manual of Mental Disorders* (DSM). In many ways the content of the books published by the press provides a more accurate portrait of American psychiatry than other definitions of the field, which stress the dominance of biological psychiatry. Of course, the press reaches a wider audience than the journals, but the range of implicit definitions of the field as reflected in the varied content of the publications is an important indicator of the full scope of American psychiatry at the beginning of the twenty-first century.

Of all the APA publications, the most radical and dramatic changes during the last half century have occurred in the *American Journal of Psychiatry*. A comparison of the current journal to those of the immediate postwar years reveals the enormity of the changes in the field. High-powered multi-authored papers on neuroscience, genetics, psychopharmacology and nosology dominate the pages. During the tenure of Dr. Nancy Andreasen as editor-in-chief (1993–2005), AJP achieved a very high level of scientific respect and authority. One result of Andreasen's establishment of a very high scientific standard for publications accepted by the journal is that there have been fewer psychodynamic articles, even though the deputy editor of the journal, Arnold Cooper, has made a strong effort to publish high-quality papers on the subject. As editor-in-chief, Andreasen helped to make the journal's appearance much more appealing, with its attractive covers, but she also insisted on the best of science inside the covers. Psychiatry needed to change its image in the scientific world, and there is no better indicator of this change than a comparison of AJP's content during Andreasen's tenure with articles published 50 years ago. According to the *Science Citation Index*, which ranks journals by the number of times they are cited by other publications, AJP is one of the most cited journals in the world. Implicitly, Andreasen's management of the journal indicates her strong agreement with Edward Shorter (1997) that, after a long hiatus, psychiatry is back on scientific track consonant with the earlier work of the St. Louis group (Feighner et al. 1972; Robins and Guze 1970).

I agree that American psychiatry had to change decisively from its ideological past and adopt a new empiricism. In fact, I took the lead in the APA's shift from ideology to evidence-based practice. I am aware that some influential psychiatric leaders believe that we still have not moved far enough and that we should, in fact, merge with neurology to become a new clinical "neuroscience" profession. In this book, however, I am suggesting that steps need to be taken in support of new, scientifically based studies of the psychosocial aspects of psychiatry, complementing the biological base in a new "bio-psycho-social" psychiatry. As editor-in-chief, Andreasen originally indicated her interest in publishing high-quality psychosocial papers. Unfortunately, the weaker scientific quality of many of these papers made it impossible to publish them. I believe that the journal, now under the leadership of Editor-in-Chief Robert Freedman, should initiate policies that give more help to the publication of psychological and social hypotheses potentially important for the field.

I believe that it was vital that Andreasen took a harder line than might be necessary today. Her elegant and carefully chosen language in an article in *Science* is quoted in part in an anonymous editorial, entitled "The Crisis in Psychiatry" (1997), published in *The Lancet*, the journal of the British Medical Association:

> Convergent data, using multiple neuroscience techniques, indicate that the neural mechanisms of mental illnesses can be understood as dysfunctions in special neural circuits and that functions and dysfunctions

can be influenced or altered by a variety of cognitive and pharmacological factors....These advances have created an era in which a scientific psychopathology that links mind and brain has become a reality.

In the article in *Science* (Andreasen 1997), Andreasen does say that neural functions and dysfunctions can be "influenced and altered by a variety of cognitive and pharmacological factors." To use the word "cognitive" is technically correct to describe the final common pathway. Does that statement reflect insufficient attention to the specificity of the psychological, social, and economic factors that bear down upon the cognitive pathways? Does the employment of psychosocial language in defining the salient variables necessarily imply a Cartesian dualism? How much attention needs to be given to the variables including what they signify to the "cognitive system"? I hope that Andreasen and others might agree that the language describing the psychological and social factors might be quite significant when formulated as hypotheses.

The anonymous writer of the *Lancet* editorial is critical of Andreasen's statement as being irrelevant for most of the developing world. Her approach, it is alleged, is exclusively that of the world of new technology. He or she would also be critical of my book's concentration upon many of the recent changes in American psychiatry. The editorial writer cites the work of Kleinman and Cohen (Kleinman and Cohen 1997), who advocate a more rational global perspective on dealing with the purported "crisis in psychiatry." The particular need of psychiatry in America to replace ideology by science was not then the concern of *The Lancet*.

From my perspective, there are important questions about the basic definition of psychiatry relevant to this discussion of AJP. Some favor a "neuroscience" field linking neurology and psychiatry (Kandel 2005). Others envisage a biopsychosocial definition to differentiate psychiatry from neurology on the one side and clinical psychology on the other. In the concluding chapter of this book, I discuss why I favor the latter model.

Whatever the long-term outcome of this debate, it might be useful for the AJP to consider finding an appropriate way of publishing work in progress on new hypothesis generation without lowering its scientific status. Highlighting new hypothesis development could be an important encouragement for future change. Ultimately these new hypotheses, when tested, could improve the reliability and validity of our scientific base. There is strong indication that the new editor-in-chief of AJP, Robert Freedman, understands these issues; it will be interesting to follow his editorial decisions on the subject.

Tracing the history of AJP reveals a great deal about the profession's priorities, concerns, and capacities. During the tenure of its first editor, Amariah Brigham, the journal closely reflected the major interests of the association. Mental hospitals and their progress were the key questions for the medical superintendents and their journal. In pre–World War II days, before the APA moved to its Washington headquarters, AJP's office was located in Toronto. Its editor, Clarence Farrar, with prodigious energy, decisiveness, and talent, somehow managed to perform heroically from 1931 to 1965. By 1965, the APA was able to house the journal in its Washington headquarters, and Francis Braceland was appointed editor. Braceland had been president of the APA in 1956–57 and was thoroughly familiar with every nuance and context affecting psychiatry. He was the director of a prestigious private psychiatric hospital, The Institute for Living, in Hartford, Connecticut, which had a long and distinguished history. Braceland, in contrast to many psychiatric leaders at the time, was not a psychoanalyst, but his thorough respect for analysis was significant. As an important Catholic layman, Braceland helped to fend off prejudicial attacks on analysis by, for example, then Monsignor Fulton Sheen, who was highly critical of its premises. Braceland broadened the scope of the journal and encouraged the acceptance of many papers on psychiatric education.

AJP gave special attention to several important conferences on training by publishing part of the deliberations and conclusions. It also gave much attention to psychodynamic clinical formulations and community psychiatry. Braceland's appointment of Evelyn Myers as managing editor of AJP was particularly important. With her superb command of the English language, her background in economics, her policy awareness, and her administrative skills, she played a key role in the journal's progress and its adaptation to the Washington scene. During Braceland's tenure the journal reflected psychiatry's interests at that time, but it was balanced and not imbued with the prevalent ideological fervour of many in the field.

When Braceland retired in 1978, he was succeeded by John Nemiah, an academic psychoanalyst from Massachusetts General Hospital and the Harvard complex. Nemiah was particularly interested in psychosomatic medicine and applied psychodynamic concepts to it with diligence but without an overarching desire to convert others to accept his viewpoint. Above all, he loved the English language, and his editorial role included special attention to style and tone. He was also a dedicated academic (Nemiah 1973). Like his predecessor, Francis Braceland, he worked well with Evelyn Myers, making a most effective team.

By 1978, when Nemiah was appointed editor, psychoanalysis had begun to decline in its powerful impact upon American psychiatry. That decline affected many leadership appointments, including fewer appointments of analysts to academic posts. But Nemiah's extraordinary talents as a writer and as academic clinician were so impressive that they outweighed biases against his analytic background. Above all, he wanted a balanced journal that included well-written, high-quality papers. He appointed Morris Lipton as deputy editor to facilitate the choice of good papers on neuroscience. Nemiah was mindful of major policy questions, and during his tenure there were significant debates and policy discussions published in AJP. His fondness for "good English" also seemed to make him attentive to British psychiatry, so that he built up a close relationship between AJP and the *British Journal of Psychiatry*.

By the time Nemiah retired in 1992, American psychiatry was struggling even more to cope with the powerful new managed care system that dominated the reimbursement climate for all of medicine. DSM-III (American Psychiatric Association 1980) had demonstrated a new approach for psychiatry, as had the new work on Practice Guidelines. Psychiatry was implementing its new commitment to empiricism and evidence-based practice. The editor-in-chief of AJP needed to be a powerful advocate of the new direction. Nancy Andreasen was passionately committed to neuroscientific research. Her appointment marked a new era for AJP. She was a brilliant neuroscientific investigator at the University of Iowa, a prolific author of textbooks and scientific papers, and a former English teacher. In addition, Andreasen was a determined policy leader and a powerful advocate for biological psychiatry.

With the appointment of Sandra Patterson as managing editor, much additional attention could be paid to the format of the journal and its literary style. The selection of Jack Gorman and Arnold Cooper as deputy editors helped Andreasen to publish the best and brightest new research.

When Andreasen's term ended in 2005, the APA selected another brilliant scientific researcher as editor-in-chief. Robert Freedman continues the tradition of keeping AJP in the vanguard of the frontiers of science. Whether it is now the right time to consider more policy papers on psychiatric research or the inclusion of more "hypothesis generating" research is a question that, I believe, merits discussion.

The comparison of AJP with *Archives of General Psychiatry* is particularly interesting. Published by the American Medical Association (AMA), *Archives of General Psychiatry* is a most significant part of the AMA's contribution to specialty medicine. While the three editors of the *Archives* in the last half of the twentieth century had significant personal and professional differences from the editors of AJP, both journals have accurately reflected the changes in American psychiatry. Roy Grinker, editor of the *Archives* from 1959 to 1970, had been my director and an important model for me. He was a major contributor to the understanding of psychiatric casualties during War War II, as discussed in Chapter 1 ("Post–World War II Scene in American Psychiatry"). He was also a theoretician, a psychosomatic researcher, and a psychoanalyst, though often critical of that field. His "transactional" approach stimulated many policy and philosophical discussions in the *Archives* in addition to its clinical content (Grinker 1959).

Daniel Freedman, editor of the *Archives* from 1970 to 1993, was one of the major leaders of psychiatric research of his time, and his presidency of the APA (1981–82) was very important for the support of new research. He was also chair of a major Department of Psychiatry (at the University of Chicago). He had enormous energy and worked hard to make the *Archives* a premier champion of research. Jack Barchas, the scholarly chair of psychiatry at Cornell, continued the empirical perspective as the editor from 1994 to 2001. In a modest but persistent fashion, he shaped the *Archives* into a modern protagonist and conveyor of advanced research. Joseph Coyle has continued in that leadership role since 2002. The AJP and the *Archives* together tell the story of a powerful new identity of psychiatry at the beginning of the twentieth-first century.

The journal *Psychiatric Services* has had a different history. Having evolved under the leadership of Daniel Blain, it told the story of America's mental hospitals. Donald Hammersley, Deputy Medical Director of the APA, took over editing the journal (then called *Hospital & Community Psychiatry*) in 1970 and worked hard to continue the traditions of the old *A.P.A. Mental Hospital Service Bulletin* and *Mental Hospitals* in the new journal. Hammersley carried out his many responsibilities quietly and energetically. He had been effective in dealing with a major part of APA's administrative activities as they had been organized before my arrival on the scene in 1974. He tried very hard to adapt to a changing APA after my appointment. Loyal to a fault, he never criticized the new priorities but did his best to keep the APA active in hospital and community care. I believe that my appointment as medical director was not altogether a happy event for Hammersley, although he never expressed his disappointment directly to me. At *Psychiatric Services,* Hammersley was assisted by a strongly committed managing editor, Teddye Clayton. She believed passionately that *Psychiatric Services* represented the heart and soul of the APA and was sensitive and resistant to any attempts to alter its priorities. After Hammersley's retirement as editor, she stayed on with John Talbott when he became editor in 1981, and they were a superb team.

Talbott, who had been president of the APA in 1984–85, embodied an integration of many late-twentieth-century psychiatric systems. He had worked at the Cornell Department of Psychiatry under the brilliant chairmanship of Robert Michels. In my judgment, Michels represented late-twentieth-century psychoanalysis very ably in his many leadership roles. Less critical of analysis than Grinker, he nevertheless sought new directions for the field (Michels 1988). At Cornell, Michels was a leading educator and statesman with extraordinary administrative talents, and he became dean of the medical school. Talbott worked with Michels and learned many of his skills, but he soon emerged on his own as a very able leader. When he became chairman of the Department of Psychiatry at the University of Maryland School of Medicine, he built an excellent system that had an exceedingly broad base, including a well-coordinated community system. Talbott's ability to build an integrated department at Maryland was superior to my efforts in Illinois much earlier, as I was able to see clearly when I joined his faculty in 1998.

Included in Talbott's plan was a special effort to coordinate his academic program with the community services. Never an easy task, this program was as good a model for a combination of academic and service programs as existed at the time. Son of a former editor of the *Journal of the American Medical Association* (JAMA), Talbott had extensive experience in such activities, having emerged as a national leader, so that he was an ideal choice for bringing a new perspective as editor. He had a long and productive tenure as editor of the journal. With the assistance of Clayton, he added many new features, including strong editorials, brief special articles, more systematic policy research, "economic" grand rounds, and the best of social and community psychiatry. When Talbott stepped down in 2004, Howard Goldman was appointed as his successor. Goldman is, in my opinion, one of America's clearest policy leaders in planning the organization of mental health services and in a modern social psychiatry.

When viewed overall, the current APA publications—the *American Journal of Psychiatry, Psychiatric Services,* APPI books and journals, and *Psychiatric News*—are an excellent reflection of what psychiatry has become in the United States. Advances in communication technology will doubtless continue to develop very rapidly along with major policy decisions in the next few decades. The APA's mammoth publishing activities seem well poised to adapt to whatever changes may occur. I cannot, however, abandon my resistance to the prediction by some younger colleagues that reading will become a nostalgic relic.

REFERENCES

American Psychiatric Association: Diagnostic and Statistical Manual of Mental Disorders, 3rd Edition. Washington, DC, American Psychiatric Association, 1980

Andreasen NC: Linking mind and brain in the study of mental illnesses: a project for a scientific psychopathology. Science 275(5306):1586–1593, 1997

The crisis in psychiatry. Lancet 349(9057):965, 1997

Feighner JP, Robins E, Guze SB, et al: Diagnostic criteria for use in psychiatric research. ArchGen Psychiatry 26:57–63, 1972

First MB, Frances A, Pincus HA: DSM-IV Handbook of Differential Diagnosis. Washington, DC, American Psychiatric Press, 1995

Gabbard GO: Psychodynamic Psychiatry in Clinical Practice, 4th Edition. Washington, DC, American Psychiatric Publishing, 2005

Gabbard GO: Gabbard's Treatments of Psychiatric Disorders, 4th Edition. Washington, DC, American Psychiatric Publishing, 2007a

Gabbard GO: Schizophrenia on filmmaker's Canvas. Psychiatr News 42(19):6–7, 2007b

Gabbard GO, Gabbard K: Psychiatry and the Cinema, 2nd Edition. Washington, DC, American Psychiatric Press, 1999

Grinker RR: A transactional model for psychotherapy. Arch Gen Psychiatry 1:132–148, 1959

Kandel ER: Psychiatry, Psychoanalysis, and the New Biology of Mind. Washington, DC, American Psychiatric Publishing, 2005

Kleinman A, Cohen A: Psychiatry's global challenge. Sci Am 276(3):86–89, 1997

Michels R: The future of psychoanalysis. Psychoanal Q 57(2):167–185, 1988

Nemiah JC: Foundations of Psychopathology. New York, Jason Aronson, 1973

Person ES, Cooper AM, Gabbard GO: The American Psychiatric Publishing Textbook of Psychoanalysis. Washington, DC, American Psychiatric Publishing, 2005

Reid WH, Wise MG: DSM-III-R Training Guide. New York, Brunner/Mazel, 1989

Robins E, Guze SB: Establishment of diagnostic validity in psychiatric illness: its application to schizophrenia. Am J Psychiatry 126:107–111, 1970

Shahrokh NC, Hales RE (eds): American Psychiatric Glossary, 8th Edition. Washington, DC, American Psychiatric Publishing, 2003

Shorter E: A History of Psychiatry: From the Era of the Asylum to the Age of Prozac. New York, Wiley, 1997

Skodol AE, Spitzer RL: An Annotated Bibliography of DSM-III. Washington, DC, American Psychiatric Press, 1987

Spitzer RL, Skodol AE, Gibbon M, et al: DSM-III Case Book: A Learning Companion to the Diagnostic and Statistical Manual of Mental Disorders (Third Edition). Washington, DC, American Psychiatric Association, 1981

Widiger TA, Frances AJ, Pincus HA, et al: DSM-IV Sourcebook, Vol 1–4. Washington, DC, American Psychiatric Association, 1994–1998

16

Governance and Leadership

*T*he changes in American psychiatry during the latter half of the twentieth century were facilitated by many institutions, organizations, and leaders. In the personal perspective of this book, I am focusing upon the role of the American Psychiatric Association, which I believe has played a decisive part in the specific alterations of the field's therapeutic practices, diagnostic formulations, public policies, educational programs, and scientific methodology. In this chapter I describe how the organization's governance structure and its diverse leadership were engaged in the process of change. The APA's policies involved more than judicious employment of an already existing administrative system to support change; they depended upon the creation of structural elements that could actually implement the new policies.

Our archives house thousand of documents that detail the the historical decisions made on behalf of the APA. Walter Barton's book The *History and Influence of the American Psychiatric Association* has an excellent and thorough review of the APA's history up to the mid-1970s (Barton 1987). My book is less of an objective or detailed account but much more focused on the processes of fundamental changes in postwar American psychiatry and the possibilities of future changes in the profession. Clearly, there is a need for objective historical scholars to examine the evolution of American psychiatry. Nevertheless, I have found some of the recent historical accounts of the period (e.g., Shorter 1997) to be questionable at several levels, and I have expressed what may be controversial opinions on the new directions in the field (Kandel 2005). My emphasis in this chapter is on what I perceive to be the major leadership and governance factors involved in achieving modification of the field as a whole. I begin with executive functions and then branch out to include a variety of relevant organizational systems and processes.

MEDICAL DIRECTOR AND PRESIDENTS

The relationship between the APA's medical director and its presidents is a fascinating example of how structural guidelines as written in administrative manuals may often be unofficially superseded by personal styles and negotiations that may be more relevant to leadership than what is prescribed in the official documents. My interactions with the presidents of the APA have been a clear example of this principle. Appendix 6 lists all the APA Presidents since the formation of the APA in 1844. I have also listed, in Appendix 13, the six medical directors of the organization.

During my tenure as medical director, which began in September 1974 and ended in 1997, I worked directly with 23 presidents. My relationships varied considerably in personal closeness, style, mood, and level of policy agreement. I have summarized some of the factors affecting the relationship in a published article and an unpublished paper. In the article, entitled "Administering a National Medical Association: The Joys, the Sorrows, and Other Challenges" (Sabshin 1991), I discussed a wide range of organizational issues, including my interaction with many officers. In an unpublished lecture in 1993 on presidential transitions, I reviewed some of the specific factors that affected my relationship with the presidents. As I write, I am struck by the fact that I have never received a comment about the published paper from anyone. In this chapter I discuss some of the broad issues first and then make brief comments about working with individual presidents.

My own stage of life at various phases of being the medical director made a big difference. In the early years, several presidents were older, experienced leaders who were almost uniformly helpful in my continuing education for the leadership role. As time passed, many of the presidents were much younger than I and often used me as a consultant for what they might do after their presidency. Some of them, when elected, were extremely well organized and had long-range plans for what they wished to do during their period as president-elect, their year of presidency, and the subsequent three years as voting members of the Board of Trustees. Toward the end of my time at the APA, two of the three last presidents were clearly looking forward to the appointment of a new medical director, and my authority had diminished, but not as much as they thought.

The fact that the president was officially designated as the chief executive officer at that time was particularly important for about five of them. A few tried, without significant success, to supervise my management of the staff; some had distinct policy differences from me, and occasionally these differences flared up in a serious dispute. For example, I had a serious conflict with a president who wanted to cancel our 1981 Annual Meeting in New Orleans, because of the State of Louisiana's failure to ratify the proposed equal rights amendment, as discussed in Chapter 14 ("Annual Meetings"). Ultimately the question had to go to the membership for decision. The great majority of presidents, however, worked as colleagues with me, and most gave me as much latitude as I needed. A few, in fact, told me to feel free to suggest and to implement policies and consult them only if a problem developed. There were rare occasions when a president was more disabled than he or she realized and I had to assert more authority, without, I hope, being too obvious or embarrassing. A number complained that the one-year presidential term was much too short. The fact that the president had served as president-elect for one year and remained as a voting member of the Board for two years after his or her presidency provided some additional time for leadership. However, the potential long-term tenure of the medical director as compared with that of the president gave the former a powerful base for leadership in long-term policy change. With the great majority of presidents, the relationship was cordial, frank, and mutually respectful.

Much could be said about each of the presidents with whom I worked from 1974 to 1997. I had the honor of being asked by seven of them to present their introduction for the presidential address at the end of their term at the convocation during the APA Annual Meeting. These occasions permitted me to describe much of their personal history and their achievements during their time in office. In this chapter, I will not be able to accomplish anything close to an adequate description of each president, but I will attempt a very brief characterization of some of their roles in changing American psychiatry.

As I reflect back on the 27 presidents with whom I served as a member of the Board of Trustees, which included the 23 presidents during my tenure as medical director, several central trends seem important. Ten of the presidents served at some point in their career as chairs of academic departments of psychiatry: Ewald W. Busse (1971–2), Alfred M. Freedman (1973–4), Donald G. Langsley (1980–81), Daniel X. Freedman (1981–2), Keith H. Brodie (1982–3), John A. Talbott (1984–5), Paul J. Fink (1988–9), Herbert Pardes (1989–90), Joseph T. English (1992–3), and Jerry M. Wiener (1994–5). Taken as a whole, these chairs who have served as APA presidents represent more diverse interests than today's (2007) chairs, who are most often neuroscientific researchers. I have concerns about whether the present generation of academic leaders will be as active in APA leadership as they are in research societies. During my tenure, academic psychiatrists were central change makers for the field as a whole. I relied on their support for most of my recommendations.

Many presidents have also been pioneers and leaders in the formation and advancement of psychiatric subspecialties. Ewald Busse and Jack Weinberg (1997–8) were very active in the maturation of geriatric psychiatry. Lawrence Hartmann (1991–92), Elissa P. Benedek (1990–91), Jerry Wiener, and Mary Jane England (1995–6) were child psychiatrists. All of them were subsequently involved in many other areas of psychiatric leadership.

Alan A. Stone (1979–80) had special interests in many forensic issues in addition to his overall legal scholarship; Elissa Benedek was a distinguished national leader in forensic psychiatry itself, as was Paul S. Appelbaum (2002–3), who also was a department chair. (I was no longer medical director during Appelbaum's term.) Robert O. Pasnau (1986–7) was a significant pioneer in consultation-liaison psychiatry. It is particularly impressive to me that all these subspecialty leaders had major interests in general psychiatric issues as well as in their sub-specialty commitments. That made a big difference in retaining subspecialist membership in the APA.

Several presidents had special interests in major subsets of psychiatry that are not formal subspecialties but represent important areas of professional work. George Tarjan (1983–4) was an internationally renowned leader in work with persons with mental disabilities; Lawrence Hartmann has been a long-term advocate and leader in social psychiatry, a field that was also supported by the work of John P. Spiegel (1974–5). John Talbott has been a major national leader in community health services and has developed a model for university collaboration with state mental health systems. Judd Marmor (1975–76), Robert W. Gibson (1976–7), George H. Pollock (1987–8), Paul Fink, and Harold Eist (1996–7) had special interests in psychoanalytic issues. Pollock had been a director of a Psychoanalytic Institute, but I do not believe that he or indeed any of our analytically oriented presidents were hard-line ideologues such as I have attempted to characterize in Chapter 8 ("Psychoanalysis"). As might be expected, the ideologues I described in that chapter directed most of their attention to psychoanalysis itself; they recognized the need for allies in academic psychiatry, but they maintained a distinction between an ally and a pure devotee.

Alfred Freedman, John Spiegel, Lawrence Hartmann, and Judd Marmor were particularly strong advocates for removing homosexuality from the classification of psychiatric disorders. For Marmor, this position brought him into direct conflict with many fellow analysts; Freedman led much of the internal debate; Hartmann, as the only acknowledged gay president, has become a major contributor to the history of APA's policies on homosexuality (Hartmann 2007). Freedman, at the age of 90, has also recently revisited these dramatic debates in an interview with Michael Blumenfield (Blumenfield 2007).

Before World War II many presidents of the APA had been directors of public mental hospitals. During my tenure as medical director, no president held that role. Several presidents—including Robert S. Garber (1970–71), Perry Clement Talkington (1972–3), and Robert Gibson—were directors of private psychiatric facilities. John McIntyre (1993–4) has been director of a psychiatric department in a general hospital. By the time I became medical director, the APA's leadership mantle was no longer held by state hospital superintendents.

Two presidents have had special careers in research policy. Daniel Freedman was a national icon as an advocate for psychiatric research. Herbert Pardes served as director of the National Institute of Mental Health and played a key role in the building of a large national psychiatric research program in the latter part of the twentieth century.

Many presidents had special interests and/or roles in international psychiatry. Alan Stone and Lawrence Hartmann assumed key positions in the international investigation of psychiatric abuse. Harold Eist and Alfred Freedman have had close involvement in the World Psychiatric Association (WPA). Since my departure, two of the APA's recent presidents, Allan Tasman (1999–2000) and Pedro Ruiz (2006–7), have been elected to the WPA's Executive Committee.

APA Presidents have been major leaders as editors of journals, text books, and publication corporations. Carol C. Nadelson (1985–6) was the distinguished and innovative editor-in-chief and first chief executive officer of American Psychiatric Press, Inc. (APPI). Daniel Freedman, Alfred Freedman, and John Talbott were editors of significant textbooks; Drs. D. Freedman and Talbott were also editors of major psychiatric journals, as described in chapter 15 ("Publications").

All the presidents were involved with psychiatry's coping with economic pressures. Robert Gibson was one of our most important and knowledgeable leaders to take a major role in our adaptation to regulatory pressures. John McIntyre made a most significant contribution, with his understanding of how practice guidelines could help psychiatrists to cope with external regulatory systems. Joseph English and Mary

Jane England have also been particularly strong leaders in the APA's coping with the new economics. English's work in gaining an exemption from a payment system that would have punished psychiatric patients fiscally was extremely helpful. Since my retirement, Steven S. Sharfstein (2005–6) has been a powerful national leader in our broad activities of adapting to many social, political, and economic pressures. From his vantage point as director of a major private psychiatric system, he has been a leading figure in the economic strategies of American psychiatry for over two decades.

Several presidents have been strong advocates for particular aspects of patient care. John Talbott, Harold Eist, and John McIntyre often demonstrated this commitment. McIntyre was very important in building APA's close relationship to the National Alliance for the Mentally Ill (NAMI; now National Alliance on Mental Illness). Often the interest in patient care had special relevance to work in our public systems as well as in private practice. Talbott's editorship of *Psychiatric Services* was devoted to the improvement of patient care. George Tarjan and, after my time, Rodrigo A. Muñoz (1998–99) were particularly important in improving patient care for special populations, such as the mentally handicapped and the ethnic minority populations.

It is important to note how many of the presidents have moved on to distinguished leadership careers beyond psychiatry. Mary Jane England was appointed a college president; Keith Brodie has served as president of Duke University (and I had the privilege of attending his inauguration); Alan Stone has been a distinguished professor at Harvard Law School; and Herbert Pardes has served as vice president for health sciences and dean of the Faculty of Medicine at Columbia University College of Physicians and Surgeons and president and chief executive officer of New York–Presbyterian Hospital for many years. A substantial number of psychiatrists have become deans of medical schools.

My discussion of the APA's presidency has focused mainly upon those who served during my tenure. Occasionally, but not systematically, I have made a brief comment about more recent presidents. It is particularly important to me that the current president (2007–8), Carolyn B. Robinowitz, has been a close colleague for many years. An extraordinary educator and academic leader, she worked previously as APA's deputy medical director and as treasurer of the APA before her presidency. I believe that her leadership will be particularly important for the future direction of our organization. That Robinowitz, Sharfstein, and Scully worked with me on the APA staff before they assumed subsequent major leadership responsibilities is of course very gratifying to me.

COORDINATION OF
THE GOVERNANCE STRUCTURE

Details of the overall governance structure and history of the APA would be an interesting topic for students of administrative systems, but that is not the basic purpose of this chapter. If it was the primary focus, at this point in my life I probably could not accomplish this task objectively and succinctly. Therefore, I have been highly selective and arbitrary in choosing examples of decisions and structures that seem best to illustrate some of the historical changes in governance and leadership. Other chapters in this book cover most of these actions, including the key decisions on the *Diagnostic and Statistical Manual of Mental Disorders* (DSM) and Practice Guidelines (Chapter 10, "Evidence-Based Diagnosis and Treatment"); development of a new educational system for students and members at all levels and the creation of new subspecialties (Chapter 12, "Psychiatric Education"); the establishment of the APA offices for government, public, and economic affairs; the shift from ideology to science and the establishment of a research and educational corporation, the American Psychiatric Institute for Research and Education (APIRE) (Chapter 11, "Psychiatric Research"); the enormous strengthening of publications (Chapter 15, "Publications"); and the organization of major scientific meetings (Chapter 14, "Annual Meetings"). Working with the Board of Trustees, the Assembly, and our committee structures, our staff have played an important role in coordinating, in suggesting action, in implementing policy, and in retaining our unity of purpose. (The APA governance system during the last year of my tenure is depicted in Appendix 14.) Each of these issues required extensive policy debate, gradual clarification, and decision making. From my perspective the ultimate membership decisions taken on with each of these questions supported scientific and educational progress for the field.

The two chief financial challenges to the APA during my tenure were the fiscal threats emanating from the malpractice programs and, equally important, the potential lawsuits against the APA if we were to cancel the Annual Meeting in New Orleans in 1981. Deft administrative handling by Joseph English and other leaders averted a malpractice crisis. A membership referendum that kept the meeting in New Orleans saved us, in my judgment, from a perilous suit, as discussed in Chapter 14 ("Annual Meetings").

While the APA had many debates on substantial policy issues, we held together despite sharp differences. The adoption of DSM-III (American Psychiatric Association 1980) caused us some membership losses, but we remained unified and secured our scientific status.

In previous chapters, I have discussed some of the organizational changes during my early years as medical director. It was clear that the complexities of many newly formed entities required careful coordination and boundaries. I appointed Jeanne Robb to head an office to coordinate the Board and the Assembly. The latter two governance systems had been carefully established during the post–World War II decades to represent somewhat different segments and perspectives of the membership. The Board in the postwar years tended to include a large number of academic chairs and educational leadership. The Assembly was primarily composed of active practitioners who represented the heart and soul of our membership. The Assembly mainly consists of representatives from each District Branch; currently, it also includes a small number of representatives from other psychiatric organizations and psychiatric residents. It has been a large group (250 total members, 170 voting members) and has acted primarily like a legislative body, with presiding officers, committee structures, and geographically based subdivisions called *Area Councils*. These councils are organized regionally into seven areas (see Appendix 10), and representatives from these areas meet during the two annual Assembly meetings and also several times during the year in their home regions. To a significant extent the areas were also organized along the lines of membership size so that they might have approximately similar numbers of members. Given the higher concentration of members when the system was established, New York and California were each designated as separate areas (Area 2 and Area 6). The South (Area 5), the Midwest (Area 4), and the West (Area 6) were very large geographically; the Mid-Atlantic States (Area 3) and New England (Area 1), were middle sized. In Chapter 13 ("A Changing Membership"), I have described a few differences in policy stances in regions of the country especially on some broad social and political issues. In recent years a national consensus has developed on most policy issues; although vigorous debate is still evident in the discussions. Early in my tenure, I appointed APA staff members from the Washington, D.C., office to serve as liaison for each of the seven Area Councils. It turned out to be very useful for coordination of policy. The staff liaison members ensured faster response time after recommendations were initiated.

JOINT NATIONAL/DISTRICT BRANCH MEMBERSHIP

The APA has consistently required members to belong to the national organization as well as to a local District Branch. Each District Branch has its own officers and staff. The size of the District Branches varies considerably. They hold their own professional and business meetings, and for many members, this local work is the real essence of the APA. Some district branches became concerned with the dual membership requirement, especially when members resigned because of their dissatisfaction with the national organization's policies. A few blamed the APA for continuing fiscal discrimination against psychiatrists and their patients. Occasionally resignations occurred because the member had a problem with the local District Branch and would have preferred to stay on only as a national member. Dual membership requires constant attention, especially during this period of managed care pressures upon individual members. About 60% of American psychiatrists are members of the APA (as of 2007, 33,226 APA members; 56,000 U.S. psychiatrists), and each is also a member of a District Branch.

ASSEMBLY OF DISTRICT BRANCHES

The rapid growth of membership (see Appendix 5) in the postwar years and the changing direction of American psychiatry stimulated several decades of reorganization within the APA. In 1969, the Board of Trustees replaced the previous Council and later included area representation as well as formal Assembly membership. In the history of the Assembly during its earliest phase, when the Assembly leadership were not yet members of the Board, there are stories of Assembly leaders waiting outside the Board meeting room until they were "summoned" inside to make their presentations. There were complaints from many Assembly members that the Board was elitist and did not respect the less privileged practitioners. This changed dramatically in the last quarter of the twentieth century with the constitutional changes, new by-laws, and the recognition by the leadership that close governance cooperation was absolutely necessary. American psychiatry could not have changed dramatically if it had been mired in fundamental disagreements. Nevertheless, there were enough concerns about relative powers of decision making so that the APA's Key Conference, held in Key Biscayne in March 1975, which considered the full range of governance issues, had to make recommendations about organizational, structural and functional change. The attendees at the conference recommended a new APA structure in which the ultimate decision making would be transferred from the Board to the Assembly. Later, a series of constitutional changes was presented to the membership for their decision. A majority of voters supported the amendments, but the changes failed, in 1979, to receive the required two-thirds margin. The Board, therefore, remained the ultimate formal decision-making body— an arrangement that continues today (as of 2008).

The Assembly, however, has become much more active in policy formation. Mechanisms for the Assembly to review Board actions have subsequently been established, and the Assembly is very often the source of major policy items put forward for Board deliberations. Officers of the APA make regular presentations at the Assembly, as does the medical director. In recent years, I have begun again to attend the plenary sessions of the Assembly. During the tenure of my successor as medical director, Steve Mirin, and some other leaders of the organization at that time, I was somewhat uncomfortable about attending APA business meetings. Now, attending the Assembly is again a pleasurable experience. I find it to be a lively event that does indeed reflect the "real world" of practice.

The representatives of other psychiatric groups are now highly visible in the Assembly. Presentations by American Medical Association leadership are particularly well received, as are those from the leadership of NAMI. For the past decade a new type of session on policy considerations has supplemented the Area Council meetings; these sessions, which have been called "reference committees" of the Assembly, deal with major policy issues. The Assembly meetings are now composed of plenary sessions, reference committee deliberations, and Area Council meetings.

I have been impressed by the leadership quality of Assembly officers. They are knowledgeable and practical. The annually elected Speakers of the Assembly who preside at the meeting have organized a group that they proudly and significantly call "the Knights of the Roundtable," and they meet annually, bringing in the new Speaker (called "the knave") at each meeting. The "knights" group was initiated in 1989 by past Speaker Alfred Auerback (1959–60). The gallantry of the "knights" is still visible, but the effectiveness of their leadership has grown considerably, and they are more comfortable with the Board's rules of engagement. A number of Assembly Speakers have subsequently been elected president of the APA. These include Robert Garber (Speaker in 1963–4 and President in 1970–1), Perry Talkington (Speaker in 1969–70 and President in 1972–3), Robert Pasnau (Speaker in 1979–80 and President in 1986–7), Lawrence Hartmann (Speaker in 1981–2 and President in 1991–2), John McIntyre (Speaker in 1988–9 and President in 1993–4) and, after my tenure, Richard Kent Harding (Speaker in 1995–6 and President in 2001–2). These Speaker-Presidents have a unique and valuable knowledge of the inner workings of the APA and of its full range of issues.

When I attend the Assembly, I see the enormous progress that has been made in its deliberations and its forcefulness. I do occasionally note, however, some concern about receiving the Board's full attention and understanding. The APA governance is close to being a bicameral system, but the Board still possesses the final authority.

I also have noted the Assembly's respect for and support of Jay Scully in his CEO's responsibilities as part of being medical director. His commitment to the Assembly is visible and very important.

BOARD OF TRUSTEES

The Board of Trustees meets several times during the year, including one three-day session for an annual policy review. Most of the decisions discussed throughout this book are the products of Board action. The Board pays close attention to budget committee proposals, recommendations from the Assembly and the staff, and the overall committee structure of the APA. In an attempt to make the Board more efficient in the early postwar years, a small executive committee of the Board was established. Nonmembers of the Executive Committee objected to being "excluded," and the Board reverted to consistent full meetings. Each year the Board holds closed sessions in order to deliberate confidential matters such as ethical charges against members. In recent years the Board has invited presentations from district branch presidents, from leaders of other organizations, and from government officials. The Board's relationship with NAMI has also become quite close.

The active participation by elected members-in-training has been notable. A cadre of future national leaders is being prepared, and the current leadership of the trainees is already making an important contribution. They are extremely active!

The medical director provides a detailed report at every meeting of the Board and most often leads the implementation of Board action. Dr. Scully's recent appointment as CEO is significant; it is a vote of confidence and a more realistic definition of responsibility. I was fortunate that I could negotiate with the presidents in order to achieve most of my goals. During my time at the APA, the organization adopted an emergency action procedure for decisions that needed to be made between Board meetings. An action could be taken if agreed upon by the president, the speaker of the Assembly, and the medical director. These actions were reviewed at the next Board meeting, and, with very rare exceptions, they were endorsed.

The APA has a vast number of component task forces, committees, commissions, joint commissions, and councils. Like all other large organizations, it employs its own bureaucratic language. The word *joint*, as used by the APA, refers to dual reporting lines to both the Board and the Assembly. The Councils refer to the major topical areas (e.g., child, research), with numerous task forces and committees under each Council's jurisdiction. Task forces are time-limited components; committees are not so limited. During the fall, all the component groups meet together; some meet on several other occasions in addition to the fall meeting. Through this system a constant flow of new recommendations are proposed for action by the Board and the Assembly.

JOINT REFERENCE COMMITTEE

To facilitate consideration and coordination of new recommendations from a variety of sources, the APA established a Joint Reference Committee (JRC), co-chaired by the president-elect and the speaker-elect, with members including the chairs of the Councils and the medical director as a voting member. I was particularly proud of this capacity, it being the only component on which the medical director had a formal vote. To have such a vote was a special opportunity to take part in debates—a function in contrast to my usual role, which heavily depended on my capacity to persuade. The distinction was less important in reality, but it seemed to satisfy some inner need for me. The JRC operated primarily as an inflow apparatus and facilitator for the Board and the Assembly. It could anticipate what might be discussed and clarify the decision-making process. Staffed very ably during my tenure by Claudia Hart, it was a focal point for coordinating governance on issues formulated by our committee structure to be considered by our Assembly and Board. For some leaders of the APA, the need for these discussions at the JRC slowed the process of decision making. On frequent occasions, efforts were made to bypass the JRC and go directly to the Board or the Assembly. After I left the APA, I was told about many efforts to improve the JRC system. Whatever means are employed, large organizations need specific mechanisms to coordinate diverse governance systems.

APA STAFF

The APA staff has been discussed in several chapters of this book. Its primary responsibilities involved implementing governance decisions under the direction of the medical director. By and large, I have been enormously pleased with staff; there were inevitably a few appointees who did not achieve what I expected, and occasionally I had to make changes. I have been criticized by some for making too many changes, and by others for not making changes quickly enough, especially during my last two years. Fortunately, in the overwhelming majority of cases, the staff was excellent, with a very high retention rate. I am pleased that

I was able to augment the staff with several new offices and functions (i.e., government affairs, public affairs, research, education, publishing, Annual Meetings, and business administration) (see Appendix 7 for APA organizational charts from 1986 and 2008). All chiefs of departments met with me each week in a group that I called "The Cabinet." For me, and I think for all the participants, the system worked well and was indispensable for carrying out the organizational changes.

Many staff responsibilities involved complex administrative arrangements. The journal editors-in-chief, for example, reported directly to the Board and supervised the work of journal staff; the Medical Director determined the salaries and promotions for the journal staff in conjunction with the editors-in-chief.

The APPI system involved a separate administrative structure. I was president of the APPI Board for many years and appointed its Editor. After my departure a new system of administering APA research and educational grants, through the American Psychiatric Institute for Research and Education (APIRE), was established; this enabled the APA to receive research contracts more efficiently.

Occasionally, the APA developed new and often complex administrative systems that were helpful for certain sections of our membership. Some of these programs did well for several years but could not be maintained permanently. In the late 1970s CHAMPUS, the medical insurance component of the Department of Defense, negotiated a contract with the APA to help in administering peer review of the practice of many psychiatrists. In order to get reimbursement for their patient care, a practitioner would submit his bill to CHAMPUS, which then asked the APA office for its recommendation about payment. Norman Penner, who administered that very large project, was able and knowledgeable; ultimately, however, there were problems with the APA administering a program that required taking increasingly restrictive action about its own members' reimbursement. The project was useful for many practitioners but problematic for others. Can a national membership organization be a proper reviewer of its members' practice without alienating many of them? Ultimately, the Department of Defense did not renew APA's contract, awarding it to another agency, perhaps better able to be objective.

At one stage we attempted to provide malpractice insurance for our members when few other providers were available. The program, which was administered by Beverly Patrick, was helpful, but the complexity of dealing with large malpractice suits made this task very difficult. These programs also required special governance systems and reporting mechanisms. For years, Alan Levenson, chairman of the Department of Psychiatry at the University of Arizona, who worked with our supervisory malpractice board, reported at every Board and Assembly meeting. He was extremely knowledgeable, but the administrative tasks required much explanation and occasional debate. Ultimately, with the leadership of Joseph English and others, the APA was able to terminate the program, with other insurance groups taking over the responsibility.

Our ethics system also needed unique reporting mechanisms and confidentiality. The APA investigated ethics charges against our members more assiduously than did any other medical specialty. Ultimately we used a quasi-legal system to investigate ethical complaints. On two occasions serious complaints were made against APA former presidents, with the complainants publicizing their allegations. These newspaper and television exposés gave rise to some of the most difficult situations of my tenure as medical director. We had to protect the APA and our profession against the claims of some critics that the ethical violations typified the behavior of most psychiatrists. At the same time we needed to assure the public that there would be no tolerance for any unethical behavior in our profession. Carol Davis, my administrative assistant, was the staff person responsible for coordinating the ethics program and did a magnificent job, often working closely with our legal counsel and our Ethics Committee. It has not been easy to maintain appropriate confidentiality in a ethics system embedded within a large medical association. Nevertheless, I was proud of our accomplishments in this difficult area. In Chapter 9 ("Forensic Psychiatry") I discuss some issues about unethical behavior that overlapped with legal questions.

The APA's constitution, by-laws, and operations manual are also very important standards in shaping our policies and determining our boundaries. During the first two post-war decades, much was accomplished to establish these documents. The APA Board of Trustees, formerly known as the Council of the APA, held a meeting in 1969 initiated by President Blain. He asked, "Is the American Psychiatric Association organized to play its appropriate role in dealing with existing problems and pressures which confront the profession of psychiatry as a whole and if not what changes could be made?" Ultimately, the conference recommended a series of constitutional changes that achieved a new organizational structure (see Appendix 14) Later, with the recommendations of the Key Conference and clarification of the role of the Assembly, the current governance system was put into place. Occasionally, some of the most controversial issues of the organization were dealt with by membership referenda. The decision to maintain the 1981 Annual Meeting in New Orleans was upheld by a membership referendum. The decision to delete the classification of homosexuality as a mental disorder was also upheld by a referendum, as discussed in Chapter 13. During the postwar years, constitutional changes were also voted on by the general membership. As already discussed, efforts to make the Assembly the ultimate decision maker failed to achieve the required two-thirds majority.

For all the problems, some ambiguities, and occasional conflict about policy, the APA has been able to carry out basic changes in the profession. Determined leadership and a democratic governance system have created a stronger American psychiatry.

REFERENCES

American Psychiatric Association: Diagnostic and Statistical Manual of Mental Disorders, 3rd Edition. Washington, DC, American Psychiatric Association, 1980

Barton WE: The History and Influence of the American Psychiatric Association. Washington, DC, American Psychiatric Press, 1987

Blumenfield M: Interview with former APA President Alfred M. Freedman, M.D. July 14, 2007. Available as Shrinkpod podcast at: http://www.shrinkpod.com/index.php?post_id=235177. Accessed December 19, 2007.

Hartmann L: Homosexuality and ignorance. The John Fryer Award Lecture, presented at the 160th annual meeting of the American Psychiatric Association, San Diego, CA, May 23, 2007

Kandel ER: Psychiatry, Psychoanalysis, and the New Biology of Mind. Washington, DC, American Psychiatric Publishing, 2005

Sabshin M: Administering a national medical association: the joys, the sorrows, and other challenges. New Dir Ment Health Serv 49:31–39, 1991

Shorter E: A History of Psychiatry: From the Era of the Asylum to the Age of Prozac. New York, Wiley, 1997

17

Management of External Relationships

*T*he pattern, intensity, and the management of relationships held by an organization with other groups are often more revealing indicators of basic priorities than any other measure. These relationships have been discussed in other chapters in the book; in this chapter the emphasis is upon how a profession manages these interactions and decides their relevance. While the American Psychiatric Association has devised, from time to time, a membership administrative structure to coordinate these external relationships, the staff also has had the major responsibility for implementing the full range of these liaison activities. The medical director has been, in effect, the primary facilitator of these connections on a de facto basis, since his or her relationship with other organizations' staff and membership is most prolonged and visible. For other organizations it is practical to keep one person in mind as the key liaison official. Of course, the medical director must delegate most of the day-to-day responsibilities to other APA staff, but it is he who must make the ultimate decision about how much staff time and resources are appropriate. He must also decide where he should play a personal role in these activities and how much time he should allocate to them. I was, for example, an elected officer of the World Psychiatric Association and found that to be a useful way to keep informed and play an active role in international work. However, I refused to be considered as a presidential candidate of that organization, as I believed that holding such an office would require too much of my time and also could constitute a conflict of interest. In the chapter on international affairs (see Chapter 7), the APA's relationship with international organizations is described as an area of special importance to many areas of APA's goals, such as education, research, and fiscal issues, that are not fully appreciated by the membership as a whole but that are high on my list of priorities. It was quite a struggle to maintain our international activities, and I regretted that the Office of International Affairs, which had been extremely important in developing and coordinating that area of our work, was closed soon after my retirement.

I maintained close ties with the leadership and staff of the American Medical Association (AMA). Later, in parallel with the remedicalization of psychiatry, APA leadership became much more active in the AMA and in other medical organizations. As of 2008, APA membership leaders and staff (e.g., Jeremy Lazarus, Jay Scully) have assumed major leadership roles in the AMA. The present medical director has wisely chosen to give this area high priority. The close liaison relationships with the AMA and other specialty groups are a significant sign of the changes in psychiatry during the last quarter of the century. While there have been exceptional individuals who have represented psychiatry in the AMA (e.g., Lindsey Beaton), the current number of psychiatric leaders at local, state, and national levels of the AMA is much larger, and their influence is stronger than ever. The relationship is broadly systemic and not based on personal ties. Our alliance with the AMA is a major example of how the APA has changed in recent times. In turn, the AMA's increasing support of parity for reimbursement for psychiatric patients has been integral in the achievement of success in this important goal.

The remedicalization of the psychiatric profession has also strengthened the APA's close relationship with other medical specialties and societies. With the development of several psychiatric subspecialties, the organizations representing these subspecialties have become central to the liaison functions with related medical organizations. The child psychiatry–pediatrics relationship has many nuanced implications, including preparation of a new combined specialty of pediatrics and psychiatry. Geriatric psychiatrists are closely allied with several geriatric medical groups. Forensic psychiatry is an important part of forensic medicine, and addiction psychiatry is a central part of the work of many groups involved with addiction treatment and management. Psychosomatic medicine (formerly psychosomatic psychiatry or consultation-liaison psychiatry) is now much more relevant to and intertwined with many medical speciality societies and functions. The APA has close ties with the American Board of Medical Specialties and is a respected participant in its deliberations. The remedicalization of psychiatry is well illustrated by its strong links with the rest of medicine at many levels. The current APA medical director is particularly active in monitoring these relationships and following up on the policy questions arising from the discussions.

A much smaller number of psychiatric patients are now hospitalized in state mental health facilities than during the peak period of the 1970s. The length of stay in private psychiatric hospitals is now much reduced from that time (Hudley et al. 1998), and more psychiatric patients are hospitalized in general hospital units than ever before (Mechanic et al. 1998).

The net effect of the changes in the meaning of psychiatric hospitalization have many implications for current organizational relationships as well as for psychiatric practice patterns. The APA works very closely with the American Hospital Association to monitor the new relationships. It also keeps close ties to organizations representing general hospital psychiatric groups and private psychiatric hospital associations.

In 1974, when I became the APA's medical director, our liaison functions with state hospital and community center psychiatrists were particularly close. There was a very special role at the APA for psychiatrists who served as state commissioners of mental health (Ulett et al. 1971). Over time, however, psychiatrist commissioners have been replaced by nonmedical administrators; this change in the role of administrators has also occurred at the level of single-hospital directorship. Many psychiatrists, of course, continue to work as salaried employees in community clinics and state hospitals, but their *formal* relationship to the APA is not quite as intense as it once was. In Chapter 18 ("Social and Community Psychiatry"), there is a more detailed discussion of psychiatry's relationship with social and community organizations, including the possibilities of a revitalization of these fields. Many of the liaison functions with these groups are now provided by the relevant APA committee and Council structure. When the APA had a Council on Professions and Associations, it kept track of the interactions. Today, it is the medical director who manages most of the contacts.

Psychiatrists' status in leadership roles at medical schools has increased during recent decades. A significant number have been appointed as deans of medical schools during the last quarter of a century. Previously, a few extraordinarily able psychiatrists had become deans. In most cases their selection was based more on their individual leadership talents than on systemic issues such as the integral importance of the department of psychiatry to the school. Today, many departments of psychiatry play a powerful role in the overall administration of the school. Psychiatrists have also been increasingly active on Admission Committees for selecting medical students. Their involvement in research policy has also increased considerably in recent years. Our Office of Education and Office of Research work in close coordination with academic medical systems and many organizations that relate to them.

As discussed in the chapter on research, one of the most interesting developments in American psychiatry during the last 25 years has been the change in the choice of chairpersons for academic departments of psychiatry. By the 1960s more than half of the departmental chairs had formal training as psychoanalysts (Eckhardt 1978). Currently, very few have such credentials. Search committees for new chairs of academic departments of psychiatry value research expertise in biological and neuroscientific areas as the cardinal criteria for choosing a chairperson. It should be noted that occasionally the number of chairs occupied by analysts from 1945 through 1975 has been exaggerated. For example, Eysenck contended, in 1952, that most chairs were held by analysts (Eysenck 1952). As important as psychoanalysis was in medical school education and in psychiatry as a whole, Eysenck's claim was not entirely accurate. A few medical schools in the postwar period—for example Washington University and the University of Iowa—chose leaders from biological psychiatry. Psychodynamic educators did have a dominant role, however, during the postwar years. Conferences in academic psychiatry clearly reflected the intense commitment to psychodynamic education by psychiatric departments (Mitchell and Whitehorn 1952, 1953; Krug and Lourie 1964). It was a unique and very special opportunity for a major role in psychiatric education. Today, the department chairs group has changed considerably, and the neuroscientific dominance in academic psychiatry has affected the ties of chairs to the APA. APA Medical Director Scully has worked hard to maintain the APA linkage with academic psychiatry, and the APA's organizational closeness is also augmented by our Department of Government Relations, Division of Research, and Division of Education.

Relationships with several other organizations are also good examples of a changing American psychiatry. For about 25 years after World War II, many psychoanalysts served in major leadership roles in the APA itself. The APA and the American Psychoanalytic Association maintained joint leadership consultations on a very close basis. For many years, their leadership held meetings during the annual Mid-Winter Convention of the American Psychoanalytic Association in New York. In more recent years, reflecting changes in the relationship between psychoanalysis and psychiatry, these special meetings were discontinued. While the American Psychoanalytic Association accepted representation in a newly reorganized APA Assembly, this was no longer an exclusive role. Analysts are still important for the APA, but a very special attachment is no longer present. In 1991, the American Psychoanalytic Association opened up full membership to nonphysicians, which reduced the unique tie that it had held with the APA (Gifford 2005). The changed relationship between psychiatry and psychoanalysis is explored in detail in Chapter 8 ("Psychoanalysis").

Relationships with the American Psychological Association also changed significantly after the 1970s. As discussed in Chapter 6 ("En Route to Equity"), clinical psychology became much more competitive with psychiatry throughout the last quarter of the twentieth century. Formal relationships with the American Psychological Association have become strained, although many cooperative relationships continue at APA district branch levels and in some areas of advocacy. However, the psychologists' efforts to obtain prescription privileges prevent the establishment of an even more cooperative program.

Our relationship with psychiatric nursing has also been an important reflection of changing times. During the postwar years the ties between psychiatrists and psychiatric nurses were significant especially in the hospital management context. Even during the era of psychodynamic dominance, the doctor–nurse relationship in a psychiatric context paralleled that relationship in the rest of medicine; the nurse was subordinate and followed the "doctor's orders." Over time, however, psychiatric nursing became increasingly sophisticated and independent; no one knew the ward milieu better than the nurses on duty in the psychiatric unit; they often were the chief organizers of the ward. As psychopharmacology grew in importance, psychiatric nurses played a key role in the entire medication process. Nursing education in pharmacology and many other medical subjects has been superior to that of most clinical psychologists. Psychiatrists have been less opposed to nurses having some prescription privileges than they have been to such privileges these being given to psychologists. Recently, academic activities of psychiatric nurses have become much stronger than ever before. Psychiatric nursing has also assumed new administrative roles in outpatient and community clinics. In addition, nursing groups have significantly increased their influence in government affairs. During the post–World War II years, the relationship between the APA and major nursing associations—the American Nursing Association and the National League of Nursing—were closer than they are today, but many policy alliances have continued in joint legislative efforts.

Psychiatric social work has also achieved a much more independent status in the last quarter of a century. During the era of the powerful influence of psychoanalysis upon psychiatric institutions, many social workers strongly adhered to this trend and assumed major leadership roles in analytically oriented clinics. Occasionally, they balanced psychoanalysis with a special blend of "real world" acuity in placements for patients and fiscal support. In recent years, psychiatric social work has assumed diverse functions in psychiatric systems. Many psychiatric social workers have continued to demonstrate interest in psychoanalytic training, aided recently by the changes in psychoanalytic institute admission practices, and have contributed significantly to the psychoanalytic literature.

Psychiatry still holds important ties with other mental health organizations but is no longer the undisputed leader of a constellation of mental health disciplines. New alliances have been established, and APA's relationship with the National Alliance on Mental Illness (NAMI) is closer than ever before. The award presented to NAMI's president, Suzanne Vogel-Scibilia, at the APA 2007 Annual Meeting in San Diego (see Plate 14) reflects APA's respect for and reliance on NAMI.

The conflict with clinical psychology over prescription privileges is still active, but there are new ties between psychiatry, cognitive psychology, and neuropsychology. Psychiatrists' relationships with psychoanalysis and social psychiatric groups have weakened. On the other hand, psychiatry's relationship with the rest of medicine has improved dramatically in recent times. Psychiatry's current organizational relationships reflect its stronger medical identity and clearer professional boundaries. I believe that many of the APA liaison functions can be decentralized to our relevant committee structures and our various office staffs. It is an area, however, that requires special attention and coordination by the medical director. In selecting future medical directors, the capacity to work in many areas of liaison relationships should be explicit. Dr. Scully is a superb model for how the job should be done.

REFERENCES

Eckhardt MH: Organizational schisms in American psychoanalysis, in American Psychoanalysis: Origins and Development. Edited by Quen JM, Carlson ET. New York, Brunner/Mazel, 1978

Eysenck HJ. The effects of psychotherapy: an evaluation. Journal of Consulting Psychology 16:319–324, 1952

Gifford S: Psychoanalysis in North America from 1895 to the present, in The American Psychiatric Publishing Textbook of Psychoanalysis. Edited by Person ES, Cooper AM, Gabbard GO. Washington, DC, American Psychiatric Publishing, 2005, pp 387–405

Hudley D, Cho D, Christman J, et al: Predicting length of stay in an acute psychiatric hospital. Psychiatr Serv 49:1049–1053, 1998

Krug O, Lourie RS (eds): Career Training in Child Psychiatry. Report of the Conference on Training in Child Psychiatry, Washington, DC, January 10–15, under the auspices of the American Academy of Child Psychiatry and the American Psychiatric Association. Washington, DC, American Psychiatric Association, 1964

Mechanic D, McAlpine DD, Olfson M: Changing patterns of psychiatric inpatient care in the United States, 1988–1994. Arch Gen Psychiatry 55:785–791, 1998

Mitchell J McK, Whitehorn JC (eds): Psychiatry and medical education. Report of a conference held at Cornell University in 1951 under the auspices of the American Psychiatric Association and the Association of American Medical Colleges. Washington, DC, American Psychiatric Association, 1952

Mitchell J McK, Whitehorn JC (eds): The psychiatrist: his training and development. Report of a conference held in at Cornell University in 1952 under the auspices of the American Psychiatric Association and the Association of American Medical Colleges. Washington, DC, American Psychiatric Association, 1953

Ulett GA, Schnibbe H, Ganser LJ, et al: Mental health director: bird of passage. Am Jo Psychiatry 127:1550–1554, 1971

18

Social and Community Psychiatry

*D*uring the 1960s and 1970s I became a strong advocate for social and community psychiatry, perhaps bordering on being an ideologue. Throughout my early career, I had been impressed with the insufficiently acknowledged impact of social factors on much of psychopathology. The pioneering work of Hollingshead and Redlich on the relationship between social class and mental illness (Hollingshead and Redlich 1958) reaffirmed my belief that the prevailing psychoanalytic focus upon intrapsychic phenomena underestimated the social system's role in pathogenesis. The demonstration by these distinguished authors that the prevalence of mental illnesses such as schizophrenia correlated with patients' social class was strong evidence of a perspective that should be investigated further. The presence of poverty, recent immigration, deleterious educational practices, and disordered family interaction all affected who became mentally ill. During my psychiatric residency at Tulane I was impressed by Kardiner's transcultural findings that diverse social patterns of child rearing and the presence of primitive religious beliefs, for example, had a profound effect on subsequent adaptation and maladaptation (Kardiner 1945; Kardiner and Linton 1939; Kardiner and Ovesey 1951). The work of Stanton (Stanton and Schwartz 1954) and of Caudill (Caudill et al. 1952) also shaped my opinion that individual psychotherapy could be significantly influenced by its social context. The social milieu of the psychiatric hospital, for example, could facilitate or hinder the patient's progress in

244 Changing American Psychiatry: A Personal Perspective

psychotherapy. It could even affect the choice and evaluation of psychopharmacological medication (Sabshin and Ramot 1956).

The impact of economic factors on mental illness has also been recognized to be of fundamental importance (Brenner 1973). For years in the Soviet Union and China it was asserted that all mental illnesses were a product of economic conditions. That opinion has changed considerably in Russia and in China with all the social changes and the introduction of modern psychiatric services. Global economic conditions, however, are essential for the understanding of mental illness in many parts of the world (Kleinman and Cohen 1997). Even in the relatively affluent United States, our own history of neglect and warehousing of patients had a profound effect on the psychiatric care available to the poor (Deutsch 1948).

When community psychiatry first became a popular national movement, it made a lot of sense. My own somewhat idiosyncratic concept of community psychiatry emphasized its role as an application of social psychiatric principles within a defined geographic area. Social psychiatry in that context was primarily a theoretical field that postulated the relevance of social variables to the causes of mental illnesses and their treatment and prevention (Sabshin 1966). These concepts never really prevailed in the organization of the community programs that were implemented in the 1970s. In fact, community psychiatry essentially became a system to provide varying levels of mental health services closer to the patient's living area to which many of them had returned after massive deinstitutionalization. That aim was worthwhile in itself, but even the less complex goal of basic service provision rather than a community-wide mental health delivery system was only partially implemented. The idea of understanding the impact of each community's particular social structure on the mental health needs of its population was a lofty goal but not a practical target in mid–twentieth century United States. It is an idea that, if it had been attempted, would have been very expensive, and its effectiveness would have been limited by the absence of clear scientific principles. Furthermore, many states that tried to reduce the number of hospitalized patients in the 1970s were primarily interested in lowering their mental health expenditures by caring for fewer patients, and the creation of a fully functioning community system would have been much too expensive. I did not grasp then that social psychiatry was not well understood and also that my definitions of social and community psychiatry were somewhat naïve.

I did play a role in assisting in the organization of an innovative and successful community program. The fascinating work of Kellam, Schiff, and Futterman in developing a project in the Woodlawn neighborhood in South Chicago was a good example of an imaginative, well-planned program. With my support, the Yale-trained group moved to Chicago from New Haven, and I participated in their decision to focus heavily on a systematic public school intervention. They identified children vulnerable to having problems in school and provided various types of social psychological support. They evaluated their results carefully (Kellam et al. 1975). Ultimately, the program was transferred from the University of Illinois to the University of Chicago and served as a national model of a significant type of community psychiatric service with an emphasis on prevention. Select programs, like this one in Chicago, were more feasible than a multipurpose complex system. Kellam, Schiff, and Futterman were pioneers in evidence-based social psychiatric intervention. In my later years I have thought more of what they accomplished in their project, and I will describe one aspect of this achievement later in the chapter.

When I left Chicago to become medical director of the APA, I did not maintain the special personal involvement in creating new social and community psychiatry projects that I had supported earlier. I was deeply involved in decisions about the APA's journal *Hospital and Community Psychiatry* and our annual Institute meeting on that subject. The renaming of the journal as *Psychiatric Services* aptly reflected efforts for more effective integration of care. My interest in the full panoply of issues relevant to social psychiatry was still high, but my major attention had to be given to the promotion of what I conceived to be an evidence-based nosological and therapeutic system of psychiatry. In all likelihood, however, my ideological fervor had cooled.

The work on DSM-III (American Psychiatric Association 1980) and DSM-IV (American Psychiatric Association 1994) was illustrative of the major areas of the APA's programmatic goal during the 1980s and 1990s. There was substantial interest in the inclusion of social psychiatric and transcultural data, but our capacity to employ the available data in those DSM volumes within the new multiaxial system was somewhat limited at that time. It is to be hoped that we have now reached the point where more appropriate emphasis in the upcoming DSM-V can be placed on transcultural and social factors relevant to nosology.

Just as the consideration of how psychological variables affected mental illness, social psychiatry in the postwar period had been mired in ideological conflicts. Specific data were not central to some of the stances that the APA advocated. Our social policy positions sometimes included moral righteousness, but the research evidence was not strong enough to buttress our specific positions on poverty, on the quality of public education, on health system reform, and on the Vietnam war. Many of us behaved as if social psychiatry were defined as the professional opinions by psychiatrists on current social issues.

At present, the convergence of several factors has helped to transform social psychiatry into to a more evidence-based field. Psychiatric epidemiology has changed dramatically in the latter part of the twentieth century. Nosological clarification has increased the reliability of prevalence and new incidence data collection round the world. Forty years ago, the report of a very high rate of neuroses in the United States and their near absence in Chinese studies was questioned by many observers.

The addition of "and Psychiatric Epidemiology" to the title of the journal *Social Psychiatry* was another sign of the importance of comparative data. The journal, edited in Germany, has been a strong bastion of social psychiatry. For many years European psychiatry has been more receptive to the field in a practical empirical fashion (Hafner and Heiden 1978). Darrel Regier's appointment to the journal's Editorial Board was an important sign that his major research role could also facilitate a new scientific advance of social psychiatry in the United States (Regier et al. 1993). Support by other American psychiatric leaders, such as Lawrence Hartmann and Zebulon Taintor in the American Society of Social Psychiatry, will also be very important.

From my perspective there are many vital issues in American psychiatry that include plausible hypotheses about the role of social variables. If we can accept and vigorously implement a biopsychosocial model, we can begin more systematic efforts to explore the relevant social psychiatric hypotheses. Perhaps we might also begin to formulate new theoretical models to link precisely the relevance of these variables to particular mental illnesses and their treatment. There are many examples of areas where social psychiatric hypotheses at various levels could have potential importance in psychiatry.

The impact of poverty on mental illness is best investigated by a biopsychosocial model. Indeed, I believe that it cannot be studied adequately without such a model. The transaction of social factors with biological and psychological variables in poverty will be important for the elucidation of etiology, for planning for the most effective treatment, and, ultimately, for the primary prevention of mental illness. Under conditions of poverty, there is clearly a higher prevalence of mental illness; by and large poor people seek help later than those with more resources. They are also less capable of compliance with appropriate treatments, primarily but not exclusively because of medication costs. These social class distinctions exist in all of medicine in the United States, but it is plausible to hypothesise today that social variables are even more directly and predictably related to the pathogenesis of mental illness. During this phase of hypothesis development, the understanding of macro and micro social variables should become increasingly important to investigators. To what extent did social isolation, poverty, and poor education in the presence of certain personality configurations contribute to the "hysterical" paralyses of the early twentieth century in France and Austria? (see Micale 1993). How do we explain the lower prevalence of the symptomatology today in Western Europe? Progress in genomic understanding is not likely to provide the total answer.

A higher prevalence of major mental illnesses in immigrant families (Kinzie 2006) poses a serious research question for some neuroscientific investigators. Most of them, however, recognize that sociocultural problems play a role in pathogenesis. The question is how do these systems interact? Why some children of vulnerable immigrant families adapt very well throughout their lives is a question that will also attract increasing attention. Resilience in these families may be determined by genetic influences, but social psychological hypotheses about factors that facilitate resilience are also relevant.

Gender differences in prevalence and symptomatology of mental illness are biologically induced by their basic definition. For most of history, the social roles of women were affected by blatant biases and discrimination that affected prevalence and incidence of mental disorders. To what extent will this change as biases decrease and glass ceilings begin to be broken? How much are so-called gender differences in certain intellectual activities a product of biological destiny and/or the complex result of social psychological phenomena? For centuries it has been assumed that superb skills in playing chess were genetically determined. Up until recently, despite intense efforts to educate many young girls in chess theory and practice, there were very few female grandmasters. Now it appears that a proportionately larger number of young women grandmasters are competing in China. How can this higher rate of superb competence be explained? Will increasing numbers of superbly gifted women mathematicians and physicists also result from long term social change?

Males have also been more vulnerable to some mental illnesses. How much these vulnerabilities are products of social expectations and conflicts about prevailing values is a fundamental question. Has the masculine role function of being the sole breadwinner changed in a way that decreases the self-esteem of some men? How do such reactions precipitate a clinical depression? Equally important is how some men experience the loss of self-esteem but "adapt" without less effective defensive manoeuvres.

There are biological tendencies that have a major impact on families and group phenomena. Attachment between mother and baby is genetically influenced, but here few would argue that social psychological variables are not also of major importance. Research on the long-term consequences of attachment is extremely important. The drive to congregate in groups varies among individuals, but it is also influenced by cultural patterns. Family and group approaches to treatment should remain very important to psychiatrists, even if most of such treatment today is conducted by other mental health therapists. The relevance of group and family systems to psychiatric disorder is still vital for psychiatrists to understand and to employ. A psychiatry that abandons such an interest could be neglecting important elements of hypothesis generation about etiology and therapy.

The role of the family in causing an increase in the prevalence of certain mental illnesses has become somewhat controversial during the last thirty years. Reacting in part to the highly questionable allegations about "schizophrenogenic" mothers, a large group of family members of schizophrenia patients, The National Alliance on Mental Illness (NAMI; formerly National Alliance for the Mentally Ill) has successfully organized a powerful group to advocate a genetic theory of etiology for the better understanding and treatment of their children's severe disorders. To be effective in this advocacy, they have found it valuable to emphasize that the parents' behavior, especially that of the mother, did not cause the illness; genetic factors were responsible. I believe that NAMI has been a powerful and effective research force, but the possible role of family members in their child's development whether positive or negative should not be restricted because of its previous misuse. The genetic factors are vital, but they may not always provide the total answer. Of course, the position opposite to NAMI's stance had been dominant and damaging for a long time and required a strong counter measure. Nevertheless, the APA and NAMI should support unfettered evidence-based understanding of severe mental illness. In the long run, this commitment will be even more effective for the best treatment of the severely mentally ill.

The genetic and biological factors governing sexual behaviour are predominant today, as is proper. Nevertheless social psychological variables are important for a more complete understanding of the subject. Freud's basic concepts of psychosexual development were heavily influenced by his cultural milieu. He stressed the power of "instinctive" forces, but his theories were affected by his society's strong prohibitions. How would he deal with today's much more explicit discussion of sexuality? Would he acknowledge that social factors were underestimated in his theories? I doubt that there would be a full acknowledgment. I believe that Freud would question whether the alleged "freedom" is a type of reaction formation in which people are still dealing with sexual anxieties but perhaps in a different way than in 1890s Vienna. From my perspective, however, to neglect the social psychological aspects of sexual behavior would be unscientific.

The basic causes of homosexuality are genetic. The movement to liberate homosexuals from restrictive and other abusive treatment has depended a great deal on being able to explain the behavior as induced by inherited, irrepressible biological drives. Even with this dominant biological perspective, the biopsychosocial approach has relevance. Under certain social conditions, such as prisons and boarding schools, homosexual tendencies may become more overt. What role exactly do the social variables play in this process? How much of the behavior is dependent on release of inhibitions, or is there a new drive stimulated by the milieu? This is still a tender question but I hope that when less defensiveness is required, all relevant biopsychosocial variables might be explored. I am proud that I was a leader in the removal of homosexuality from the DSM, and I recognize the social and the political consequences of the decision in addition to its scientific importance. But I believe that research on the sociopsychological aspects of homosexual development should not be forbidden territory.

Studies of a full life cycle also require an approach that includes the exploration of social variables relevant to each phase of life. Childhood and adolescent psychiatry need to be closely tied to social psychiatric understanding as well as to their relationship to rapidly changing biological systems. Teenagers are indeed influenced by peer culture in their basic attitudes toward the use of addictive drugs, alcohol, sexual behavior, and education. Biological destiny for the prevalence of psychiatric disorders during adolescence has dominated American psychiatry. Biology must be taken into account in any explanation of pressures on teenagers, but understanding how some adolescents cope resiliently with these pressures may be very significant for new hypotheses (Offer and Offer 1973; Offer and Sabshin 1966).

The social psychological aspects of geriatric psychiatry are also vital for the progress of that field. With the ever-increasing average life expectancy, great changes have occurred in the image of the American elderly population. The very meaning of the word "old" is decidedly different today. Many 60-year-olds currently behave as 40-year-olds did half a century ago. The biological aspects of aging still, of course, are central, but the social psychological supports for coping have become increasingly pertinent. Communities supporting retirement age living demonstrate patterns of social and sexual behavior that were not prevalent half a century ago. Geriatric psychiatry is a rapidly growing field, but the importance of its biopsychosocial perspective has become increasingly apparent. Social factors have had a powerful effect on the entire life cycle and need special attention at each phase.

My work with Kellam, Schiff, and Futterman thirty years ago taught me how important a school system could be in a community psychiatry program. In recent years I have learned a great deal from my wife, Marion Bennathan, about the possibilities of schools being helpful to vulnerable children in a group setting by providing them with specific help for various developmental deficits. A number of psychiatrists and psychologists have made significant contributions to the overlapping fields of education and mental health.

James Comer of Yale University, in his School Development Program, has for many years been demonstrating how helping teachers to understand the meaning of their pupils' behavior, to see how the world of school looks to the child, can transform the management and teaching of children at risk of failure and help them to succeed (Comer 2005). William Granatir, a distinguished psychoanalyst in Washington, D.C., already in his eighties, has taught me a great deal about providing services in the school system. He has founded a charity to bring psychiatric support to troubled adolescents in Washington's inner-city schools. Young people in danger of social exclusion, who would certainly not of their own or their families' accord have sought help, responded to his counseling in their own socially familiar school setting (Granatir 2004). Other psychiatrists have expressed interest in this type of work, but it is a field that is yet to be fully developed.

In the United Kingdom, John Bowlby's attachment theory (Bowlby 1965) has been made widely known to educators by the work of "nurture groups." These are small classes in well over a thousand mainstream schools where children at risk of exclusion or academic and social failure are taught by two staff members, trained to offer emotional acceptance and to teach at the developmental stage the child has reached. The skills of relating positively to adults and to other children are demonstrated. Parents are welcomed into the classroom and family relationships improve (Bennathan and Boxall 2000). An extensive research project has shown remarkable gains for children in the group in attainment, in self-esteem, in attendance, and in family relationships. There is also a "whole school effect" as the entire staff group, who have been involved from the beginning in the setting up of the groups, understand better the origins of maladaptive behavior and begin to use the strategies they see succeeding in the group (Cooper and Whitebread 2007).

In the future of social and community psychiatry, the educational system can play a particularly valuable role in complementing the family's primary responsibility of facilitating healthier maturation of their children.

For most adults, the work environment plays an important role in mental health in addition to its basic economic function. The world of psychopathology has been enriched by a vocabulary of work stress and its consequences for physical and mental health. Does the word *burnout* have implications for a psychological meaning beyond physical exhaustion or a biological meaning beyond depression? How do problems in a marriage or in a family affect adaptation at work and vice versa? Coping with management styles, boredom, promotion strategy, gender, age and racial biases, and the threat of unemployment are examples of common problems that illustrate the biopsychosocial aspects of work. For many, however, work is gratifying, stimulating, and vital for their self esteem. As with the educational context for children, work experience is central to the well-being of men and for a rapidly increasing number of women.

A broader definition of community psychiatry includes schools, work settings, and place of residence. Social psychiatry has relevance for macro- and micro-organizational and group variables that can be related to the understanding of adaptation and mental disorder. Psychiatrists should continue to be actively involved in the inclusion of these variables as highly relevant to our understanding of mental illness. Genes, neurons, transmitters, and complex neural pathways are vital, but they respond to a changing context.

REFERENCES

American Psychiatric Association: Diagnostic and Statistical Manual of Mental Disorders, 3rd Edition. Washington, DC, American Psychiatric Association, 1980

American Psychiatric Association: Diagnostic and Statistical Manual of Mental Disorders, 4th Edition. Washington, DC, American Psychiatric Association, 1994

Bennathan M, Boxall M: Effective Intervention in Primary Schools: Nurture Groups, 2nd Edition. London, David Fulton, 2000

Bowlby J: Child Care and the Growth of Love, 2nd Edition. Chichester, UK, Penguin, 1965

Brenner MH: Mental Illness and the Economy. Cambridge, MA, Harvard University Press, 1973

Caudill W, Redlich FC, Gilmore HR, et al: Social structure and interaction processes on a psychiatric ward. Am J Orthopsychiatry 22:314–334, 1952

Comer JP: Leave No Child Behind: Preparing Today's Youth for Tomorrow's World. New Haven, CT, Yale University Press, 2005

Cooper P, Whitebread D: The effectiveness of nurture groups on student progress: evidence from a national research study. Emotional and Behavioural Difficulties 12(3):171–190, 2007

Deutsch A: The Shame of the States. New York, Harcourt, Brace, 1948

Granatir WL: A retired psychoanalyst volunteers to promote school-based mental health, in Analysts in the Trenches: Streets, Schools, War Zones. Edited by Sklarew B, Twemlow SW, Wilkinson S. Hillsdale, NJ, Analytic Press, 2004, pp 137–168

Hafner H, Heiden W an der (eds): Psychiatrische Epidemiologie : Geschichte, Einführung und ausgewählte Forschungsergebnisse. Berlin, Springer, 1978

Hollingshead AB, Redlich FC: Social Class and Mental Illness: A Community Study. New York, Wiley, 1958

Kardiner A: The Psychological Frontiers of Society. New York, Columbia University Press, 1945

Kardiner A, Linton R: The Individual and His Society: The Psychodynamics of Primitive Social Organization. New York, Columbia University Press, 1939

Kardiner A, Ovesey L: The Mark of Oppression: A Psychosocial Study of the American Negro. New York, WW Norton, 1951

Kellam SG, Branch JD, Agrawal KC, et al: Mental Health and Going to School: The Woodlawn Program of Assessment, Early Intervention, and Evaluation. Chicago, IL, University of Chicago Press, 1975

Kinzie JD: Immigrants and refugees: the psychiatric perspective. Transcult Psychiatry 43(4):577–591, 2006

Kleinman A, Cohen A: Psychiatry's global challenge. Sci Am 276(3):86–89, 1997

Micale MS: On the "disappearance" of hysteria: a study in the clinical deconstruction of a diagnosis. Isis 84(3):496–526, 1993

Offer D, Offer J: From Teenage to Young Manhood. New York, Basic Books, 1973

Offer D, Sabshin M (eds): Normality: Theoretical and Clinical Concepts of Mental Health. New York, Basic Books, 1966

Regier DA, Farmer ME, Rae DS, et al: One-month prevalence of mental disorders in the United States and sociodemographic characteristics: the Epidemiologic Catchment Area study. Acta Psychiatr Scand 88:35–47, 1993

Sabshin M: Theoretical models in community and social psychiatry, in Community Psychiatry. Edited by Roberts LM, Halleck S, Loeb M. Madison, University of Wisconsin Press, 1966

Sabshin M, Ramot J: Pharmacotherapeutic evaluations and the psychiatric setting. AMA Archives of Neurology and Psychiatry 75:342–373, 1956

Stanton AH, Schwartz MS: The Mental Hospital: A Study of Institutional Participation in Psychiatric Illness and Treatment. New York, Basic Books, 1954

19

Conclusions

*T*his book is a personal perspective on two periods of decisive change in American psychiatry since World War II. As I have stressed throughout the book, we are now entering a significantly new phase of decision making about American psychiatry's future course. As an active leader in the changes starting in the 1970s, I have attempted to formulate some of the basic reasons for the changes. In some cases I have differed from the historical accounts of other authors. I have expressed a preference for one of the options in the current debate about psychiatry's future, namely, a reformulated biopsychosocial model.

American psychiatry has survived a crisis that peaked in the 1970s. With the resolution of that conflict, the field has become a more respected part of medicine and its scientific credentials are now higher than ever before. For all the gains, however, American psychiatrists are severely challenged today, and no simple solutions are in sight. If we had not taken decisive action 30 years ago, I believe that the profession would have become isolated and marginalized. I recognize that most American psychiatrists practising today cannot empathize easily with a "What would have happened if we hadn't changed?" scenario. What they perceive are the harsh and occasionally irrational restrictions of today's managed care systems that limit whom they can treat, what therapies they can employ, and whether or not they will be reimbursed. Psychotherapy practice has been particularly discouraged under the new regime. The use of medication is encouraged but only in the context of the most efficient way to produce a rapid stabilization. Managed care does not facilitate a systematic approach for what is most important to the patient and his or her family in the long run. For many psychiatric patients such focus on shorter-term symptomatic relief may be inadequate for overall long-term improvement. The present care of the mentally ill is, in my judgment, superior to care based on previous ideological approaches, but America still lacks a mental health system that can genuinely serve the entire population.

It will be very difficult to change our current focus on immediate results. To change, we must first understand how we have reached the present system—its advantages and disadvantages—and how we might proceed to find better solutions. In this book I have concentrated on how we have previously addressed major problems, but I am also discussing how we might begin to deal with the current set of dilemmas.

Ebullience, optimism, and pride are not prominent features of today's psychiatric practitioners. There is a longing by many for an unfettered practice that might permit more time with patients without omnipresent restrictions. There is also a pervasive fantasy that in the distant past there was once a golden age during which psychiatrists were unregulated and free to choose their own type of practice.

In this book I have attempted to place our fantasies about the past and our dissatisfaction with the present in a historical context. For a brief time after World War II, there was indeed a period of special hope that most people with mental illness, especially veterans with traumatic neuroses, might be understood and helped. It was an exciting and happy time, during which massive increases occurred in the number of physicians entering psychiatry. It was also a period in which academic psychiatry grew exponentially. Influential psychiatrists addressed state legislatures about the importance of mental health and the message was heard. The National Institute of Mental Health (NIMH) was established and at first generously increased support for training. Jurists such as Judge David Bazelon made decisions based on optimistic interpretations of the status of psychiatric research. Psychoanalysis grew rapidly across parts of the country, accompanied by its open discussion of sexuality and aggression and its dynamic formulations of mental structure and disorder. The public seemed sympathetic.

That enormously exciting period stimulates the current fantasies of a golden age. As with most fantasies, however, there is a tendency to focus on the pleasurable features but to overlook aspects of reality that were problematic or contradictory. For most psychiatric patients the state mental health facilities, including its massive hospitals, were the chief providers of custodial mental health care. There were few evidence-based effective treatments available for the seriously ill, although electroconvulsive therapy, insulin, and fever therapy might be helpful for some patients (Noyes and Haydon 1940; Strecker et al. 1947). Psychoanalysis broadened its base, but its utilization was limited, and ultimately its formulations, brilliant and stimulating as they were, began to be seriously criticized by the families of mental patients, by policy makers, by investigators, and by many clinical psychiatrists, for their lack of objective scientific evidence. Psychiatry had become segmentalized into competing factions. The golden age in reality was a period in which ideologies prevailed and, eventually, the absence of the "emperor's clothing" became evident.

Most often, fantasies preserve hope and reduce dissatisfaction with the present. However, their distortions of reality may also contribute in the long run to an underlying pessimism, inhibiting long-term efforts at problem solving. Ultimately, American psychiatry recognized that it had fallen into an ideologically fashioned trap that required drastic change. It needed to extricate itself from a cultish morass and become an accountable, evidence-based part of medicine. Psychiatry changed itself radically, and its scientific status improved considerably. Description of that purposeful transition is the major aim of this book. But soon the profession faced new realities of a restrictive managed care system.

In presenting my perspective on a half century of change in psychiatry in the United States, I have criticized specific ideologies with a special emphasis on psychoanalysis and its ambiguous implications for policy. This book, however, takes a different position from that of Shorter, Andreasen, Torrey, Insel, and others who criticize psychoanalysis, describing it primarily as a "hiatus" or a false theory. These authors tend to dismiss the postwar psychodynamic psychiatry completely and to deny any of its relevance to the future. This rejection is easily extended by the critics to fundamental questions about the importance of psychological and social experiences in the etiology and treatment of mental disorders.

This point of view facilitates the belief of influential leaders that psychiatry should join with neurology in a new specialty of neuroscientific medicine. Kandel makes a very strong case for such a merger and believes that it is the only way to ensure a future for psychiatry (Kandel 2005). His eminent scientific status gives special weight to his recommendations. In my view, however, despite Kandel's fond reminiscences of his early psychodynamic training and his brilliant neuroanalytic research, his model would marginalize social and psychological variables in psychiatry. It would leave them as only occasional reminders of possible factors secondary to the primacy of disorders within the central nervous system. Other mental health professionals might be available to provide some psychological services, but psychiatrists would focus upon the fundamental brain dysfunctions that define mental illness. The psychiatrist would establish the diagnosis and then provide the appropriate medication or newer methods of clinical neuroscientific care.

There is an alternative model that employs a formerly compounded word, "bio-psycho-social" (Engel 1977, 1980). This approach to psychiatry is under attack today, especially by those who question the scientific relevance of the "psycho" and "social" parts of the model. I would agree with some of this criticism if "psycho-social" aspects of the field were still dominated by ideologues, but this is no longer predominantly the case. In fact, during the past two decades a scientific renaissance has begun at both the psychological and social level. Social psychiatry in Europe and the United States has progressed from an ideology to a much more empirically based field. I doubt, however, that a clinical neuroscientific speciality would focus adequately on social psychiatric systems. Social variables would be investigated primarily by specialists outside the field as is the case in most of social medicine. The powerful impact of social influences on every part of human development and psychopathology would inevitably be given less attention. Group structure, family dynamics, subcultures of addiction, school environments, social attitudes to aging, and a host of other macro- and microsocial systems would not easily fit into a clinical neuroscience model.

Enormous change is also occurring in the understanding of psychological variables. Psychoanalysis has begun to arouse itself from its prolonged clinging to old theories and is beginning to create new formulations and therapies (Fonagy and Target 2006; Gabbard 2007; Person et al. 2005). Fonagy's mentalization concept, for example, has interesting applications far beyond classical psychoanalysis. His ideas about the neuroanalytic scientific basis for mentalization could lead to a number of new hypotheses about pathogenesis and therapy. In addition, the recently developed *Psychoanalytic Diagnostic Manual* (Alliance of Psychoanalytic Organizations 2006) could open up new directions for psychodynamic models, but it also raises many questions. There is still insufficient acknowledgement or recognition of the weaknesses in hypothesis testing of many basic psychoanalytic principles. In Chapter 8 ("Psychoanalysis"), I indicated my hope that during the next two decades a new generation of analysts will begin to modify their field from one still dominated by many untested theoretical formulations to one that emphasizes hypothesis testing and the formation of new hypotheses. Psychiatry achieved a scientific transformation in the last few decades and is still recalibrating its impact. Psychoanalysis could also try to achieve a higher scientific status by supporting its own research and developing many research alliances. Whatever pathway is taken by psychoanalysis, psychiatry should attempt to strengthen its own efforts in psychosocial research and practice.

The increased interest in combining psychotherapy and pharmaco-therapy and the development of new forms of psychotherapy by psychiatrists and psychologists are indicators of continued progress, and they are full of promise for generating new hypotheses. I believe that support for this approach will grow considerably when the treatment limitations of pharmacotherapy alone become clearer. For each disorder, future evidence-based practice guidelines will presumably include more specific psychotherapeutic complements to medication. In some disorders after empirical studies the medication might even be utilized as a supplement to the basic psychotherapy.

Psychiatry must be able to play a central role in such a new, combined diagnostic and therapeutic system. It should not abandon its commitment to psychosocial aspects of etiology and therapeutics, which I believe might occur in a newly formed neuroscience profession. A psychosomatic system without the "psycho," a child psychiatry without the school or the family environment, and inattention to the culture of aging and addiction would weaken the advances in hypothesis development. A psychiatry without a psychological approach to childhood history and without an evidence-based psychotherapy would be as incomplete as would be a psychiatry without a fundamental neuroscientific base. Eisenberg's caution in 1986 against the dangers of a "mindless" and "brainless" psychiatry is quite relevant to today's debates (Eisenberg 1986). Joining neurology in a neuroscientific specialty could facilitate our understanding of the brain but could also fatally weaken the resurgence of a psychosocial psychiatry. For all of psychiatry's advances toward parity and equity in American medicine, its future progress will depend heavily on the evolution of a more rational health system. The current emphasis upon biological psychiatry and the limitations of psychotherapy are facilitated to a significant extent by systemic reimbursement practices within American medicine as a whole. The same regulatory pressures so visible in psychiatry are also seen in other parts of medicine. Sadly, a majority of physicians today are somewhat pessimistic and would prefer their children not to enter careers in medicine. The golden era of unfettered practice has vanished in most parts of American medicine, which is ironic when we consider that the brilliance of the field's research has improved treatment results and lengthened the life of many people.

Just as we demonstrated in changing psychiatry decisively during the 1970s, the field must become much more oriented toward the future. We need to take resolute action to increase our commitment to a broadly defined evidence based anchor for the next period of change to help us to overcome the constrictive pressures of today.

Changing our field so that it can employ an empirically based biopsychosocial model could revitalize the next phase of American psychiatry. To employ this model fully would probably require a newly trained generation of clinicians and researchers who could actually comprehend and utilize a newly formulated biopsychosocial approach. Playing an active role in producing a more rational health care system will be central to psychiatry's achievement of genuine equity in a truly brave new world.

REFERENCES

Alliance of Psychoanalytic Organizations: Psychodynamic Diagnostic Manual. Silver Spring, MD, Alliance of Psychoanalytic Organizations, 2006

Eisenberg L: Mindlessness and brainlessness in psychiatry. Br J Psychiatry 148:497–508, 1986

Engel GL: The need for a new medical model: a challenge for biomedicine. Science 196:129–136, 1977

Engel GL: The clinical application of the biopsychosocial model. Am J Psychiatry 137:535–544, 1980

Fonagy P, Target M: The mentalization-focused approach to self pathology. J Personal Disord 20:544–576, 2006

Gabbard GO: Gabbard's Treatments of Psychiatric Disorders, 4th Edition. Washington, DC, American Psychiatric Publishing, 2007

Kandel ER: Psychiatry, Psychoanalysis, and the New Biology of Mind. Washington, DC, American Psychiatric Publishing, 2005

Noyes AP, Haydon EM: A Textbook of Psychiatry, 3rd Edition. New York, Macmillan, 1940

Person ES, Cooper AM, Gabbard GO: The American Psychiatric Publishing Textbook of Psychoanalysis. Washington, DC, American Psychiatric Publishing, 2005

Strecker EA, Ebaugh FG, Ewalt JR: Practical Clinical Psychiatry, 6th Edition. Philadelphia, PA, Blakiston, 1947

Appendix 1

Selected Papers

Appendix 1A

Turning Points in Twentieth-Century American Psychiatry

Melvin Sabshin, M.D.

*I*n 1966, on the occasion of the centenary of Adolf Meyer's birth, Theodore Lidz delivered the Meyer lecture, entitling it "Adolf Meyer and the Development of American Psychiatry."[1] He concluded the published version of the paper by saying, "In commemorating him, we can do much for ourselves and for psychiatry by recognizing and utilizing the heritage he left us." Analogously, in 1980 John Neill reviewed Meyer's contributions in a paper on

Presented as the Adolf Meyer lecture at the 142nd annual meeting of the American Psychiatric Association, San Francisco, May 6-11, 1989. Received Nov. 21, 1989; revision received April 23, 1990; accepted June 1, 1990. From the American Psychiatric Association. Address reprint requests to Dr. Sabshin, APA, 1400 K St., N.W., Washington, DC 20005.

A slightly modified version of this article was published in German by Georg Thieme Verlag in 1990.

"Adolf Meyer and American Psychiatry Today."[2] He stated, "Meyer's times were similar to ours in many ways. In a curious fashion our professional wheel has come full circle to where it was in 1900, and we are again in need of the Meyerian spirit, a holistic perspective. Acquainting ourselves with the wisdom in his legacy is an important first step on the journey forward." In the 1985 Adolf Meyer lecture, Michael Rutter[3] pointed out the relevance of Meyer's work to major current issues in psychiatry. His paper, entitled "Meyerian Psychobiology, Personality Development, and the Role of Life Experiences," clearly enunciated the fundamental implications of the psychobiological concept. In this paper, I wish to follow my eminent predecessors but also to delineate in my own way how a reexamination of these Meyerian concepts might point the way toward the next turning point in American psychiatry. Indeed, I perceive subtle signs of the early phases around which the next stage might coalesce, and I anticipate that by the beginning of the twenty-first century, the developmental lines will be much clearer.

To be the Medical Director of APA is in itself a remarkable honor, and I have consistently relished the opportunity to be part of the profession's adaptation to new forces from within and outside of its changing boundaries. Lidz stated that "Adolf Meyer virtually identified himself with psychiatry,"[1] and I empathize with that position as long as it is understood that I have also maintained the differentiation.

Of late I have noted the tendency (not yet a symptom) to reminisce and reflect about the broader sweep of events; indeed, I have been a participant and observer in remarkable changes in our field. In this paper, I wish to review some of these events with emphasis upon the post–World War II changes that have been part of my personal experience. The scientific program of APA's 1989 annual meeting is an excellent symbol of our current status—quite different from the symbols and substance of the meetings of a quarter of a century ago. In this paper, I wish to highlight four turning points: 1) the rise of Meyerian psychobiology and its peak impact in the second quarter of the twentieth century, 2) the dominance of divergent therapeutic ideologies, including the important impact of psychoanalysis in the post–World War II years, 3) the current surge of neuroscience and psychopharmacology along with empiricism and logical positivism, 4) a predicted reemergence of analogues of Meyerian psychobiology at the turn of the twenty-first century accompanied by a) a new systematized psychobiology of coping, of adaptation, and of active efforts by persons to deal with multileveled stresses, b) an increased knowledge base in life course transactions converting the elaborate Meyerian history taking system to a more dynamic and relevant process, c) a trend toward a new nosological system that will give life and greater utility to the current axis IV and V systems (DSM-III and DSM-III-R) and will deal more effectively with the boundaries between health and disorder, d) with a, b, and c (coping, life history, and boundaries between health and illness), and accompanied by appropriate professional leadership, the reemergence of a vital new clinical psychiatry, e) a more balanced overall approach using psychoanalytic, social psychiatric, and biological concepts that have become clear enough to test empirically, and f) a more rational therapeutic system emphasizing new combinations and transactions between pharmacotherapy and psychotherapy—along with a new generation of educators experienced in these combinations.

THE RISE OF MEYERIAN PSYCHOBIOLOGY AND ITS PEAK IMPACT IN THE SECOND QUARTER OF THE TWENTIETH CENTURY

I entered psychiatry in the decade after World War II. The winds of change had already altered the psychiatric landscape, and almost all of my clinical supervisors and teachers espoused the new "dynamic psychiatry." The textbooks of psychiatry, however, were still dominated strongly by the prewar developments, and my introduction to Adolf Meyer was influenced primarily by written words rather than by clinical interactions and case conferences or personal contact. In retrospect, I understand that this was unfortunate because it was not easy to grasp Meyer's ideas from his written words alone. Henderson[4] said that "Adolf Meyer had to surmount language difficulties affecting his speech and his writing which made it far from easy to get his meaning and rendered his ideas more obscure than they really were." Ebaugh[5], commenting on the same subject, stated that "It was frequently difficult to grasp the full import of Dr. Meyer's formulations. It was his tendency to be elliptical or to verbalize incomplete thoughts which meandered in the direction of his own special interest of the moment. This may account, in part, for the fact that his theories are not fully recorded, or are, at best, inadequately understood." (It is hoped that late twentieth-century technology will afford subsequent generations an opportunity to learn from current theorist leaders by ways other than written words.) Over time, however, I have become increasingly knowledgeable about the basic tenets of Meyer's ideas and understand better what a pervasive influence he exerted. Even more important for me, I began to understand why his ideas were so important. It is hoped that others will find it rewarding to make their own judgments on this matter.

On several occasions, Meyer sketched his own perception of the historical phases of psychiatry in the United States.[6] He tended to call the first phase "the time of the Thirteen," honoring the founders of APA. He then described the second phase as "the preoccupation with the brain (a mere word with most) as the palpable issue in the disorder, when the workers actually looked for new emphases and concrete methods having to regulate complex organismal wholes, and the rising of competition from outside after the Civil War." That prototypic Meyerian description, with all of its ambiguity, lies at the heart of his concerns, namely, that the biological reductionism in the late nineteenth century was, at least in part, a defensive maneuver against the influx of immigrants into the United States. The "moral psychiatry" of the earlier part of the nineteenth century was fine with Yankee patients and doctors but somehow less appropriate with postindustrial America. In characterizing a third phase of American psychiatry from the 1890s to World War I, Meyer essentially described a period of increased systematization of research, followed by a fourth phase that was a description of some of his hopes and aspirations. Meyer highlighted the development of special psychiatric centers (research oriented institutes) that could be models for an advancing science of psychiatry. His thoughts about psychosomatic processes and psychiatry's role in medicine were enunciated with emphasis upon "the person" and strong criticism of dualism and reductionism.

From our late twentieth century vantage point, the nuances of changes in the first part of this century are overshadowed by a dominant trend symbolized by Meyer himself. Indeed, the turning point that peaked in the second quarter of this century can be characterized as a gradual shift from the prior biological reductionism and its attendant practices and value systems to a phase where clinical psychiatry took on new aspirations, new methods, and new interests. While Meyer characterized his major approach as psychobiology, his personal style reflected the biopsychosocial model as enunciated much later by Engel.[7] When finally ensconced in his pivotal professorship at Johns Hopkins (Phipps Clinic), Meyer maintained a profound interest in clinical practice, carried out experimental procedures in the anatomical laboratories adjacent to his office, became the preeminent educator of the psychiatric leaders of the next generation, and continuously served as an ardent advocate of community programs. Simultaneously, he collaborated with leaders in other clinical departments to develop psychosomatic programs (including liaison activities) and also kept abreast of larger philosophic, social, and political events. Keeping abreast was not an extraneous abstraction but involved friendship and collaboration with an impressive array of scholars, politicians, and moral philosophers.

It is likely, of course, that American psychiatry would have changed direction even without Meyer, but its contour and evolution were deeply influenced by him. It took a very special leader, however, to effect a turning of psychiatry toward a new direction. His solid biological roots gave special credence to his emphasis upon the patient as a person; simultaneously, his interest in social and community phenomena could not be brushed away as irrelevant abstractions. Kraepelin and his American counterparts had been challenged by a worthy critic who shook the lugubrious roots of the concept of dementia praecox. S. Weir Mitchell's 1894 challenge[8] to psychiatry to solidify its scientific and medical foundations was being answered by a leader with impeccable medical and scientific credentials. A mood of hope and of increasing capacity to cope with the enormous problems began to spread through the new scientific and academic institutes created by Meyer and his students. Many of these students became the directors and chairs of the major psychiatric departments across the country and also overseas. As they began to confront the many issues, however, progress was not easy. Hundreds of thousands of patients were housed in deteriorating institutions; treatment techniques and methods were unspecific; and the number of trained practitioners was much too small for the demands upon them. Just as the first rays of light began to seep through the end of the tunnel, World War II occurred and American psychiatry became absorbed in a momentous maelstrom that challenged many fundamental tenets.

THE DOMINANCE OF DIVERGENT THERAPEUTIC IDEOLOGIES INCLUDING THE IMPORTANT IMPACT OF PSYCHOANALYSIS IN THE POST–WORLD WAR II YEARS

World War II produced massive upheavals beyond the preemptive political and military events that changed the future course of history. In the wake of larger changes, old boundaries and barriers between nations became more permeable so that both people and ideas moved from one part of the world to another. The movement included the emigration of brilliant psychoanalysts to Western Europe, the United States, and Canada.

For American psychiatry these events precipitated significant qualitative changes that have been well documented in many excellent publications. In this paper I wish to emphasize a few aspects of these changes, which, at least in part, have not been emphasized enough.

The large number of American psychiatric casualties among our troops had riveted public attention to what began to be understood as a serious national problem. Wide publicity about new techniques to deal with traumatic neuroses, as developed by an able cadre of military psychiatrists, also had a significant impact. (I was fortunate enough to work for many years with Roy Grinker[9] and learned much about those heady days.)

What I wish to emphasize in this paper is that all of these postwar changes were engrafted upon the predisposing tendencies engendered during the Meyerian turning point. The uncompleted psychobiological revolution had opened new possibilities to concentrate upon the person and upon the individual clinical case. Biological psychiatry had not met the earlier challenges fully and gradually began to feel isolated. The dawn of a more concentrated effort at social and community psychiatry had been encouraged by Meyer himself. Most important, Meyer had directly and indirectly supported the development of psychoanalysis in the United States; but by the early 1950s psychoanalysis superseded psychobiology and in fact paid only cursory attention to it.

In some quarters (Sargant[10] in the United Kingdom, among others) it was believed that psychoanalysis had taken over United States psychiatry lock, stock, and barrel. This perception was incorrect because, in fact, it overlooked competing ideologies (e.g., in social and biological psychiatry) that frequently challenged psychoanalysis, adding to the siege mentality that consistently pervaded the field. Nevertheless, psychoanalysis developed enormous academic institutional power and affected significant hospitals, associations, and their leaders. Equally, perhaps even more important, ideas and practices throughout the field were profoundly influenced. Repeatedly, I have emphasized one change that is only beginning to be understood by decision makers. Psychoanalysis altered the boundaries of psychiatry radically in terms of its implicit definition of psychopathology and its implicit concepts of what psychiatrists should do and should not do. Freud's *Psychopathology of Everyday Life*[11], in the context of his brilliantly written clinical examples and structural concepts, led to an assumption of the near universality of psychopathology. When psychoanalytic theory was coupled with equally profound changes in child and adolescent psychiatry, the world of nosology was given a near-mortal wound.

In previous publications, I have described these events in detail; in this paper I wish to emphasize a few salient points. Psychoanalysts and psychiatric leaders influenced significantly by analysis failed to perceive the enormous policy influence exerted by psychoanalytic theory and practice. With only rare exceptions, they did not demonstrate an interest in these implications. Epidemiology was essentially ignored as much as nosology, although without the opprobrium that many analysts cast upon classificatory systems. While some psychoanalysts manifested interest in treatment of psychotic patients (and some hospitals demonstrated special interest in psychotherapeutic work with severely ill populations), the predominant interest shifted away from the severely ill patient.

Furthermore, the overwhelming majority of psychoanalysts demonstrated minimal interest in exploring the relationship between intrapsychic process and new biological concepts. Fixated on hydraulic physical models of energy distribution and mechanics, relatively few analysts became involved in transactional systems, cybernetics, or new systematized field models. For all the neglect of modern biological psychiatry, the attitudes of analysts toward social and community psychiatry were even more negative. In contrast to Meyer's reaching out to develop new community approaches, the dominant pattern of psychoanalysts involved reiteration of the intrapsychic as much more significant than the interpersonal or the social interactional field. To be involved in social psychiatry was seen as diluting the basic concentration.

Increasingly, psychoanalysts manifested a dominant ideological approach based on deductions, belief systems, and therapeutic values. To a significant extent, these patterns related to a need to defend against critics of psychoanalysis. Simultaneously and, in part, reactively, biological and social psychiatry developed their own ideological systems which differed markedly with each other and with analysis. In turn, psychoanalysts surrounded themselves with siege wagons even during a phase when many outside the wagons thought that the analysts held the real power. There is, of course, much truth in the analysts' belief that they were, at best, ambivalently received by colleagues in psychiatry. Nevertheless, the proclivity to be a besieged minority cannot be entirely explained by external attack. It was ingrained into the core functions and psychological structure of many analysts.

By the middle 1960s, American psychiatry was characterized by multiple ideological divisions in which little communication occurred between or among the various groups. While the biological psychiatrists tried to cling to their medical roots, they often became rigid in this defense and were not very persuasive. Limited as they were to unspecific medications and such treatments as ECT, insulin, and even lobotomy, they often found themselves regarded poorly within their profession and by the public at large. The psychoanalysts and the social psychiatrists, on the other hand—each in their own fashion—moved away from a medical model. Their demonstration of only minimal interest in systematic, empirically based etiology, nosology, and epidemiology and in development of treatments based on nosology marked the nadir of psychiatrists' demedicalization in the United States. Simultaneously, it also marked a period of massive public confusion about the differences among clinical psychologists, psychiatric social workers, and psychiatrists. The key paradigm here is that the broader the boundaries of psychiatry and the broader the definition of what a psychiatrist can and should do, the more overlap there is, for example, between clinical psychology and psychiatry. While the emphasis here is on the impact of boundary problems upon differentiation of mental health professionals, many other factors contributed to role blurring. The shortage of psychiatrists in World War II and in the postwar period led many within psychiatry and outside the profession to support treatment roles of other disciplines.

During the 1950s and most of the 1960s, public demand for psychiatry's accountability had been slow in developing. (Of course, there were many countertrends and exceptions.) Gradually, however, warning signals began to appear on the horizon. While Bailey's scholarly but tendentious critique of psychoanalysis at our 112th annual meeting in 1956[12] was offset by Ernest Jones's equally eloquent statement at the same meeting[13], the drumbeat of criticism began to mount a decade later. By the late 1960s, a confluence of trends became clear. The combination of psychiatry's boundary expansion, the predominance of ideology over science, and the field's demedicalization began to produce a vulnerability. Many decision makers became skeptical about psychiatrists' capacity to diagnose and treat patients. Criticism of psychiatry began to mount to a level beyond general criticism of weaknesses in medicine as a whole. A new form of stigmatization of psychiatrists gradually emerged. When these developments were perceived in the face of the continuing "shame of the states"[14] and psychiatry's relatively low status in medical schools, and with little demonstration of accountability, a crack in important segments of public support began to widen.

Simultaneously, criticism of institutionalization of psychiatric patients began to reach a zenith. Civil rights activists pointed out that patients had often been hospitalized without sufficient guarantee against abuse. Commitment procedures began to be altered, and a massive movement toward deinstitutionalization began. With the introduction of new psychotropic medication, deinstitutionalization accelerated rapidly. It was hoped that community mental health centers (CMHCs) would meet the needs of their patients, and the legislation developing these centers became a focal point for development in the 1960s. In retrospect, the resources for these centers were not adequate; furthermore, the centers did not concentrate their efforts sufficiently on severely ill individuals.

Superimposed upon deinstitutionalization, revolutionary changes in payment for all medical services had an early impact on psychiatry, given the continuing stigmatization of patients and practitioners. A demand for cost-effective services based on objective data increased steadily. Justification for increased manpower production became required. With the expansion of CMHCs and economic constraints, competition between and among mental health practitioners emerged as a publicly visible reality. The torrid relationship between psychiatry and psychoanalysis started to cool. More and more decision makers and payers of psychiatric services began to visualize the field as a bottomless pit requiring unlimited resources. Steadily, regulation began to replace the free market, and the cottage industry proved inadequate to meet the new regulatory and economic challenges. By 1970, the critics were joined by those who perceived previous promissory notes, including those made for CMHCs, as having been unmet. We found ourselves caught in the vortex of a crisis. We had difficulty in coping with the new economics, and the bottomless pit was sucking us in.

THE CURRENT SURGE OF NEUROSCIENCE AND PSYCHOPHARMACOLOGY ALONG WITH EMPIRICISM AND LOGICAL POSITIVISM

Biological psychiatry had become isolated in the decade after World War II and had retreated into ideological sparring with the psychotherapeutic boom of the 1950s. Nevertheless, a rising from the ashes was reflected in the clinical trials of chlorpromazine. Practical use of psychotropics soon emerged, and while resistance to pharmacotherapy was distinct in the 1950s, the dawn of the next turning point was strongly influenced by the new science and the new economics. In other presentations, I have emphasized the interaction between the two; some preferred to pay attention to only the science, while others paid attention to the economics.[15] The profession must be mindful of both, including their interdependence.

During the past two decades, research in the neurosciences has advanced at a dizzying pace. (It has been especially dizzying to older practitioners whose world seemed to be so markedly changed.) While the advances have affected many medical specialties, the impact on psychiatry had been prodigious. For the scientists working in the laboratories and for many of those engaged in clinical research, the new knowledge emerged because of the freedom of scientists to develop their own hypotheses and to test them objectively. From my perception, social, political, and especially economic forces have also played a critical role in the new research developments. Decision makers on Senate and House appropriation committees have commented frequently that they are now more willing to support the Institutes of the Alcohol, Drug Abuse, and Mental Health Administration because they can understand the palpable outcomes of the new generation of research. The development of public support groups has had enormous significance in accelerating the momentum. The National Alliance for the Mentally Ill has grown rapidly in size and power; its passionate espousal of biological psychiatry will be of great interest to psychiatric historians in the next century. The families of severely ill mental patients, rightly or wrongly, felt attacked by psychotherapeutic and sociotherapeutic concepts in psychiatry. To the extent that genetic, biological variables became preemptive etiologically, the families' poignant struggles to deal with severely ill family members became more easily explainable. The support of the National Alliance for the Mentally Ill for research helped to reinvigorate the National Mental Health Association and facilitated the formation of disease oriented advocacy groups that demanded advances in treatment of manic-depressive illnesses, phobias (and panic disorders), obsessive-compulsive neuroses, Alzheimer's disease, schizophrenia, and other psychiatric disorders.

Before this late-century turning point, the public image of psychiatry had begun to sour. Public perceptions of the field have always included gross stigmata, but in the heady post–World War II decade, a window of opportunity developed. For me, Ingrid Bergman's portrayal of the psychiatrist in the movie *Spellbound* symbolized a willingness to perceive that psychiatrists could be helpful under most difficult circumstances. At the opposite extreme, Michael Caine's more recent portrayal of the psychiatrist as psychotic murderer in *Dressed to Kill* reflected a composite of negative stigmatized perceptions. The public's negative perception of psychiatry also was a response to unmet expectations, anger at purported abuse of patients, and ridicule of psychiatrists arguing with each other in the courtroom. The reaction to John Hinckley's being determined not guilty by virtue of insanity symbolized the vulnerability of psychiatry far beyond the courtroom. The national firestorm after the Hinckley decision traduced our diagnostic capacities, treatment techniques, and basic competence in every other way. The need to answer these criticisms has affected our policies more forcefully than many of us realize.

During this past decade, the best stories about psychiatry in print and electronic media have involved the scientific advances in the field. As these stories have increased, they have begun to offset the continuing negative stories and may be moving to a point where they will go beyond offsetting. The need to change the public image of psychiatry has also played a key role in producing the current turning point. For some of my research colleagues, this effect is passionately denied as if it meant that their work is designed to influence the public. Just the opposite is true; high-quality work affects the public because it is high quality. But we must want to seek public support while reducing the stigma against patients and practitioners. In this process, a tendency to overcorrect for previous errors is inevitable. A focus upon genetic markers for manic-depressive illness gets much more attention than stories about the less fashionable reports of successful psychotherapy. This attention and the resultant allocation of resources affect many segments of our training programs, certification procedures, and accreditation processes. The overreaction certainly has many practical consequences.

One of the best symbols of late-century American psychiatry has been the increasing centrality of nosology in our scientific and clinical work. From the depths of the 1950s when nosology was perceived by many as an esoteric nonentity, DSM-III and DSM-III-R have influenced American psychiatry profoundly, but they have also been influenced by forces outside the field. By the middle 1970s, key decision makers not only perceived psychiatry as a bottomless pit but also began to take steps to limit reimbursement for psychiatric treatment. Publicity about psychiatrists testifying on opposite sides of insanity defense pleas brought out enormous criticism about the unreliability of psychiatric diagnosis. By the time of the Hinckley decision, the peak criticism of psychiatry occurred. By then, however, countermoves had already commenced. The nosologists who had created DSM-III attempted to shield themselves from political forces, although they could not maintain this stance consistently, and they were simultaneously criticized by social activists (concerning sexism and racism) and by other scientists. Despite this sniping, the DSM-III committees and task forces of APA produced amazing documents that did indeed change the shape of American psychiatry. While it was a brilliant tour de force, its acceptance was deeply influenced by the dire need for objectification in American psychiatry. We needed to prove to many people that psychiatric disorders could be diagnosed and that a rational basis for determining how to deal with psychiatric patients could be developed. Thus, there has been great pressure to follow DSM-III with treatment guidelines—objective guidelines for when hospitalization becomes necessary and for how long we need to keep people in the hospital. Quantification and objectification moved rapidly, perhaps at times too rapidly, across our entire field. Implicitly, theory building receded and an effort was made to move toward an empirical, quantitative direction where logical positivism and its empirical modes prevailed. Precise thinking could only be said to occur when we used our sensory capacities to observe and measure objectifiable data. This position has been extremely helpful in obtaining research funding and has been adaptive in work with industry and their insurance carriers.

Simultaneously with these sweeping changes, a number of other related developments have occurred. Epidemiology has also moved to center stage from its earlier isolation. The need to collect broad population data to aid in the formulation of psychiatric policies has become obvious. The universality of psychopathology hypothesis extant in Freud's *Psychopathology of Everyday Life*[11] or in Erikson's normal late adolescent crisis[16] could not be afforded—even in affluent America.

The nadir of demedicalization of American psychiatry of the mid-1960s is about to be replaced in the early 1990s by an apogee of remedicalization. It is a structural remedicalization manifested by the emphasis upon etiology, diagnosis, rational choices of treatment, psychobiological approaches to prevention, and the importance of epidemiology. It also is reflected in psychiatry's alliance with other medical specialties and medical organizations.

In this context, the borders and boundaries of psychiatry that seemed infinite in the 1960s became somewhat narrower; we promised much less to be all things to all people and we limited both our declared areas of expertise and our definitions of disorder.

In the 1960s, our field had been dominated by boundary expansion and by predominance of ideology over science and demedicalization. By 1989, our field is dominated by a remedicalization, a predominance of science over ideology, and a tendency toward boundary circumscription. While DSM-III and DSM-III-R are still very broad in scope, they attempt to provide objective criteria for diagnosing each disorder. Psychiatrists have also tended to focus much more on clearly defined role functions than they assumed in the 1960s. Explicit and implicit action was taken to respond to those critics who had described psychiatry as a bottomless pit in the 1960s. Nevertheless, there are signs that the remarkable correction that has taken place in the last two decades has overcorrected in some areas. Fears of losing vitality in clinical psychiatry have been expressed by an increasing number of observers. Caricatures of a "mindless" psychiatry[17] have replaced the previous "brainless" psychiatry and are drawing increased attention. I believe that these forces and others will begin to combine at the beginning of the next century and I will conclude this paper by predicting another turning point by the first decade of the twenty-first century.

THE REEMERGENCE OF ANALOGUES OF MEYERIAN PSYCHOBIOLOGY AT THE TURN OF THE TWENTY-FIRST CENTURY: A PREDICTION

The point and counterpoint of current American psychiatry include predecessors of changes that I believe will gather momentum to become the next turning point. Rutter[3] has pointed out frequently that we must study the large population who do not become ill when facing the genetic and life-stress factors that induce illnesses in so many others. Along with a number of distinguished observers, he has emphasized the remarkable individual variations in coping with high-risk variables. Meyer had discussed this phenomenon on many occasions, and leaders of psychosomatic medicine have repeatedly called attention to such variations. While these questions have been given attention, I believe that a confluence of factors will elevate the questions about adaptation and coping to a pivotal position in psychiatry.

To predict that issues which have been in the penumbra of psychiatry for over a century will move to center stage may be risky, but I do believe that there are good reasons to make this prediction. By the beginning of the twenty-first century, I believe that the adaptability of many individuals with apparent high-risk loading for psychiatric illness will not be able to be ignored. In addition to scientific development, I believe that economic forces will be at play and policy makers will want to know why large segments of the population fail to become ill. The capacity to cope and hence to reduce risk of illness will be very important in the actuarial world of the early twenty-first century.

Simultaneously, the technological advances of the late twentieth century will be applied to determine markers of adaptability just as we now study markers of disease proclivity. When our technology permits longitudinal studies of biological systems and adaptability, we will be in an advantageous position for new hypotheses. In effect, I am saying that the psychobiology of coping and adaptability will become a major part of psychiatric research and practice. Modern technology will permit us to take Meyer's old concepts and apply them (as well as the best of psychosomatic medicine) in a variety of new ways. Integral to this new emphasis will be the transactions and interactions between psychological adaptation and biological systems. Both pathology and health will need to be explained in psychobiological terms.

The increased interest in adaptation could have a direct influence on the clinical practice of psychiatry in the early part of the twenty-first century. At present, there is a decline in interest in taking a full psychiatric history; establishing criteria for a DSM-III diagnosis has become the current cornerstone of psychiatric history taking. With a decline in psychodynamic formulations, the excitement in looking for historical and other clinical nuances has almost been lost. Many clinician educators have talked about loss of clinical vitality in the profession. I am convinced that revived interest in adaptation could help to reverse this trend. Currently, axes IV and V of the DSM are primarily research tools, but I believe that scientific and economic forces will increase our attention to the field of stress and adaptation. To the extent that clinicians as well as researchers see the value in documenting these data, collecting and interpreting such information will become a major part of day-to-day clinical practice. I am hopeful that the process of collecting such data will stimulate a new interest in history taking. The psychodynamic formulation of the 1950s might be replaced by a psychobiological (or biopsychosocial) formulation of the year 2010. This formulation will involve more than historical data, since laboratory findings (measuring both adaptational and pathological elements) should also become very important.

For many years I have been interested in psychiatrists' involvement in research on normal populations.[18, 19] In part, this interest has been based on a wish to find empirical bases to distinguish normal from pathological conditions in psychiatry. I am convinced that such efforts will ultimately help to define the scope and boundaries of psychiatry. There is every reason to believe in much greater variety of normal development than there is in pathological sequences. Longitudinal studies of life-course adaptation will catalyze our knowledge in this arena, and I look forward to exciting progress that will attract the next generation of investigators and clinicians. As I have studied Meyer's efforts in history taking, he was seeking a way to follow "persons" (to use his term) throughout successive developmental stages, but he lacked the tools and measurements to make it practical. His vision on this matter, however, deserves to be studied in preparation for a new kind of history taking that will seek to ascertain both adaptational and pathological elements.

With increased emphasis upon coping, the boundaries between health and illness, and life histories, I believe that the clinical psychiatry of the early 21st century can be revitalized without becoming vitalistic. The new clinical psychiatry can lift us from the potential reductionism, mechanization, and trivialization that weaken current clinical psychiatry. It can also keep open lines to develop new hypotheses rather than seeking dynamic formulations that follow established theoretical constructs.

The revitalization of clinical psychiatry should also permit us to find a new synthesis of psychoanalytic, social psychiatric, and biological psychiatry. In the years after World War II, American psychiatry has oscillated widely between dominant concepts and practices. A more steady, empirically driven phase should modulate and temper the current overcorrection. As the tempering occurs, new ideas about comorbidity and multimodal treatment should develop. Indeed, I anticipate that most psychiatric patients early in the next century will be treated by combinations of psychotherapy and somatic therapies. These combinations will be based on empirical clinical trials, and a generation of clinician-educators experienced in such combinations will become the modal supervisors and textbook writers.

My predictions are based on both scientific and economic indicators. I am, of course, hopeful that leaders in psychiatry will see the new opportunities in the next phase. I am also hopeful that decision makers and the general public will support these efforts.

Adolf Meyer was not born in the United States, but he helped to create an indigenous psychiatry, the first American psychiatry since the moral reform period early in the nineteenth century. After the turbulence of the last half of the twentieth century, we may have an opportunity to reflect on what Meyer accomplished and find a new balance. We can build on his base but we must also take advantage of new technology, new methods, new public support, and new partnerships with patients and their families to facilitate and support the next turning point.

REFERENCES

1. Lidz T: Adolf Meyer and the development of American psychiatry. Am J Psychiatry 123:320–332, 1966
2. Neill JR: Adolf Meyer and American psychiatry today. Am J Psychiatry 137:460–464, 1980
3. Rutter M: Meyerian psychobiology, personality development, and the role of life experiences. Am J Psychiatry 143:1077–1087, 1986
4. Henderson D: Adolf Meyer: a tribute from abroad. Am J Psychiatry 123:332–334, 1966
5. Ebaugh FG: Adolf Meyer: a tribute from home. Am J Psychiatry 123:334–336, 1966
6. Meyer A: Presidential address: thirty-five years of psychiatry in the United States and our present outlook. Am J Psychiatry 85:1–31, 1928
7. Engel GL: The unified concept of health and disease. Perspect Biol Med 3:459–485, 1960
8. Mitchell SW: Address before the fiftieth annual meeting of the American Medico-Psychological Association, held in Philadelphia, May 16th, 1894. J Nerv Ment Dis 21:413–437, 1894
9. Grinker R: Psychiatry rides madly in all directions. Arch Gen Psychiatry 10:228–237, 1964
10. Sargant WW: Battle for the Mind: A Physiology of Conversion and Brain-Washing. London, Heinemann, 1957
11. Freud S: The Psychopathology of Everyday Life. New York, Macmillan, 1915
12. Bailey P: The great psychiatric revolution. Am J Psychiatry 113:387–406, 1956

13. Jones E: Psychiatry before and after Freud, in The Scientific Papers of the 112th Annual Meeting of the American Psychiatnc Association in Summary Form. Washington, DC, American Psychiatric Association, 1956
14. Deutsch A: The Shame of the States (1948). New York, Arno Press, 1973
15. Sabshin M: Science, pragmatism and the progress of psychiatry, in Contemporary Themes in Psychiatry: A Tribute to Sir Martin Roth. Edited by Davison K, Kerr A. London, Gaskell (Royal College of Psychiatrists), 1989
16. Erikson E: Identity and the Life Cycle. Psychol Issues 1(1), 1959
17. Eisenberg L: Mindlessness and brainlessness in psychiatry. Br J Psychiatry 148:497–508, 1986
18. Offer D, Sabshin M: Normality and the Life Cycle. New York, Basic Books, 1984
19. Sabshin M: Normality and the boundaries of psychopathology. J Personal Disord 3:259–293, 1989

Appendix 1B

The Future of Psychiatry

Melvin Sabshin, M.D.

*T*he last quarter century has been characterized by enormous changes in almost every aspect of psychiatry in the United States. From my perspective, many of these changes have resulted from the interaction of new research and new economics. Although this interaction between science and economics has been most dramatic in North America and western Europe, similar changes have begun to occur throughout the world. Certainly, economic pressures have had a great impact on psychiatry throughout the twentieth century. At times, the field has grown in influence and power with surges of fiscal support. In the United States, such a spurt occurred after World War II. Both public and private support grew rapidly; many people sought treatment, and plans for reformation of our mental health care system began to take shape. During that time, however, the field of psychiatry in the United States was subdivided among several divergent treatment ideologies. Each point of view was advocated by separate leadership, and these leaders rarely consulted with each other. The charisma of much of this leadership sometimes obscured the fact that the therapeutic approaches were often not founded on good evidence, and ultimately confidence in the field began to weaken (Sabshin 1990).

During the past quarter century, the domination of American psychiatry by ideological groupings began to change. Evidence-based psychiatry became more powerful, and empirically based treatment became the rule rather than the exception. These changes occurred in the context of radical changes in the economic principles affecting our entire medical system. Health care in the United States has changed from being offered through an almost free market to being heavily regulated. Today, for treatment to be reimbursed, approval of the treatment must be obtained in advance from the managed care company. Length of hospitalization is severely limited and alternative care systems are preferred. In the mental health field, an effort is often made by these intermediaries to have treatment conducted by psychologists or social workers, who, it is assumed, will charge less than psychiatrists.

The pressure to limit length of hospital stay and the pressure to produce more rapid results in outpatients have reinforced the use of psychopharmacological agents in clinical practice. Recent developments in psychopharmacology have supported psychiatry's efforts to cope with the external economic pressures. On the other hand, psychosocial treatments have been made more difficult to support in the world of managed care. The future of psychotherapeutic work by psychiatrists is under attack from several fronts, and strong efforts will need to be made to prevent atrophy of psychiatrists' psychotherapeutic skills. Several other danger signals to American psychiatry have appeared; indeed, this chapter on the future of psychiatry is being written at a time when much of American psychiatry faces irrational external regulation and constraint.

When I first came to the American Psychiatric Association in 1974, I had a vision concerning how the field might be united and how we as psychiatrists might deal with the many challenges of that time (Sabshin 1976, 1977). Similarly, in this chapter I have emphasized steps that psychiatry might take to facilitate coping with the new challenges. Some of the predictions are based on developments already in progress. Others represent aspirations of new directions that will require much work if they are to be achieved. The list is not intended to be a complete formulation; rather, I have chosen several areas in which I have a special interest.

DEVELOPMENTS IN DIAGNOSIS AND RELATED MEASURES

American psychiatrists' interest in nosology has undergone dramatic change during the last quarter of the twentieth century. The status of nosology in the United States was somewhat de-emphasized following World War II, but interest in diagnosis has now become a central feature of American psychiatry (Frances et al. 1989). Indeed, DSM-III (American Psychiatric Association 1980), DSM-III-R (American Psychiatric Association 1987), and DSM-IV (American Psychiatric Association 1994) have had enormous worldwide impact and, along with ICD-10 (World Health Organization 1992), have contributed to a scientific resurgence in the entire nosological arena. No issue dramatizes change in American psychiatry more than the relative importance of diagnostic methodology in the past half century. Psychiatrists' capacity or incapacity to make reliable diagnoses had become a matter of public policy concern. The great scientific progress during the last 25 years has increased the credibility of psychiatry for the general public and for decision makers.

Much work remains to be done in refining the diagnostic categories. It is to be hoped that by the second half of the twenty-first century there will have been more progress in developing an etiologically and pathogenetically based nosology. Such a nosology has been a fundamental goal of psychiatry for a long time, and its systematic evolution will help to define an evidence-based psychiatry.

An important step in achieving greater scientific precision will involve increased use of all of the multiaxial categories in diagnosis. I believe that psychobiological understanding of adaptation will be enhanced in the first quarter of the twenty-first century and will help researchers and clinicians to explain why some people are more or less vulnerable to disorder. Those individuals who have greater psychobiological predilection to cope will be less vulnerable. More attention to data about the best level of adaptation experienced by patients should also be helpful in understanding the clinical implications of adaptation.

One of the most important current needs involves an understanding of the level of disability found in patients with each psychiatric disorder (Massel et al. 1990). The development of disability indices should indeed be a high priority for American psychiatry; such assessment has notable social and economic implications, as well as clinical importance.

DEVELOPMENT OF PRACTICE GUIDELINES AND NETWORKS

During the last decade, much progress in American psychiatry has occurred with the publication of practice guidelines. These efforts will continue in the twenty-first century, and it is anticipated that such guidelines will be formulated for almost all nosological entities. The interaction between nosological advances and guidelines is vital, and evidence-based treatment has depended on systematic evolution of a modern diagnostic system. After their original formulation, these guidelines will continue to be amended as new methods are introduced and new results are determined for each treatment.

In addition to the development of practice guidelines, the organization of a practice research network in the United States has great potential (Zarin et al. 1997). Such a network will complement the traditional methods of evaluating new treatments under controlled conditions. This control may make it necessary to concentrate on conditions in which patients have one clear diagnosis and are treated by one specific approach. Given the prevalence of comorbidity in the case of psychiatric conditions and given the need to test treatments in a variety of contexts, a treatment network may provide much additional information. I look forward to the organization of such networks in many specialties and many countries. Each of them will be composed of practitioners representing multiple areas of interest. Embedded within this concept is the concern that current systems of assessing treatment may, in some cases, be somewhat constrained and insufficiently reflective of actual practice. Clearly, both controlled and network-generated data have special purposes and should complement one another.

The emergence of networks across the world will be a major step toward a more sophisticated transnational comparative analysis of psychiatry. Similarities and differences of findings by different networks will be very important. The maturation of an evidence-based international psychiatry will be one of the most exciting aspects of our field throughout the twenty-first century.

I predict a continued evolution of nosology, which, in turn, should facilitate a rational evolution of treatment guidelines. The emergence of treatment research networks will reflect and facilitate the new guidelines and the new treatments. Ultimately, new treatments will evolve in a more sophisticated manner.

COMBINED USE OF PSYCHOTHERAPY AND PHARMACOTHERAPY BY PSYCHIATRISTS

Many patients with psychiatric disorders are now treated with a combination of medication and psychotherapy (Beitman and Klerman 1991). Often, however, these treatments are provided by different therapists and there is relatively little communication about the therapeutic interactions. When a single therapist employs both psychopharmacotherapy and psychotherapy today, most often these treatments are used additively rather than integratively. The future practice of psychiatry will be influenced meaningfully by efforts at genuine integration of these treatments.

Traditionally, pharmacotherapy and psychotherapy have developed under separate auspices. Indeed, in the era of ideological domination, there often were conflicts between proponents of pharmacotherapy and those who advocated psychotherapy (Klerman 1991). More recently, many psychiatrists have recognized that patients may require medication before they can respond adequately to psychotherapy. Conversely, many psychopharmacologists have recognized that psychotherapy may enhance and prolong the effects of medication. In my judgment, this recognition is an early step in understanding that many types of interaction between the treatments are possible. The effects of psychotherapy and pharmacotherapy, when better understood, should be complementary and reinforcing. Various types of medications will have different kinds of effects when used with different types of psychotherapy, and various types of psychotherapy will have different effects when used with different kinds of medication.

The current separation of psychotherapy and pharmacotherapy reflects their divergent historical roots. Integration will require educational programs in which the teaching of both is combined. Ultimately, individual educators should be able to teach about the combined treatment and individual psychiatrists should be able to provide integrated rather than separate or additive treatment.

Most current discussion of psychiatrists' role in providing psychotherapy fails to include consideration of the implications for combined use of psychotherapy and pharmacotherapy.

The psychiatrist who is untrained in psychotherapy will not, of course, be able to provide the combined treatment. It should be obvious that a psychiatrist without experience in psychotherapy will not be able to supervise treatment by this method. Nevertheless, it has been advocated that such supervision could be provided by psychiatrists even if they do not conduct psychotherapy themselves.

The combined treatment will have many economic implications. One psychiatrist providing such combined treatment will increase his or her efficiency and, I believe, will also have better long-term results. I predict that this kind of integrated treatment will become the type of service provided by the psychiatrist by the middle of the twenty-first century. I also predict that the combined treatment will differentiate the psychiatrist from colleagues in primary care medicine and colleagues in other mental health fields. To accomplish this goal in a successful fashion, a large number of educational and service delivery changes will be required. It is hoped that some of these changes will begin now with efforts designed to preserve and improve psychiatrists' skills in various kinds of psychotherapy. These skills will be the bedrock for the combined treatments.

BIOLOGICAL AND PSYCHOLOGICAL MARKERS

In medical specialties other than psychiatry, predilection or vulnerability to various illnesses may be ascertained by specific tests long before signs or symptoms of the disorder make their appearance. In psychiatry, such accurate predictions of vulnerability are rare (Bunney et al. 1986). In part, the paucity of specific markers relates to our lack of information about the pathophysiology of most psychiatric disorders. At times, however, we have come close to proposing hypotheses about blood tests, radiographic signs, or identification of genetic findings that might predict the later emergence of specific disorders or parts thereof. Unfortunately, we have not yet found reliable predictors.

I have already mentioned that a nosological system based on pathogenesis or etiology should be present by the latter part of the twenty-first century. Such a system should facilitate the discovery of laboratory findings that precede and hence predict the onset of disorder. Of course, relevant prediction should lead to preventive steps that might be taken to block the pathological tendencies. These biological markers will include indicators of genetic predilection to disorder as well as vulnerabilities that develop later. Molecular genetics will become an even more important basic science for psychiatric progress.

One variant of these markers will involve measurement of factors that may reduce the chance for a specific disorder or disorders to develop. For example, those processes that enhance coping and/or adaptation may also be measurable and this measurement may become one of the most important aspects for the future of psychiatry. Markers indicating lowered vulnerability to disorders may be as important as those predicting the development of disorders.

In psychiatry, psychological markers should also emerge in conjunction with biological and physical markers. The subject of psychological markers has been very much affected by theories and hypotheses throughout the twentieth century that have formulated a relationship between childhood trauma and adult illnesses. Psychiatric researchers have often questioned the scientific basis of many of these earlier hypotheses and prefer to emphasize the need for hypotheses that can be tested and validated or invalidated. Psychobiological markers that predict vulnerability to disorder or predict capacity to deal effectively with impending disorder will become a major part of psychiatry by the middle of the twenty-first century. The psychological component of those markers will include personality traits, subsyndromal symptomatology, and developmental deficits. These psychological markers should also include a new language of coping and adaptational criteria.

The biopsychosocial psychiatry (some prefer the term *psychobiological*) of the latter part of the twenty-first century will also lend itself to a different kind of nosological system for psychiatry that takes etiology and pathogeneses into consideration. The markers used in predicting vulnerability and immunity will be important in the new etiologically based diagnostic system. Studies of markers that may indicate a capacity to reduce vulnerability to illness have important theoretical as well as practical implications. The psychosomatic medicine of the twenty-first century may be affected substantially by study of these mechanisms. The knowledge that some people are highly unlikely to develop peptic ulcers or hypertension, for example, may be as important as good predictors of specific vulnerability.

STUDIES OF THE LIFE CYCLE

During the twentieth century, it has been logical to separate child/adolescent psychiatry as a subspecialty of psychiatry. Subsequently, it also was logical that geriatric psychiatry became a subspecialty. It was not logical, however, to think of general psychiatry simply as psychiatry geared toward the time between adolescence and old age. General psychiatry always included chronological components, but time did not necessarily serve as the central feature of general psychiatry, even when the term *adult psychiatry* was employed. Adulthood does not have the same relatively clearly delineated chronological characteristics as do childhood and older age. I predict, however, that there will be a better formulation of adult development in the twenty-first century.

I believe that the total life cycle will be reexamined in the twenty-first century, with the development of new hypotheses related to vulnerabilities and also the capacity to deal with these vulnerabilities. Throughout the twentieth century there have been important debates about the continuity or discontinuity of psychopathology (Chess and Alexander 1990). Continuity or discontinuity of adaptive methods and styles has undergone less study but should become a much more important topic. Adaptation will be studied directly, not simply through studying people who demonstrate low scores on a scale of maladaptation. Understanding why and how some people adapt over a full life cycle should have many implications for new types of treatment and prevention of illness. New types of treatment that facilitate adaptation rather than combat illness, as in the approach taken in oncology, could become a central part of psychiatry. Also, the understanding of chronic illness should be facilitated by data about the continuity or discontinuity of symptomatology during various phases of the life cycle.

TECHNOLOGICAL ADVANCES

There are several contexts in which new technology will have a notable impact on the field of psychiatry.

The technology of psychopharmacology has had a remarkable developmental history in the last four decades. There is good reason to expect that developments in neuroscience and psychopharmacology will continue. As the underlying psychobiological basis of disorders unfolds, new forms of psychopharmacological treatment will be developed. The psychopharmacological treatments facilitating adaptation will also become a new form of therapy. I predict an emerging psychopharmacological industry with a new model, one emphasizing reinforcement of adaptive capacity rather than the combating of disorder.

A variety of new approaches and hypotheses will also refine the current techniques employed in psychotherapy. Combined use of pharmacotherapy and psychotherapy will facilitate the focusing of attention on new possibilities in psychotherapy. In the past, psychotherapeutic techniques have been used to support "defenses" (e.g., rationalization); the implicit concept of this approach is a method to shore up less than optimal techniques. The concept of adaptation is different from the concept of defense mechanism, and this concept should affect psychotherapeutic techniques substantially. A new technology of psychotherapy should emerge.

New technology can also have other special implications for psychotherapy and psychiatric rehabilitation. Telepsychiatry and cyberspace techniques will probably revolutionize interpersonal treatment during the next quarter century. The therapist's office has been the site of much outpatient treatment. Twenty-five years from now, therapist and patient will have many other options. It will be possible to treat a patient by therapeutic techniques in settings almost fully approximating current sensory reality—even when the patient is thousands of miles away from the therapist. It may also be possible to administer medication and perform other medical treatments through cyberspace. The implications for follow-up treatment after patient or therapist changes residence are enormous, as is the problem of licensing and credentialing. All of these new techniques may seem somewhat strange for those raised earlier in the twentieth century but will be easier for those raised in an environment in which such use of the Internet and of telemedicine is much more common.

Telepsychiatry is already useful for reminding people to take their medications and for reinforcing treatment. The use of such methods for elderly and incapacitated patients has begun but has many implications that will be expanded as new techniques are implemented. There are many practical implications of these new technological advances, including increase in efficiency and cost-effectiveness.

PREVENTION OF MENTAL ILLNESS

Throughout the twentieth century there have been many programs designed to prevent the onset of mental illness (primary prevention) or intended to provide effective therapeutic early intervention (secondary prevention). Some of these programs have been very effective. For example, the psychoses associated with vitamin deficiency have been prevented by better nutrition, and pellagra has become less common as well. In the middle of the twentieth century, syphilis had a major impact and affected psychiatry throughout the world. Tertiary syphilis was associated with psychotic syndromes that were common and diverse. The effectiveness of penicillin in treating central nervous system syphilis, and, even more important, in preventing tertiary symptoms, has been one of the great preventive achievements of the century. Indeed, the decrease in prevalence of many infectious diseases has had important ramifications for psychiatry. However, new infectious diseases have now emerged that have a powerful impact on the central nervous system. HIV infection has had a major effect on the psychiatry of the turn of the century (Checkley et al. 1996; Rosenbaum 1994).

General principles of better child care, adequate education, better treatment for many medical illnesses, careful attention to a variety of toxic reactions (including the effects of many medications), and better public health have had a positive impact on mental illnesses with generic types of primary prevention. In some countries, after social upheaval or revolution, it was hoped that improvement in the implementation of these measures would eradicate mental illness. Unfortunately, even after effective general preventive actions, severe mental illnesses continue to occur, as do some less severe illnesses, and many of these illnesses continue to create major health problems throughout the world.

Primary prevention of most severe mental illnesses is limited without better understanding of their causes and also awaits improvement of methods for early diagnosis and early intervention. Schizophrenia has been studied intensively, but achieving a full understanding of its pathogenesis will require much work in the new century; in many cases, however, reduction of residual symptomatology in schizophrenic patients is now possible. Further, once a diagnosis of depression has been made, secondary preventive treatment results in patients with this disorder are very good ("Health Care Reform for Americans With Severe Mental Illnesses" 1993). Primary prevention for most severe mental illnesses, however, is a goal that will not be attained until late in the twenty-first century. I anticipate that a resurgence of preventive psychiatry will occur by the first quarter of the century and that preventive psychiatry will gain a more solid footing as the century goes on.

INTEGRATION OF THEORY AND PRACTICE

During the third quarter of the twentieth century, there was an efflorescence of theoretical concepts, many of which were attached to specific ideologies within psychiatry. In the last 25 years, however, there has been a marked tendency toward a pragmatism almost devoid of theory. In my judgment, American psychiatry has attempted to compensate for its earlier immersion in theory by emphasizing an evidence-based approach in developing new hypotheses. I believe that the current lack of theory will begin to have a negative impact when new efforts are made to integrate biological, psychological, and social data. Throughout this chapter, I have discussed the need for a scientific rationale of treatment. New theoretical formulation of levels and sequences of integration between biological and psychological data will be very important as long as they lead to hypotheses that can be tested. It is my opinion that there will be a gradual increase in willingness and ability to formulate new psychosomatic theories and new theories designed to help the understanding of the interaction between vulnerability and adaptation.

There is already some increased interest in psychiatric theory. The new journal *Philosophy, Psychiatry, & Psychology* has gained many subscribers in both the United Kingdom and America. I believe that the journal's popularity will increase and will help lead us out of the current atheoretical period.

GRADUAL DECLINE OF STIGMA

In the United States, there has been a substantial decline in stigma against psychiatric patients and psychiatrists in the last 25 years. Various surveys have indicated that the majority of the public now believes that mental illness is diagnosable and treatable (Clements 1993). In the middle of the twentieth century, by contrast, there was much skepticism about diagnosis and treatment. Even earlier in the century, much more stigma existed, represented by gross distortions of psychiatric illness. There was also gross distortion about what psychiatrists actually did with patients.

During the 1990s, extensive debate took place in the United States Congress regarding legislation designed to provide parity of care for patients with psychiatric illness (Mental Health Parity Act of 1996). The arguments against this legislation involved concern about increased costs of such efforts. Connected with this concern, however, was old-fashioned stigma. It was asserted repeatedly that mental illness could not be diagnosed accurately, and it was also stated that treatments had little success and tended to be employed interminably. These allegations illustrate that progress against stigma may be reversed under the stress of seeking parity of care for the mentally ill. Furthermore, the Domenici-Wellstone amendment did not provide for parity for those who engage in substance abuse. A very special kind a stigma still exists in the arena of care for substance abusers.

Stigma against psychiatrists has also been reduced in the last decade. The fact that a substantial number of psychiatrists have become deans of American medical schools demonstrates that there is widespread respect for certain psychiatrists. Nevertheless, among the medical colleagues of psychiatrists, substantial stigma still exists against most psychiatrists. When a medical student tells classmates or professors that he or she plans to seek a residency in psychiatry, the reaction is often negative.

As widespread awareness of psychiatric research spreads in many sectors of public understanding, however, stigma against psychiatric patients and psychiatrists diminishes. I believe that this trend will continue into the twenty-first century and that there will be a continuing gradual decline of stigma. There still will be some stigma, however, even at the end of an enlightened new century. Dealing with irrational and occasionally unpredictable behavior will always stir up questions and misunderstanding.

Psychiatrists' alliances with patients and family groups will become stronger, and such alliances will play a beneficial role in many areas and will also play a role in reducing stigma. The continuing reduction of stigma will occupy much attention of the mental health/mental disorder/brain disease alliances of the twenty-first century.

CHANGES IN DELIVERY OF PSYCHIATRIC SERVICES

There is enormous variation in the way in which psychiatric services are delivered in different countries today. In some nations, primitive systems continue and reform will take many years to accomplish. In the United States, during the past decade, there has been tremendous change in the regulation of all medical care, including psychiatric treatment. A determined effort has been mounted through managed care to control health costs; included in this effort is an attempt to limit reimbursement to those clinical approaches that are perceived to be efficient and/or cost-effective (Bartlett 1994). There is currently a backlash against managed care. Some practitioners stay outside the system by limiting their practice to patients who pay for care entirely out of their own pockets. I predict that there will also be increased attempts at local levels to regulate and control egregious practices of managed care. Suits initiated by practitioners to combat bad managed care will be another effort to combat bad practice.

One of the most important political and economic developments related to care of psychiatric patients in the United States has been the parity movement. The middle 1990s saw the emergence of a determined effort to raise the level of reimbursement for psychiatric treatment so that the reimbursement was equivalent to that for treatment of other medical illnesses. The Domenici-Wellstone amendment was a major step toward achieving partial parity (Sabshin 1997). Although the amendment's provisions were limited and involved annual and lifetime caps for psychiatric care to become equivalent, under certain conditions, to other medical caps, the passage of the amendment was notable. In the debate before the president signed the legislation, those opposing the Domenici-Wellstone amendment used old-fashioned, stigma-related approaches, including questioning the reliability of psychiatric diagnoses and the effectiveness of psychiatric treatment. Those arguments failed.

I believe that parity legislation at the national level will continue to be passed and will bring about equality for psychiatric treatment compared with the rest of medical treatment by the second decade of the twenty-first century (Sabshin 1997). The implication of this prediction is that a majority of decision makers will join together to support parity despite residual opposition by a strong group who will nevertheless find themselves in a minority. For the first time in history, a series of political decisions will be made supporting parity of care for the mentally ill in the face of vigorous public discussion, including opposition.

In the United States, the debate regarding parity will also occur in each state. Support for the mentally ill will spread throughout the United States by the end of the first decade of the new century. In accomplishing this purpose, families of the mentally ill will join with citizens' groups and professional groups. The increasing effectiveness of this coalition will have much impact on the parity movement. In addition, I predict that this coalition will ultimately make a difference in the debate about equity in reimbursement for treatment of mental illness.

One of the most important current questions involves how mental illness is defined for purposes of reimbursement. Some groups advocate the limitation of reimbursement to those with severe and persistent mental illness. I believe that this approach will dominate the national and state parity efforts for the next decade. I also predict that by the second decade of the twenty-first century, there will be a resurgence of interest in those people with less severe mental illnesses that nevertheless have a substantial impact in the workplace and in family life. Also, those disorders that affect children will receive increased attention. The fact that many individuals who engage in substance abuse also have a comorbid mental illness will receive much more attention as better treatments are more widely appreciated early in the new century.

PSYCHIATRIC WORKFORCE

Projections regarding the number of psychiatrists needed in particular countries depend on a variety of assumptions and definitions (Scully 1995). When a limited definition of mental illness is employed and when it is assumed that most of the less severely ill patients will continue to be treated by nonpsychiatrists, the projected number of psychiatrists needed is low.

Projections based on just the opposite assumptions are also made today. These assumptions include a very broad definition of mental illness that encompasses substance abuse and the treatment of notable comorbidity. Under these conditions the need for psychiatrists is greater. There is also the question of the extent of needs in the subspecialty areas of psychiatry; the demand for practitioners increases with the increase in needs across many subspecialties. Very much related to these projections is how the definition of mental illness is handled in particular reimbursement schemes. As demand for treatment for those individuals with psychiatric problems affecting work and family life increases, the need for psychiatrists to be part of these treatment efforts will rise. Of course, other mental health workers will be involved in such programs as well, but psychiatrists will provide very special combinations of psychotherapy and pharmacotherapy. Earlier in this chapter I discussed this increased use of conjoint psychotherapy and pharmacotherapy by one practitioner—namely, the psychiatrist. If this prediction is correct, the need for psychiatrists will be greater.

The potential workforce in mental health is diverse and large. I believe that physicians other than psychiatrists will become increasingly involved in providing pharmacotherapeutic care for many psychiatric patients. I believe also that mental health workers other then psychiatrists will provide psychotherapeutic care for a larger sample of the population. Psychotherapy and pharmacotherapy will, however, become even more integrated, and psychiatrists will be especially qualified for providing such combined treatment.

Workforce projections will also be affected by new technological possibilities—namely, those of treating people who reside in other parts of the world. Licensing and credentialing will be important issues in telepsychiatry. Nevertheless, workforce demands in the United States will be affected by worldwide psychiatric needs in the twenty-first century.

In the United States, there is one area in which there is an enormous need for psychiatrists, and this need is likely to grow in the next two decades. Forensic psychiatry has expanded far beyond previous projections in almost all of its divisions. Policy decisions will determine what kind of support will be provided for prisoners with overt and serious mental problems. Provision of psychiatric treatment to prisoners is a major societal issue, one that will demand discussion and could affect educational programs and workforce projections.

RIGHTS OF PSYCHIATRIC PATIENTS

Human rights issues have very special meaning for psychiatric patients and for the individuals who treat them. When psychiatric patients are treated under authoritarian conditions, numerous problems affect the process and the outcome. The authoritarianism may result from political, religious, economic, or other social circumstances. All of these variables affect the confidentiality of treatment, the conditions under which treatment is administered, the relationship between the patient and the persons and institutions providing treatment, and the basis for hospitalization and discharge. Democracy and human rights have particular impacts on the mental health field, more perhaps than on any other area of medicine (Sabshin 1995). It is to be hoped that in the twenty-first century a broader understanding of this relationship will exist and efforts will be made around the world to guarantee the rights of patients with mental illness.

At the same time, there needs to be an awareness that antipsychiatry groups have entered this arena of patients' rights. These groups argue for human rights from a libertarian or scientology perspective. Scientologists are very much against psychiatry and have tended to portray psychiatrists as despicable villains. The problems with psychiatry, from this group's perspective, are the providers and the treatment itself, and scientologists are a strong force in the struggle against all mental health care. Libertarians also argue against treatment (especially involuntary treatment) and question whether commitment to mental institutions is still necessary. Despite antipsychiatry, democratic principles have been promulgated widely to support better psychiatric treatment in many countries. Psychiatric abuses still occur, however, and efforts to expose these abuses and improve care will continue to make a large difference. Rights for psychiatric patients are fundamental to good practice and development of these rights will be part of psychiatric advances in the twenty-first century.

CONCLUSIONS

This chapter has included discussion and future projections of some of the major issues facing psychiatry. Some predictions have been made as well. I have focused on an increasingly evidence-based psychiatry that will recognize its dependence on a good mixture of science, humanistic clinical practice, and democratic conditions. New technology could help psychiatric patients and psychiatrists in a number of ways—for example, through provision of treatment to patients living far from their therapists. The psychiatrist in the twenty-first century might concentrate on providing combined psychotherapy and pharmacotherapy, an exciting area of psychiatry that awaits additional refinement. Many economic constraints have recently been placed on the psychiatrist and psychiatric patients. It is to be hoped that these constraints will diminish with the advent of more enlightened policies of parity and equity regarding psychiatric treatment.

REFERENCES

American Psychiatric Association: Diagnostic and Statistical Manual of Mental Disorders, 3rd Edition. Washington, DC, American Psychiatric Association, 1980

American Psychiatric Association: Diagnostic and Statistical Manual of Mental Disorders, 3rd Edition, Revised. Washington, DC, American Psychiatric Association, 1987

American Psychiatric Association: Diagnostic and Statistical Manual of Mental Disorders, 4th Edition. Washington, DC, American Psychiatric Association, 1994

Bartlett J: The emergence of managed care and its impact on psychiatry. New Dir Ment Health Serv 63:25–34, 1994

Beitman BD, Klerman GL (eds): Integrating Pharmacotherapy and Psychotherapy. Washington, DC, American Psychiatric Press, 1991

Bunney WE, Garland-Bunney B, Patel SB: Biological markers in depression. Psychopathology 19 (suppl 2):72–78, 1986

Checkley GE, Thompson SC, Crofts N, et al: HIV in the mentally ill (review). Aust N Z J Psychiatry 30:184–194, 1996

Chess S, Alexander T: Continuities and discontinuities in temperament, in Straight and Devious Pathways From Childhood to Adulthood. Edited by Robins LN, Rutter M. Cambridge, England, Cambridge University Press, 1990, pp 205–220

Clements M: What we say about mental illness. Parade, October 31, 1993, pp 4–6

Frances AJ, Widiger TA, Pincus HA: The development of DSM-IV. Arch Gen Psychiatry 46:373–375, 1989

Health care reform for Americans with severe mental illnesses: report of the National Advisory Mental Health Council. Am J Psychiatry 150:447–465, 1993

Klerman GL: Ideological conflicts in integrating pharmacotherapy and psychotherapy, in Integrating Pharmacotherapy and Psychotherapy. Edited by Beitman BD, Klerman GL. Washington, DC, American Psychiatric Press, 1991, pp 3–19

Massel HK, Liberman RP, Mintz J, et al: Evaluating the capacity to work of the mentally ill. Psychiatry 53:31–43, 1990

Mental Health Parity Act of 1996. U.S. Public Law 104-204, 1996

Rosenbaum M: Similarities of psychiatric disorders of AIDS and syphilis: history repeats itself. Bull Menninger Clin 58:375–382, 1994

Sabshin M: Medical Director's Report. Am J Psychiatry 133:1236–1240, 1976

Sabshin M: Medical Director's Report. Am J Psychiatry 134:1194–1199, 1977

Sabshin M: Turning points in twentieth-century American psychiatry. Am J Psychiatry 147:1267–1274, 1990

Sabshin M: Authoritarianism and the practice of psychiatry. Paper presented at the Institute on Psychiatric Services, October 1995

Sabshin M: Parity for mental illness: the half-full glass. Mol Psychiatry 2:177, 1997

Scully JH: Determining workforce needs. Paper presented at the 148th annual meeting of the American Psychiatric Association, Miami, FL, May 20–25, 1995

World Health Organization: International Classification of Diseases, 10th Revision. Geneva, World Health Organization, 1992

Zarin DA, Pincus HA, McIntyre JS: Practice based research in psychiatry. Am J Psychiatry 154:1199–1208, 1997

Appendix 2

American Psychiatric Association Speakers of Assembly of District Branches

TERM	NAME
1955–1956	Addison M. Duval
1956–1957	Mathew Ross
1959–1960	Alfred Auerback
1960–1961	John R. Saunders
1963–1964	Robert S. Garber
1964–1965	Philip B. Reed,
1966–1967	Hamilton Ford
1967–1968	John R. Adams
1969–1970	Perry C. Talkington
1970–1971	John S. Visher
1971–1972	Harry H. Brunt Jr.
1972–1973	James C. Johnson Jr.
1974–1975	Robert B. Neu
1975–1976	Miltiades L. Zaphiropoulos
1976–1977	Irwin N. Perr
1977–1978	Daniel A. Grabski
1978–1979	Robert J. Campbell III
1979–1980	Robert O. Pasnau
1980–1981	Melvin M. Lipsett
1981–1982	Lawrence Hartmann
1982–1983	William Sorum
1983–1984	Harvey Bluestone
1984–1985	Fred Gottlieb

1985–1986	James M. Trench
1986–1987	Roger Peele
1987–1988	Irwin M. Cohen
1988–1989	John S. McIntyre
1989–1990	Gerald H. Flamm
1990–1991	Edward Hanin
1991–1992	G. Thomas Pfaehler
1992–1993	Ronald A. Shellow
1993–1994	Richard M. Bridburg
1994–1995	Norman A. Clemens
1995–1996	Richard K. Harding
1996–1997	R. Dale Walker
1997–1998	Jeremy A. Lazarus
1998–1999	Donna M. Norris
1999–2000	Alfred Herzog
2000–2001	R. Michael Pearce
2001–2002	Nada L. Stotland
2002–2003	Albert C. Gaw
2003–2004	Prakash N. Desa
2004–2005	James E. Nininger

Appendix 3

Presidential Themes for American Psychiatric Association Annual Meetings, 1984–2008[1]

---

[1]Presidential themes were begun in 1984.

YEAR	CITY	PRESIDENT	THEME
1984	Los Angeles, CA	George Tarjan, M.D.	American Psychiatry: A Dynamic Mosaic
1985	Dallas, TX	John A. Talbott, M.D.	Our Patients in a Changing World
1986	Washington, DC	Carol C. Nadelson, M.D.	Unity Admist Diversity: Future Challenges
1987	Chicago, IL	Robert O. Pasnau, M.D.	Psychiatry in Medicine Medicine in Psychiatry
1988	Montreal, Canada	George H. Pollock, M.D.	Theme: Opportunities and Challenges for Psychiatrists and Psychiatry: 1988–2000
1989	San Francisco, CA	Paul J. Fink, M.D.	Overcoming Stigma
1990	New York, NY	Herbert Pardes, M.D.	The Research Alliance: Road to Clinical Excellence
1991	New Orleans, LA	Elissa P. Benedek, M.D.	Our Children, Our Future
1992	Washington, DC	Lawrence Hartmann, M.D.	Humane Values and Biopsychosocial Integration
1993	San Francisco, CA	Joseph T. English, M.D.	Patient Care for the Twenty-First Century: Asserting Professional Values Within Economic Constraints
1994	Philadelphia, PA	John S. McIntyre, M.D.	Our Heritage Our Future
1995	Miami, FL	Jerry M. Wiener, M.D.	Encompassing Diversity: Demanding Equity
1996	New York, NY	Mary Jane England, M.D.	America's Mental Health: Partnerships, Equity, Quality, Outcomes

Year	Location	Name	Theme
1997	San Diego, CA	Harold H. Eist, M.D.	Strengthening Psychiatry's Dedication and Commitment to Compassionate Care, Educational Excellence, Creative Research
1998	Toronto, Canada	Herbert S. Sacks, M.D.	New Challenges for Proven Values: Defending Access, Fairness, Ethics, Decency
1999	Washington, DC	Rodrigo A. Muñoz, M.D.	The Clinician
2000	Chicago, IL	Allan Tasman, M.D.	The Doctor–Patient Relationship
2001	New Orleans, LA	Daniel B. Borenstein, M.D.	Mind Meets Brain: Integrating Psychiatry, Psychoanalysis, Neuroscience
2002	Philadelphia, PA	Richard K. Harding, M.D.	The Twenty-First Century Psychiatrist
2003	San Francisco, CA	Paul S. Appelbaum, M.D.	The Promise of Science—The Power of Healing
2004	New York, NY	Marcia Kraft Goin, M.D.	Psychotherapy and Psychopharmacology: Dissolving the Mind–Brain Barrier
2005	Atlanta, GA	Michelle B. Riba, M.D.	Psychosomatic Medicine: Integrating Psychiatry and Medicine
2006	Toronto, Canada	Steven S. Sharfstein, M.D.	From Science to Public Policy: Advocacy for Patients and the Profession
2007	San Diego, CA	Pedro Ruiz, M.D.	Addressing Patient Needs: Access, Parity and Humane Care
2008	Washington, DC	Carolyn B. Robinowitz, M.D.	Our Voice in Action: Advancing Science, Care and the Profession

Appendix 4

Officers of the American Psychiatric Association

Note.   *Two Presidents–Elect, AB. Richardson (1903–1904 term) and H. Douglas Singer (1941–1942), died before assuming office. Their names have appeared on some historical rosters of Presidents.

From 1936 through 1957, the Vice-President was deleted from the APA Constitution. The Constitution was revised in 1957 to allow two vice presidents. The Bylaws were revised again in 2003 to eliminate one Vice-President beginning in 2004. One Vice-President to be elected in 2005 and then in alternate years.

The Bylaws were revised in 2003 to merge the Secretary and Treasurer positions in 2005. Treasurer elected in 2004 serves as Treasurer from May 2004 to May 2005 and as Secretary–Treasurer from May 2005 to May 2006. Secretary–Treasurer to be elected 2006 and then in alternate years.

BY NAME

NAME	OFFICE	TERM
Ackerly, S. Spafford	Vice-President	1959–1960
Adams, John R.	Speaker	1967–1968
Andrews, J. B.	President	1892–1893
Anglin, James V.	President	1917–1918
Appel, Kenneth E.	President	1953–1954
Appelbaum, Paul S.	Secretary	1997–1999
Appelbaum, Paul S.	Vice-President	1999–2001
Appelbaum, Paul Stuart	President	2002–2003
Auerback, Alfred	Speaker	1959–1960
Auerback, Alfred	Vice-President	1966–1967
Awl, William M.	Vice-President	1846–1848
Awl, William McClay	President	1848–1851
Bancroft, Charles P.	President	1907–1908
Barrett, Albert M.	President	1921–1922
Bartemeier, Leo H.	Secretary	1946–1950
Bartemeier, Leo H.	President	1951–1952
Barton, Walter E.	President	1961–1962
Bay, Alfred Paul	Vice-President	1962–1963
Beigel, Allan	Vice-President	1987–1989
Bell, Luther V.	Vice-President	1850–1851
Bell, Luther V.	President	1851–1855
Benedek, Elissa P.	President	1990–1991
Benedek, Elissa P.	Vice-President	1983–1985
Benedek, Elissa P.	Secretary	1985–1989
Bernard, Viola	Vice-President	1971–1972
Bernstein, Carol B.	Treasurer	2000–2004
Blain, Daniel	President	1964–1965
Bluestone, Harvey	Speaker	1983–1984
Blumer, G. Alder	President	1902–1903
Bond, Earl D.	President	1929–1930
Borenstein, Daniel B.	President	2000–2001
Borenstein, Daniel B.	Secretary	1995–1997
Borenstein, Daniel B.	Vice-President	1997–1999
Bowman, Karl M.	President	1944–1946
Braceland, Francis J.	President	1956–1957
Branch, C. H. Hardin	President	1962–1963

Branch, C. H. Hardin	Secretary	1958–1961
Bridburg, Richard M.	Speaker	1993–1994
Brigham, Amariah	Vice-President	1848–1850
Brodie, H. Keith H.	Secretary	1977–1981
Brodie, H. Keith H.	President	1982–1983
Brosin, Henry W.	Vice-President	1961–1962
Brosin, Henry W.	President	1967–1968
Brunt, Jr., Harry H.	Speaker	1971–1972
Brush, Edward N.	President	1915–1916
Bucke, Richard M.	President	1897–1898
Burgess, T.J.	President	1904–1905
Burr, C.B.	President	1905–1906
Busse, Ewald W.	Vice-President	1966–1967
Busse, Ewald W.	President	1971–1972
Butler, John S.	Vice-President	1862–1870
Butler, John S.	President	1870–1873
Buttolph, H.A.	President	1886–1887
Callender, John H.	Vice-President	1879–1882
Callender, John H.	President	1882–1883
Cameron, D. Ewen	President	1952–1953
Cameron, Dale C.	Treasurer	1963–1968
Campbell, C. Macfie	President	1936–1937
Campbell III, Robert J.	Speaker	1978–1979
Campbell, Robert	Vice-President	1980–1982
Carmichael, Hugh T.	Vice-President	1963–1964
Chapin, John B.	President	1888–1889
Chapman, Ross McC.	President	1937–1938
Cheney, Clarence O.	President	1935–1936
Christmas, June Jackson	Vice-President	1974–1975
Clark, Daniel	President	1891–1892
Clemens, Norman A.	Speaker	1994–1995
Cohen, Irvin M.	Speaker	1987–1988
Copp, Owen	President	1920–1921
Cowles, Edward	President	1894–1895
Curwen, John	President	1893–1894
Desa, Prakash N.	Speaker	2003–2004
Dewey, Richard	President	1895–1896
Dickstein, Leah J.	Vice-President	1991–1993

Donahue, Hayden	Treasurer	1968–1973
Drewry, William F.	President	1909–1910
Duval, Addison M.	Speaker	1955–1956
Duval, Addison M.	Treasurer	1959–1963
Duval, Addison M.	Vice-President	1964–1965
Earle, Pliny	Vice-President	1883–1884
Earle, Pliny	President	1884–1885
Ebasugh, Franklin	Vice-President	1959–1960
Eist, Harold	President	1996–1997
England, Mary Jane	President	1995–1996
England, Mary Jane	Treasurer	1990–1994
English, Joseph T.	President	1992–1993
English, Walter M.	President	1930–1931
Everts, Orpheus	Vice-President	1884–1885
Everts, Orpheus	President	1885–1886
Ewalt, Jack R.	Treasurer	1954–1958
Ewalt, Jack R.	President	1963–1964
Eyman, Henry C.	President	1919–1920
Felix, Robert H.	Treasurer	1958–1959
Felix, Robert H.	President	1960–1961
Fink, Paul J.	Vice-President	1985–1987
Fink, Paul J.	President	1988–1989
Flamm, Gerald H.	Speaker	1989–1990
Ford, Hamilton f.	Speaker	1966–1967
Ford, Hamilton F.	Vice-President	1969–1970
Frazier, Shervert H.	Secretary	1983–1985
Freedman, Alfred M.	President	1973–1974
Freedman, Daniel X.	Vice-President	1975–1977
Freedman, Daniel X.	President	1981–1982
Garber, Robert S.	Speaker	1963–1964
Garber, Robert S.	Secretary	1965–1969
Garber, Robert S.	President	1970–1971
Gaskill, Herbert S.	Vice-President	1970–1971
Gaw, Albert C.	Speaker	2002–2003
Gayle Jr., R. Finley	President	1955–1956
Gerty, Francis J.	President	1958–1959
Gibson, Robert W.	Secretary	1972–1975
Gibson, Robert W.	President	1976–1977

Godding, W.W.	President	1889–1890
Goin, Marcia	President	2003–2004
Goin, Marcia Kraft	Vice-President	2000–2002
Gottlieb, Fred	Speaker	1984–1985
Gottlieb, Fred	Vice-President	1989–1991
Gottlieb, Fred	Treasurer	1994–1998
Grabski, Daniel A.	Speaker	1977–1978
Gray, John P.	Vice-President	1882–1883
Gray, John P.	President	1883–1884
Greenblatt, Milton	Vice-President	1972–1973
Grissom, Eugene	President	1887–1888
Hall, James King	President	1941–1942
Hamilton, Samuel W.	President	1946–1947
Hanin, Edward	Speaker	1990–1991
Harding, Richard K.	Speaker	1995–1996
Harding, Richard K.	Vice-President	1998–2000
Harding, Richard K.	President	2001–2002
Harper, Edward O.	Vice-President	1969–1970
Harris, Titus H.	Vice-President	1961–1962
Hartmann, Lawrence	Speaker	1981–1982
Hartmann, Lawrence	Vice-President	1988–1990
Hartmann, Lawrence	President	1991–1992
Haviland, C. Floyd	President	1925–1926
Herzog, Alfred	Speaker	1999–2000
Hill, Charles G.	President	1906–1907
Hurd, Henry M.	President	1898–1899
Hutchings, Richard H.	President	1938–1939
Johnson, Jr., James C.	Speaker	1972–1973
Judd, Lewis L.	Vice-President	1992–1994
Kaufman, M. Ralph	Vice-President	1963–1964
Kenworthy, Marion E.	Vice-President	1965–1966
Kilbourne, Arthur F.	President	1908–1909
Kirby, George H.	President	1933–1934
Kirkbride, Thomas S.	President	1862–1870
Kirkbride, Thomas S.	Vice-President	1855–1862
Kirkpatrick, Martha J.	Vice-President	1993–1995
Kline, George M.	President	1926–1927
Kolb, Lawrence C.	President	1968–1969

Langsley, Donald G.	Vice-President	1977–1979
Langsley, Donald G.	President	1980–1981
Lazarus, Jeremy A.	Speaker	1997–1998
Lemkau, Paul V.	Vice-President	1968–1969
Levenson, Alan I.	Treasurer	1986–1990
Lipsett, Melvin M.	Speaker	1980–1981
Luton, Frank	Vice-President	1965–1966
Lymberis, Maria T.	Treasurer	1998–2000
Macdonald, A. E.	President	1903–1904
MacDonald, Carlos F.	President	1913–1914
Malamud, William	Secretary	1954–1958
Malamud, William	President	1959–1960
Margolis, Philip M.	Secretary	1989–1991
Marmor, Judd	Vice-President	1972–1973
Marmor, Judd	President	1975–1976
Martin, Peter A.	Vice-President	1979–1981
Masserman, Jules	Vice-President	1974–1975
Masserman, Jules	Secretary	1975–1977
Masserman, Jules	President	1978–1979
May, James V.	President	1932–1933
McFarland, Andrew	President	1859–1862
McIntyre, John S.	President	1993–1994
McIntyre, John S.	Speaker	1988–1989
McIntyre, John S.	Vice-President	1990–1992
McKerracher, D. Griffith	Vice-President	1960–1961
Menninger, William C.	President	1948–1949
Meyer, Adolf	President	1927–1928
Mitchell, H.W.	President	1922–1923
Mitchell-Bateman, Mildred	Vice-President	1973–1974
Modlin, Herbert	Vice-President	1971–1972
Munoz, Rodrigo A.	President	1998–1999
Munoz, Rodrigo A.	Vice-President	1995–1997
Nadelson, Carol C.	Vice-President	1981–1983
Nadelson, Carol C.	President	1985–1986
Neu, Robert B.	Speaker	1974–1975
Nichols, Charles H.	Vice-President	1870–1873
Nichols, Charles H.	President	1873–1879
Nininger, James E.	Speaker	2004–2005

Norris, Donna M.	Speaker	1998–1999
Noyes, Arthur P.	President	1954–1955
Orton, Samuel T.	President	1928–1929
Overholser, Winfred	President	1947–1948
Pardes, Herbert	Vice-President	1986–1988
Pardes, Herbert	President	1989–1990
Pasnau, Robert O.	Vice-President	1982–1984
Pasnau, Robert O.	President	1986–1987
Pasnau, Robert O.	Speaker	1979–1980
Pearce, R. Michael	Speaker	2000–2001
Peele, Roger	Speaker	1986–1987
Perr, Irwin N.	Speaker	1976–1977
Perr, Irwin N.	Vice-President	1984–1986
Pfaehler, G. Thomas	Speaker	1991–1992
Pilgrim, Charles W.	President	1910–1911
Pollock, George H.	Treasurer	1980–1986
Pollock, George H.	President	1987–1988
Potter, Howard W.	Treasurer	1947–1954
Powell, Theophilus O.	President	1896–1897
Preston, Robert J.	President	1901–1902
Prudhomme, Charles	Vice-President	1970–1971
Ray, Isaac	Vice-President	1851–1855
Ray, Isaac	President	1855–1859
Reed, Philip B.	Speaker	1964–1965
Reed, Philip B.	Vice-President	1968–1969
Riba, Michelle	President	2004–2005
Riba, Michelle B.	Secretary	1999–2001
Riba, Michelle B.	Vice-President	2001–2003
Richardson, A. B.*	President	—
Robbins, Lewis	Vice-President	1978–1980
Robinowitz, Carolyn B.	Treasurer	2004–2006
Rogers, Joseph G.	President	1899–1900
Rome, Howard P.	President	1965–1966
Ross, Mathew	Speaker	1956–1957
Ruggles, Arthur H.	President	1942–1943
Ruiz, Pedro	Vice-President	2003–2005
Ruiz, Pedro	Secretary	2001–2003
Russell, William L.	President	1931–1932

Sacks, Herbert S.	President	1997–1998
Sacks, Herbert S.	Vice-President	1994–1996
Salmon, Thomas W.	President	1923–1924
Sandy, William C.	President	1939–1940
Saunders, John R.	Speaker	1960–1961
Saunders, John R.	Vice-President	1962–1963
Searcy, James T.	President	1912–1913
Sharfstein, Steven S.	Secretary	1991–1995
Sharfstein, Steven S.	Vice-President	2002–2004
Shellow, Ronald A.	Speaker	1992–1993
Singer, H. Douglas*	President	—
Smith, Samuel E.	President	1914–1915
Solomon, Harry C.	President	1957–1958
Sorum, William	Speaker	1982–1983
Southard, Elmer E.	President	1918–1919
Spiegel, John P.	President	1974–1975
Stearnes, H. P.	President	1890–1891
Stevenson, George H.	President	1940–1941
Stevenson, George S.	President	1949–1950
Stokes, Aldwyn B.	Vice-President	1964–1965
Stone, Alan A.	Vice-President	1976–1978
Stone, Alan A.	President	1979–1980
Stotland, Nada L.	Speaker	2001–2002
Stotland, Nada L.	Secretary	2003–2005
Strecker, Edward A.	President	1943–1944
Talbott, John A.	President	1984–1985
Talkington, Perry C.	Speaker	1969–1970
Talkington, Perry C.	President	1972–1973
Tarjan, George	Vice-President	1967–1968
Tarjan, George	Secretary	1969–1972
Tarjan, George	President	1983–1984
Tasman, Allan	President	1999–2000
Tasman, Allan	Vice-President	1996–1998
Terhune, William	Vice-President	1958–1959
Tompkins, Harvey J.	Secretary	1961–1965
Tompkins, Harvey J.	President	1966–1967
Trench, James M.	Speaker	1985–1986
Visher, John S.	Speaker	1970–1971

Visotsky, Harold M.	Secretary	1981–1982
Visotsky, Harold M.	Vice-President	1973–1974
Waggoner, Raymond W.	Vice-President	1960–1961
Waggoner, Raymond W.	President	1969–1970
Wagner, Charles G.	President	1916–1917
Walker, Clement A.	Vice-President	1873–1879
Walker, Clement A.	President	1879–1882
Walker, R. Dale	Speaker	1996–1997
Weinberg, Jack	Treasurer	1973–1976
Weinberg, Jack	President	1977–1978
White, Samuel	Vice-President	1844–1846
White, William A.	President	1924–1925
Whitehorn, John C.	President	1950–1951
Wiener, Jerry M.	President	1994–1995
Wilkinson, Charles	Treasurer	1976–1980
Williams, C. Fred	President	1934–1935
Wilson, David C.	Vice-President	1958–1959
Wise, Peter M.	President	1900–1901
Wittson, Cecil L.	Vice-President	1967–1968
Wolford, Jack A.	Vice-President	1975–1976
Woodward, Samuel B.	President	1844–1848
Work, Hubert	President	1911–1912
Zaphiropoulos, Miltiades L.	Speaker	1975–1976

BY TERM

TERM	OFFICE	NAME
1844–1846	Vice-President	White, Samuel
1844–1848	President	Woodward, Samuel B.
1846–1848	Vice-President	Awl, William M.
1848–1850	Vice-President	Brigham, Amariah
1848–1851	President	Awl, William McClay
1850–1851	Vice-President	Bell, Luther V.
1851–1855	President	Bell, Luther V.
1851–1855	Vice-President	Ray, Isaac
1855–1859	President	Ray, Isaac
1855–1862	Vice-President	Kirkbride, Thomas S.
1859–1862	President	McFarland, Andrew
1862–1870	Vice-President	Butler, John S.

1862–1870	President	Kirkbride, , Thomas S.
1870–1873	President	Butler, John S.
1870–1873	Vice-President	Nichols, Charles H.
1873–1879	President	Nichols, Charles H.
1873–1879	Vice-President	Walker, Clement A.
1879–1882	Vice-President	Callender, John H.
1879–1882	President	Walker, Clement A.
1882–1883	President	Callender, John H.
1882–1883	Vice-President	Gray, John P.
1883–1884	Vice-President	Earle, Pliny
1883–1884	President	Gray, John P.
1884–1885	President	Earle, Pliny
1884–1885	Vice-President	Everts, Orpheus
1885–1886	President	Everts, Orpheus
1886–1887	President	Buttolph, H.A.
1887–1888	President	Grissom, Eugene
1888–1889	President	Chapin, John B.
1889–1890	President	Godding, W.W.
1890–1891	President	Stearnes, H.P.
1891–1892	President	Clark, Daniel
1892–1893	President	Andrews, J.B.
1893–1894	President	Curwen, John
1894–1895	President	Cowles, Edward
1895–1896	President	Dewey, Richard
1896–1897	President	Powell, Theophilus O.
1897–1898	President	Bucke, Richard M.
1898–1899	President	Hurd, Henry M.
1899–1900	President	Rogers, Joseph G.
1900–1901	President	Wise, Peter M.
1901–1902	President	Preston, Robert J.
1902–	President	Richardson, AB.*
1902–1903	President	Blumer, G. Alder
1903–1904	President	Macdonald, A.E.
1904–1905	President	Burgess, T.J.
1905–1906	President	Burr, C.B.
1906–1907	President	Hill, Charles G.
1907–1908	President	Bancroft, Charles P.
1908–1909	President	Kilbourne, Arthur F.

1909–1910	President	Drewry, William F.
1910–1911	President	Pilgrim, Charles W.
1911–1912	President	Work, Hubert
1912–1913	President	Searcy, James T.
1913–1914	President	MacDonald, Carlos F.
1914–1915	President	Smith, Samuel E.
1915–1916	President	Brush, Edward N.
1916–1917	President	Wagner, Charles G.
1917–1918	President	Anglin, James V.
1918–1919	President	Southard, Elmer E.
1919–1920	President	Eyman, Henry C.
1920–1921	President	Copp, Owen
1921–1922	President	Barrett, Albert M.
1922–1923	President	Mitchell, H. W.
1923–1924	President	Salmon, Thomas W.
1924–1925	President	White, William A.
1925–1926	President	Haviland, C. Floyd
1926–1927	President	Kline, George M.
1927–1928	President	Meyer, Adolf
1928–1929	President	Orton, Samuel T.
1929–1930	President	Bond, Earl D.
1930–1931	President	English, Walter M.
1931–1932	President	Russell, William L.
1932–1933	President	May, James V.
1933–1934	President	Kirby, George H.
1934–1935	President	Williams, C. Fred
1935–1936	President	Cheney, Clarence O.
1936–1937	President	Campbell, C. Macfie
1937–1938	President	Chapman, Ross McC.
1938–1939	President	Hutchings, Richard H.
1939–1940	President	Sandy, William C.
1940–1941	President	Stevenson, George H.
1941–1942	President	Hall, James King
1942–	President	Singer, H. Douglas*
1942–1943	President	Ruggles, Arthur H.
1943–1944	President	Strecker, Edward A.
1944–1946	President	Bowman, Karl M.
1946–1947	President	Hamilton, Samuel W.

1946–1950	Secretary	Bartemeier, Leo H.
1947–1948	President	Overholser, Winfred
1947–1954	Treasurer	Potter, Howard W.
1948–1949	President	Menninger, William C.
1949–1950	President	Stevenson, George S.
1950–1951	President	Whitehorn, John C.
1951–1952	President	Bartemeier, Leo H.
1952–1953	President	Cameron, D. Ewen
1953–1954	President	Appel, Kenneth E.
1954–1955	President	Noyes, Arthur P.
1954–1958	Treasurer	Ewalt, Jack R.
1954–1958	Secretary	Malamud, William
1955–1956	Speaker	Duval, Addison M.
1955–1956	President	Gayle Jr., R. Finley
1956–1957	President	Braceland, Francis J.
1956–1957	Speaker	Ross, Mathew
1957–1958	President	Solomon, Harry C.
1958–1959	Treasurer	Felix, Robert H.
1958–1959	President	Gerty, Francis J.
1958–1959	Vice-President	Terhune, William
1958–1959	Vice-President	Wilson, David C.
1958–1961	Secretary	Branch, C.H. Hardin
1959–1960	Vice-President	Ackerly, S. Spafford
1959–1960	Speaker	Auerback, Alfred
1959–1960	Vice-President	Ebasugh, Franklin
1959–1960	President	Malamud, William
1959–1963	Treasurer	Duval, Addison M.
1960–1961	President	Felix, Robert H.
1960–1961	Vice-President	McKerracher, D. Griffith
1960–1961	Speaker	Saunders, John R.
1960–1961	Vice-President	Waggoner, Raymond W.
1961–1962	President	Barton, Walter E.
1961–1962	Vice-President	Brosin, Henry W.
1961–1962	Vice-President	Harris, Titus H.
1961–1965	Secretary	Tompkins, Harvey J.
1962–1963	Vice-President	Bay, Alfred Paul
1962–1963	President	Branch, C.H. Hardin
1962–1963	Vice-President	Saunders, John R.

1963–1964	Vice-President	Carmichael, Hugh T.
1963–1964	President	Ewalt, Jack R.
1963–1964	Speaker	Garber, Robert S.
1963–1964	Vice-President	Kaufman, M. Ralph
1963–1968	Treasurer	Cameron, Dale C.
1964–1965	President	Blain, Daniel
1964–1965	Vice-President	Duval, Addison M.
1964–1965	Speaker	Reed, Philip B.
1964–1965	Vice-President	Stokes, Aldwyn B.
1965–1966	Vice-President	Kenworthy, Marion E.
1965–1966	Vice-President	Luton, Frank
1965–1966	President	Rome, Howard P.
1965–1969	Secretary	Garber, Robert S.
1966–1967	Vice-President	Auerback, Alfred
1966–1967	Vice-President	Busse, Ewald W.
1966–1967	Speaker	Ford, Hamilton
1966–1967	President	Tompkins, Harvey J.
1967–1968	Speaker	Adams, John R.
1967–1968	President	Brosin, Henry W.
1967–1968	Vice-President	Tarjan, George
1967–1968	Vice-President	Wittson, Cecil L.
1968–1969	President	Kolb, Lawrence C.
1968–1969	Vice-President	Lemkau, Paul V.
1968–1969	Vice-President	Reed, Philip B.
1968–1973	Treasurer	Donahue, Hayden
1969–1970	Vice-President	Ford, Hamilton F.
1969–1970	Vice-President	Harper, Edward O.
1969–1970	Speaker	Talkington, Perry C.
1969–1970	President	Waggoner, Raymond W.
1969–1972	Secretary	Tarjan, George
1970–1971	President	Garber, Robert S.
1970–1971	Vice-President	Gaskill, Herbert S.
1970–1971	Vice-President	Prudhomme, Charles
1970–1971	Speaker	Visher, John S.
1971–1972	Vice-President	Bernard, Viola
1971–1972	Speaker	Brunt, Jr., Harry H.
1971–1972	President	Busse, Ewald W.
1971–1972	Vice-President	Modlin, Herbert

1972–1973	Vice-President	Greenblatt, Milton
1972–1973	Speaker	Johnson, Jr., James C.
1972–1973	Vice-President	Marmor, Judd
1972–1973	President	Talkington, Perry C.
1972–1975	Secretary	Gibson, Robert W.
1973–1974	President	Freedman, Alfred M.
1973–1974	Vice-President	Mitchell-Bateman, Mildred
1973–1974	Vice-President	Visotsky, Harold M.
1973–1976	Treasurer	Weinberg, Jack
1974–1975	Vice-President	Christmas, June Jackson
1974–1975	Vice-President	Masserman, Jules
1974–1975	Speaker	Neu, Robert B.
1974–1975	President	Spiegel, John P.
1975–1976	President	Marmor, Judd
1975–1976	Vice-President	Wolford, Jack A.
1975–1976	Speaker	Zaphiropoulos, Miltiades L.
1975–1977	Vice-President	Freedman, Daniel X.
1975–1977	Secretary	Masserman, Jules
1976–1977	President	Gibson, Robert W.
1976–1977	Speaker	Perr, Irwin N.
1976–1978	Vice-President	Stone, Alan A.
1976–1980	Treasurer	Wilkinson, Charles
1977–1978	Speaker	Grabski, Daniel A.
1977–1978	President	Weinberg, Jack
1977–1979	Vice-President	Langsley, Donald G.
1977–1981	Secretary	Brodie, H. Keith H.
1978–1979	Speaker	Campbell, III, Robert J.
1978–1979	President	Masserman, Jules
1978–1980	Vice-President	Robbins, Lewis
1979–1980	Speaker	Pasnau, Robert O.
1979–1980	President	Stone, Alan A.
1979–1981	Vice-President	Martin, Peter A.
1980–1981	President	Langsley, Donald G.
1980–1981	Speaker	Lipsett, Melvin M.
1980–1982	Vice-President	Campbell, Robert
1980–1986	Treasurer	Pollock, George H.
1981–1982	President	Freedman, Daniel X.
1981–1982	Speaker	Hartmann, Lawrence

1981–1982	Secretary	Visotsky, Harold
1981–1983	Vice-President	Nadelson, Carol C.
1982–1983	President	Brodie, H. Keith H.
1982–1983	Speaker	Sorum, William
1982–1984	Vice-President	Pasnau, Robert O.
1983–1984	Speaker	Bluestone, Harvey
1983–1984	President	Tarjan, George
1983–1985	Vice-President	Benedek, Elissa P.
1983–1985	Secretary	Frazier, Shervert H.
1984–1985	Speaker	Gottlieb, Fred
1984–1985	President	Talbott, John A.
1984–1986	Vice-President	Perr, Irwin N.
1985–1986	President	Nadelson, Carol C.
1985–1986	Speaker	Trench, James M.
1985–1987	Vice-President	Fink, Paul J.
1985–1989	Secretary	Benedek, Elissa P.
1986–1987	President	Pasnau, Robert O.
1986–1987	Speaker	Peele, Roger
1986–1988	Vice-President	Pardes, Herbert
1986–1990	Treasurer	Levenson, Alan I.
1987–1988	Speaker	Cohen, Irvin M.
1987–1988	President	Pollock, George H.
1987–1989	Vice-President	Beigel, Allan
1988–1989	President	Fink, Paul J.
1988–1989	Speaker	McIntyre, John S.
1988–1990	Vice-President	Hartmann, Lawrence
1989–1990	Speaker	Flamm, Gerald H.
1989–1990	President	Pardes, Herbert
1989–1991	Vice-President	Gottlieb, Fred
1989–1991	Secretary	Margolis, Philip M.
1990–1991	President	Benedek, Elissa
1990–1991	Speaker	Hanin, Edward
1990–1992	Vice-President	McIntyre, John S.
1990–1994	Treasurer	England, Mary Jane R.
1991–1992	President	Hartmann, Lawrence
1991–1992	Speaker	Pfaehler, G. Thomas
1991–1993	Vice-President	Dickstein, Leah J.
1991–1995	Secretary	Sharfstein, Steven S.

1992–1993	President	English, Joseph T.
1992–1993	Speaker	Shellow, Ronald A.
1992–1994	Vice-President	Judd, Lewis L.
1993–1994	Speaker	Bridburg, Richard M.
1993–1994	President	McIntyre, John
1993–1995	Vice-President	Kirkpatrick, Martha J.
1994–1995	Speaker	Clemens, Norman A.
1994–1995	President	Wiener, Jerry M.
1994–1996	Vice-President	Sacks, Herbert S.
1994–1998	Treasurer	Gottlieb, Fred
1995–1996	President	England, Mary Jane
1995–1996	Speaker	Harding, Richard K.
1995–1997	Secretary	Borenstein, Daniel B.
1995–1997	Vice-President	Munoz, Rodrigo A.
1996–1997	President	Eist, Harold
1996–1997	Speaker	Walker, R. Dale
1996–1998	Vice-President	Tasman, Allan
1997–1998	Speaker	Lazarus, Jeremy A.
1997–1998	President	Sacks, Herbert S.
1997–1999	Secretary	Appelbaum, Paul S.
1997–1999	Vice-President	Borenstein, Daniel B.
1998–1999	President	Muñoz, Rodrigo A.
1998–1999	Speaker	Norris, Donna M.
1998–2000	Vice-President	Harding, Richard K.
1998–2000	Treasurer	Lymberis, Maria T.
1999–2000	Speaker	Herzog, Alfred
1999–2000	President	Tasman, Allan
1999–2001	Vice-President	Appelbaum, Paul S.
1999–2001	Secretary	Riba, Michelle B.
2000–2001	President	Borenstein, Daniel
2000–2001	Speaker	Pearce, R. Michael
2000–2002	Vice-President	Goin, Marcia Kraft
2000–2004	Treasurer	Bernstein, Carol B.
2001–2002	President	Harding, Richard Kent
2001–2002	Speaker	Stotland, Nada L.
2001–2003	Vice-President	Riba, Michelle B.
2001–2003	Secretary	Ruiz, Pedro
2002–2003	President	Appelbaum, Paul Stuart

2002–2003	Speaker	Gaw, Albert C.
2002–2004	Vice-President	Sharfstein, Steven S.
2003–2004	Speaker	Desa, Prakash N.
2003–2004	President	Goin, Marcia
2003–2005	Vice-President	Ruiz, Pedro
2003–2005	Secretary	Stotland, Nada L.
2004–2005	Speaker	Nininger, James E.
2004–2005	President	Riba, Michelle
2004–2006	Treasurer	Robinowitz, Carolyn B.

Appendix 5

American Psychiatric Association Membership Figures, 1873–2007

Date	Number of Members	Date	Number of Members	Date	Number of Members	Date	Number of Members
1873	93	1930	1,346	1960	11,037	1990	36,208
1885	134	1931	1,393	1961	11,637	1991	36,918
1895	300	1932	1,416	1962	12,267	1992	37,279
1896	303	1933	1,517	1963	12,872	1993	37,983
1897	312	1934	1,604	1964	13,396	1994	38,285
1898	321	1935	1,676	1965	13,853	1995	39,450
1899	376	1936	1,749	1966	14,341	1996	40,537
1900	377	1937	1,889	1967	14,935	1997	40,978
1901	366	1938	2,053	1968	16,524	1998	40,278
1902	384	1939	2,235	1969	17,050	1999	37,380
1903	402	1940	2,423	1970	18,407	2000	37,843
1904	409	1941	2,667	1971	19,037	2001	37,146
1905	424	1942	2,913	1972	19,579	2002	36,213
1906	423	1943	3,125	1973	20,261	2003	34,807
1907	451	1944	3,387	1974	20,856	2004	35,359
1908	450	1945	3,634	1975	21,251	2005	35,086
1918	901	1946	4,010	1976	22,205	2006	35,816
1920	937	1947	4,341	1977	23,301	2007	36,438
1921	1,001	1948	4,678	1978	24,210		
1922	1,063	1949	5,276	1979	24,676		

1923	1,093	**1950**	**5,856**	**1980**	**25,345**
1924	1,131	1951	6,581	1981	25,814
1925	**1,211**	1952	7,125	1982	26,470
1926	1,262	1953	7,608	1983	27,355
1927	1,282	1954	8,149	1984	29,009
1928	1,302	**1955**	**8,534**	**1985**	**30,514**
1929	1,325	1956	8,673	1986	31,837
		1957	9,247	1987	33,293
		1958	9,801	1988	34,306
		1959	10,420	1989	35,168

Appendix 6

Presidents of the American Psychiatric Association

BY TERM

No.	Term	Name
1	1844–1848	Woodward, Samuel B.
2	1848–1851	Awl, William McClay
3	1851–1855	Bell, Luther V.
4	1855–1859	Ray, Isaac
5	1859–1862	McFarland, Andrew
6	1862–1870	Kirkbride, Thomas S.
7	1870–1873	Butler, John S.
8	1873–1879	Nichols, Charles H.
9	1879–1882	Walker, Clement A.
10	1882–1883	Callender, John H.
11	1883–1884	Gray, John P.
12	1884–1885	Earle, Pliny
13	1885–1886	Everts, Orpheus
14	1886–1887	Buttolph, H.A.
15	1887–1888	Grissom, Eugene
16	1888–1889	Chapin, John B.
17	1889–1890	Godding, W.W.
18	1890–1891	Stearnes, H.P.
19	1891–1892	Clark, Daniel

*Two Presidents–Elect, A.B. Richardson (1903–1904 term) and H. Douglas Singer (1941–1942 term), died before assuming office. Their names have appeared on some historical rosters of Presidents.

20	1892–1893	Andrews, J. B.
21	1893–1894	Curwen, John
22	1894–1895	Cowles, Edward
23	1895–1896	Dewey, Richard
24	1896–1897	Powell, Theophilus O.
25	1897–1898	Bucke, Richard M.
26	1898–1899	Hurd, Henry M.
27	1899–1900	Rogers, Joseph G.
28	1900–1901	Wise, Peter M.
29	1901–1902	Preston, Robert J.
–	1902–	Richardson, A. B.[*]
30	1902–1903	Blumer, G. Alder
31	1903–1904	Macdonald, A. E.
32	1904–1905	Burgess, T. J.
33	1905–1906	Burr, C. B.
34	1906–1907	Hill, Charles G.
35	1907–1908	Bancroft, Charles P.
36	1908–1909	Kilbourne, Arthur F.
37	1909–1910	Drewry, William F.
38	1910–1911	Pilgrim, Charles W.
39	1911–1912	Work, Hubert
40	1912–1913	Searcy, James T.
41	1913–1914	MacDonald, Carlos F.
42	1914–1915	Smith, Samuel E.
43	1915–1916	Brush, Edward N.
44	1916–1917	Wagner, Charles G.
45	1917–1918	Anglin, James V.
46	1918–1919	Southard, Elmer E.
47	1919–1920	Eyman, Henry C.
48	1920–1921	Copp, Owen
49	1921–1922	Barrett, Albert M.
50	1922–1923	Mitchell, H. W.
51	1923–1924	Salmon, Thomas W.
52	1924–1925	White, William A.
53	1925–1926	Haviland, C. Floyd
54	1926–1927	Kline, George M.
55	1927–1928	Meyer, Adolf
56	1928–1929	Orton, Samuel T.
57	1929–1930	Bond, Earl D.

58	1930–1931	English, Walter M.
59	1931–1932	Russell, William L.
60	1932–1933	May, James V.
61	1933–1934	Kirby, George H.
62	1934–1935	Williams, C. Fred
63	1935–1936	Cheney, Clarence O.
64	1936–1937	Campbell, C. Macfie
65	1937–1938	Chapman, Ross McC.
66	1938–1939	Hutchings, Richard H.
67	1939–1940	Sandy, William C.
68	1940–1941	Stevenson, George H.
69	1941–1942	Hall, James King
–	1942–	Singer, H. Douglas*
70	1942–1943	Ruggles, Arthur H.
71	1943–1944	Strecker, Edward A.
72	1944–1946	Bowman, Karl M.
73	1946–1947	Hamilton, Samuel W.
74	1947–1948	Overholser, Winfred
75	1948–1949	Menninger, William C.
76	1949–1950	Stevenson, George S.
77	1950–1951	Whitehorn, John C.
78	1951–1952	Bartemeier, Leo H.
79	1952–1953	Cameron, D. Ewen
80	1953–1954	Appel, Kenneth E.
81	1954–1955	Noyes, Arthur P.
82	1955–1956	Gayle, Jr., R. Finley
83	1956–1957	Braceland, Francis J.
84	1957–1958	Solomon, Harry C.
85	1958–1959	Gerty, Francis J.
86	1959–1960	Malamud, William
87	1960–1961	Felix, Robert H.
88	1961–1962	Barton, Walter E.
89	1962–1963	Branch, C. H. Hardin
90	1963–1964	Ewalt, Jack R.
91	1964–1965	Blain, Daniel
92	1965–1966	Rome, Howard P.
93	1966–1967	Tompkins, Harvey J.
94	1967–1968	Brosin, Henry W.
95	1968–1969	Kolb, Lawrence C.

96	1969–1970	Waggoner, Raymond W.
97	1970–1971	Garber, Robert S.
98	1971–1972	Busse, Ewald W.
99	1972–1973	Talkington, Perry C.
100	1973–1974	Freedman, Alfred M.
101	1974–1975	Spiegel, John P.
102	1975–1976	Marmor, Judd
103	1976–1977	Gibson, Robert W.
104	1977–1978	Weinberg, Jack
105	1978–1979	Masserman, Jules
106	1979–1980	Stone, Alan A.
107	1980–1981	Langsley, Donald G.
108	1981–1982	Freedman, Daniel X.
109	1982–1983	Brodie, H. Keith H.
110	1983–1984	Tarjan, George
111	1984–1985	Talbott, John A.
112	1985–1986	Nadelson, Carol C.
113	1986–1987	Pasnau, Robert O.
114	1987–1988	Pollock, George H.
115	1988–1989	Fink, Paul J.
116	1989–1990	Pardes, Herbert
117	1990–1991	Benedek, Elissa
118	1991–1992	Hartmann, Lawrence
119	1992–1993	English, Joseph T.
120	1993–1994	McIntyre, John
121	1994–1995	Wiener, Jerry M.
122	1995–1996	England, Mary Jane
123	1996–1997	Eist, Harold
124	1997–1998	Sacks, Herbert S.
125	1998–1999	Muñoz, Rodrigo A.
126	1999–2000	Tasman, Allan
127	2000–2001	Borenstein, Daniel
128	2001–2002	Harding, Richard Kent
129	2002–2003	Appelbaum, Paul Stuart
130	2003–2004	Goin, Marcia
131	2004–2005	Riba, Michelle
132	2005–2006	Sharfstein, Steven
132	2006–2007	Ruiz, Pedro
133	2007–2008	Robinowitz, Carolyn

BY NAME

No.	Term	Name
20	1892–1893	Andrews, J. B.
45	1917–1918	Anglin, James V.
80	1953–1954	Appel, Kenneth E.
129	2002–2003	Appelbaum, Paul Stuart
2	1848–1851	Awl, William McClay
35	1907–1908	Bancroft, Charles P.
49	1921–1922	Barrett, Albert M.
78	1951–1952	Bartemeier, Leo H.
88	1961–1962	Barton, Walter E.
3	1851–1855	Bell, Luther V.
117	1990–1991	Benedek, Elissa
91	1964–1965	Blain, Daniel
30	1902–1903	Blumer, G. Alder
57	1929–1930	Bond, Earl D.
127	2000–2001	Borenstein, Daniel
72	1944–1946	Bowman, Karl M.
83	1956–1957	Braceland, Francis J.
89	1962–1963	Branch, C. H. Hardin
109	1982–1983	Brodie, H. Keith H.
94	1967–1968	Brosin, Henry W.
43	1915–1916	Brush, Edward N.
25	1897–1898	Bucke, Richard M.
32	1904–1905	Burgess, T.J.
33	1905–1906	Burr, C. B.
98	1971–1972	Busse, Ewald W.
7	1870–1873	Butler, John S.
14	1886–1887	Buttolph, H. A.
10	1882–1883	Callender, John H.
79	1952–1953	Cameron, D. Ewen
64	1936–1937	Campbell, C. Macfie
16	1888–1889	Chapin, John B.
65	1937–1938	Chapman, Ross McC.
63	1935–1936	Cheney, Clarence O.
19	1891–1892	Clark, Daniel
48	1920–1921	Copp, Owen
22	1894–1895	Cowles, Edward

21	1893–1894	Curwen, John
23	1895–1896	Dewey, Richard
37	1909–1910	Drewry, William F.
12	1884–1885	Earle, Pliny
123	1996–1997	Eist, Harold
122	1995–1996	England, Mary Jane
119	1992–1993	English, Joseph T.
58	1930–1931	English, Walter M.
13	1885–1886	Everts, Orpheus
90	1963–1964	Ewalt, Jack R.
47	1919–1920	Eyman, Henry C.
87	1960–1961	Felix, Robert H.
115	1988–1989	Fink, Paul J.
100	1973–1974	Freedman, Alfred M.
108	1981–1982	Freedman, Daniel X.
97	1970–1971	Garber, Robert S.
82	1955–1956	Gayle Jr., R. Finley
85	1958–1959	Gerty, Francis J.
103	1976–1977	Gibson, Robert W.
17	1889–1890	Godding, W.W.
130	2003–2004	Goin, Marcia
11	1883–1884	Gray, John P.
15	1887–1888	Grissom, Eugene
69	1941–1942	Hall, James King
73	1946–1947	Hamilton, Samuel W.
128	2001–2002	Harding, Richard Kent
118	1991–1992	Hartmann, Lawrence
53	1925–1926	Haviland, C. Floyd
34	1906–1907	Hill, Charles G.
26	1898–1899	Hurd, Henry M.
66	1938–1939	Hutchings, Richard H.
36	1908–1909	Kilbourne, Arthur F.
61	1933–1934	Kirby, George H.
6	1862–1870	Kirkbride, Thomas S.
54	1926–1927	Kline, George M.
95	1968–1969	Kolb, Lawrence C.
107	1980–1981	Langsley, Donald G.
31	1903–1904	Macdonald, A. E.

41	1913–1914	MacDonald, Carlos F.
86	1959–1960	Malamud, William
102	1975–1976	Marmor, Judd
105	1978–1979	Masserman, Jules
60	1932–1933	May, James V.
5	1859–1862	McFarland, Andrew
120	1993–1994	McIntyre, John
75	1948–1949	Menninger, William C.
55	1927–1928	Meyer, Adolf
50	1922–1923	Mitchell, H.W.
125	1998–1999	Muñoz, Rodrigo A.
112	1985–1986	Nadelson, Carol C.
8	1873–1879	Nichols, Charles H.
81	1954–1955	Noyes, Arthur P.
56	1928–1929	Orton, Samuel T.
74	1947–1948	Overholser, Winfred
116	1989–1990	Pardes, Herbert
113	1986–1987	Pasnau, Robert O.
38	1910–1911	Pilgrim, Charles W.
114	1987–1988	Pollock, George H.
24	1896–1897	Powell, Theophilus O.
29	1901–1902	Preston, Robert J.
4	1855–1859	Ray, Isaac
131	2004–2005	Riba, Michelle
–	1902–	Richardson, AB.*
133	2007–2008	Robinowitz, Carolyn
27	1899–1900	Rogers, Joseph G.
92	1965–1966	Rome, Howard P.
70	1942–1943	Ruggles, Arthur H.
132	2006–2007	Ruiz, Pedro
59	1931–1932	Russell, William L.
124	1997–1998	Sacks, Herbert S.
51	1923–1924	Salmon, Thomas W.
67	1939–1940	Sandy, William C.
40	1912–1913	Searcy, James T.
132	2005–2006	Sharfstein, Steven
–	1942–	Singer, H. Douglas*
42	1914–1915	Smith, Samuel E.

84	1957–1958	Solomon, Harry C.
46	1918–1919	Southard, Elmer E.
101	1974–1975	Spiegel, John P.
18	1890–1891	Stearnes, H. P.
68	1940–1941	Stevenson, George H.
76	1949–1950	Stevenson, George S.
106	1979–1980	Stone, Alan A.
71	1943–1944	Strecker, Edward A.
111	1984–1985	Talbott, John A.
99	1972–1973	Talkington, Perry C.
110	1983–1984	Tarjan, George
126	1999–2000	Tasman, Allan
93	1966–1967	Tompkins, Harvey J.
96	1969–1970	Waggoner, Raymond W.
44	1916–1917	Wagner, Charles G.
9	1879–1882	Walker, Clement A.
104	1977–1978	Weinberg, Jack
52	1924–1925	White, William A.
77	1950–1951	Whitehorn, John C.
121	1994–1995	Wiener, Jerry M.
62	1934–1935	Williams, C. Fred
28	1900–1901	Wise, Peter M.
1	1844–1848	Woodward, Samuel B.
39	1911–1912	Work, Hubert

Appendix 7

American Psychiatric Association Organizational Chart, 2008 and 1986

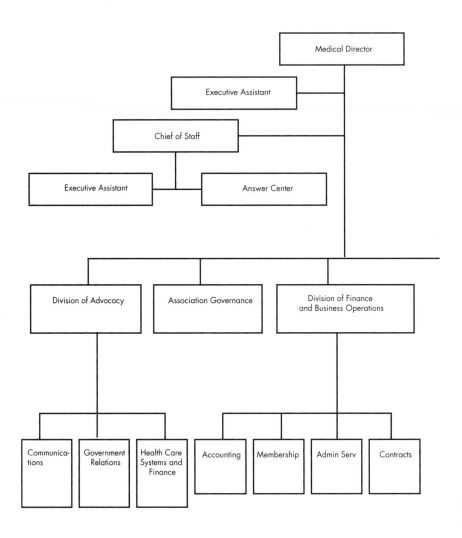

2008

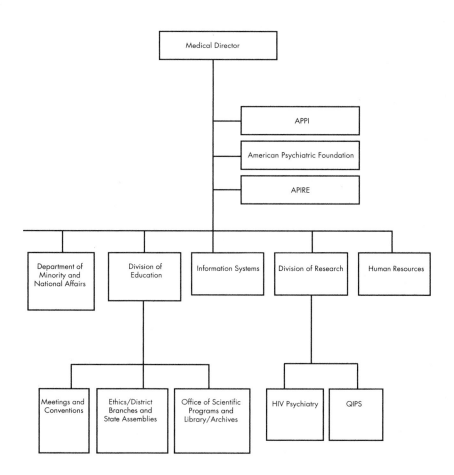

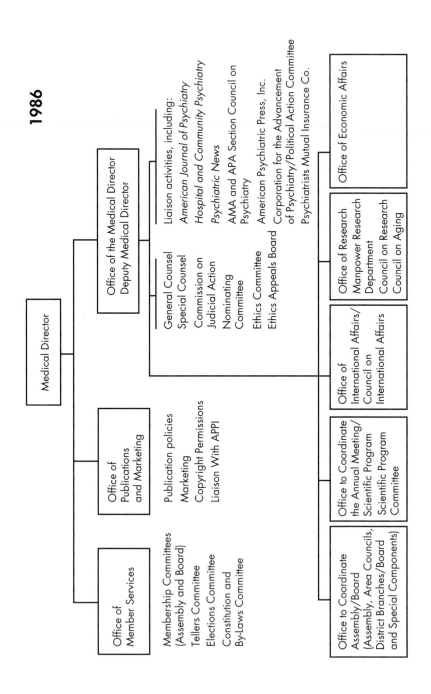

1986

Medical Director

Office of Member Services

Membership Committees (Assembly and Board)
Tellers Committee
Elections Committee
Constitution and By-Laws Committee

Office of Publications and Marketing

Publication policies
Marketing
Copyright Permissions
Liaison With APPI

Office of the Medical Director
Deputy Medical Director

General Counsel
Special Counsel
Commission on Judicial Action
Nominating Committee

Ethics Committee
Ethics Appeals Board

Liaison activities, including:
American Journal of Psychiatry
Hospital and Community Psychiatry
Psychiatric News
AMA and APA Section Council on Psychiatry
American Psychiatric Press, Inc.
Corporation for the Advancement of Psychiatry/Political Action Committee
Psychiatrists Mutual Insurance Co.

Office to Coordinate Assembly/Board (Assembly, Area Councils, District Branches/Board and Special Components)

Office to Coordinate the Annual Meeting/Scientific Program
Scientific Program Committee

Office of International Affairs/Council on International Affairs

Office of Research
Manpower Research Department
Council on Research
Council on Aging

Office of Economic Affairs

Appendix 8

American Psychiatric Association Joint Commission on Government Relations

1976–1978	Robert J. Campbell, M.D. (Chairperson), New York, NY
1975–1979	Francis L. deMarneffe, M.D., McLean Hospital, Belmont, MA. (Area I)
1975–1978	Lewis Kurke, M.D., Stonybrook, Long Island, NY (Area II)
1977–1980	John J. McGrath, M.D., Washington, DC (Area III)
1976–1979	James L. Cavanaugh Jr., Winnetka, IL (Area IV)
1975–1978	Hayden H. Donahue, M.D., Central State Hospital, Norman, OK (Area V)
1977–1980	Harold E. Mann, M.D., Berkeley, CA (Area VI)
1975–1979	Frederick A. Lewis, Denver, CO. (Area VII)
1976–1978	Shervert Frazier, M.D., McLean Hospital, Belmont, MA (liaison with Joint Commission on Public Affairs)
1977–1978	Robert W. Gibson, M.D., Sheppard & Enoch Pratt Hospital, Towson MD. (consultant)
	Jay Cutler, M.D., Washington, D.C. (staff assigned)

Appendix 9

Psychiatry Organizations of Interest

Academy for Eating Disorders
111 Deer Lake Road, Suite 100
Deerfield, IL 60015
Phone: (847) 498-4274
E-mail: info@aedweb.org
Web: www.aedweb.org

Academy of Organizational and Occupational Psychiatry
P.O. Box 343
Ridgefield Park, NJ 07660
Phone: (877) 789-2667
E-mail: aoopadmn@verizon.net
Web: www.aoop.org

Academy of Psychosomatic Medicine
Norman Wallis, Ph.D., Executive Director
5272 River Road, Suite 630
Bethesda, MD 20816
Phone: (301) 718-6520
E-mail: apm@apm.org
Web: www.apm.org

Please contact individual organizations to confirm meeting dates and locations. The information presented in this appendix may have changed since our update in January 2008.

American Academy of Addiction Psychiatry
345 Blackstone Blvd.
First Floor–Weld
Providence, RI 02906
Phone: (401) 524-3076
E-mail: info@aaap.org
Web: www.aaap.org

American Academy of Child and Adolescent Psychiatry
3615 Wisconsin Avenue, N.W.
Washington, DC 20016-3007
Phone: (202) 966-7300
E-mail: meetings@aacap.org
Web: www.aacap.org

American Academy of Clinical Psychiatrists
Beverly Davidson, Executive Secretary
P.O. Box 458
Glastonbury, CT 06033
Phone: (860) 635-5533
E-mail: aacp@cox.net
Web: www.aacp.com

American Academy of Family Physicians
Douglas E. Henley, M.D., Executive Vice President
P.O. Box 11210
Shawnee Mission, KS 62207-1210
Phone: (800) 274-2237
E-mail: fp@aafp.org
Web: www.aafp.org

American Academy of Neurology
Catherine Rydell, Executive Director and
Chief Executive Officer
1080 Montreal Avenue
St. Paul, MN 55116
Phone: (651) 695-2800
E-mail: crydell@aan.com
Web: www.aan.com

American Academy of Pain Medicine
4700 West Lake Avenue
Glenview, IL 60025
Phone: (847) 375-4731
E-mail: info@painmed.org
Web: www.painmed.org

American Academy of Psychiatry and the Law
One Regency Drive
P.O. Box 30
Bloomfield, CT 06002-0030
Phone: (800) 331-1389
E-mail: execoff@aapl.org
Web: www.aapl.org

American Academy of Psychoanalysis and Dynamic Psychiatry
One Regency Drive
P.O. Box 30
Bloomfield, CT 06002-0030
Phone: (888) 691-8281
E-mail: info@AAPDP.org
Web: www.aapdp.org

American Association of Chairs of Departments of Psychiatry
AACDP Executive Office
1594 Cumberland Street #319
Lebanon, PA 17042
Phone: (717) 270-1673
E-mail: aacdp@verizon.net
Web: www.aacdp.org

American Association of Community Psychiatrists
Frances Bell, Administrative Director
P.O. Box 570218
Dallas, TX 75357-0218
Phone: (972) 613-0985
E-mail: frda1@airmail.net
Web: www.comm.psych.pitt.edu

American Association of Directors of
Psychiatric Residency Training, Inc.
AADPRT Executive Office
1594 Cumberland Street #319
Lebanon, PA 17042
Phone: (717) 270-1673
E-mail: aadprt@verizon.net
Web: www.aadprt.org

American Association for Emergency Psychiatry
One Regency Drive
P.O. Box 30
Bloomfield, CT 06002
Phone: (888) 945-5430
E-mail: aaep@emergencypsychiatry.org
Web: www.emergencypsychiatry.org

American Association for Geriatric Psychiatry
7910 Woodmont Avenue, Suite 1050
Bethesda, MD 20814
Phone: (301) 654-7850
E-mail: main@aagponline.org
Web: www.aagpgpa.org

American Association for Marriage and Family Therapy
112 South Alfred Street
Alexandria, VA 22314-3061
Phone: (703) 838-9808
E-mail: central@aamft.org
Web: www.aamft.org

American Board of Psychiatry and Neurology, Inc.
2150 Lake Cook Road, Suite 900
Buffalo Grove, IL 60089
Phone: (847) 229-6500
Web: www.abpn.com

American College of Mental Health Administration
7804 Loma del Norte Road, NE
Albuquerque, NM 87109-5419
Phone: (505) 822-5038
E-mail: Executive.Director@acmha.org
Web: www.acmha.org

American College of Neuropsychopharmacology
545 Mainstream Drive, Suite 110
Nashville, TN 37228
Phone: (615) 324-2360
E-mail: acnp@acnp.org
Web: www.acnp.org

American College of Psychiatrists
122 South Michigan Ave, Suite 1360
Chicago, IL 60603
Phone: (312) 662-1020
E-mail: angel@ACPsych.org
Web: www.ACPsych.org

American College of Psychoanalysts
Frances Bell
P.O. Box 570218
Dallas, TX 75357-0218
Phone: (972) 613-0985
Web: www.acopsa.org

American Geriatrics Society
The Empire State Building
350 Fifth Avenue, Suite 801
New York, NY 10118
Phone: (212) 308-1414
E-mail: info.amger@americangeriatrics.org
Web: www.americangeriatrics.org

American Group Psychotherapy Association, Inc.
25 East 21st Street, 6th Floor
New York, NY 10010
Phone: (877) 668-2472 or (212) 477-2677
E-mail: info@agpa.org
Web: www.agpa.org

American Music Therapy Association
8455 Colesville Road, Suite 1000
Silver Spring, MD 20910
Phone: (301) 589-3300
E-mail: info@musictherapy.org
Web: www.musictherapy.org

American Neurological Association
5841 Cedar Lake Road, Suite 204
Minneapolis, MN 55416
Phone: (952) 545-6284
E-mail: ana@llmsi.com
Web: www.aneuroa.org

American Neuropsychiatric Association
700 Ackerman Road, Suite 625
Columbus, OH 43202
Phone: (614) 447-2077
E-mail: anpa@osu.edu
Web: www.anpaonline.org

American Occupational Therapy Association
4720 Montgomery Lane
P.O. Box 31220
Bethesda, MD 20824-1220
Phone: (301) 652-2682
Web: www.aota.org

American Orthopsychiatric Association
Department of Psychology
Box 871104
Arizona State University
Tempe, AZ 85287-1104
Phone: (480) 727-7518
E-mail: americanortho@gmail.com
Web: www.amerortho.org

American Pain Society
4700 West Lake Avenue
Glenview, IL 60025-1485
Phone: (847) 375-4715
E-mail: info@ampainsoc.org
Web: www.ampainsoc.org

American Psychiatric Association
1000 Wilson Boulevard, Suite 1825
Arlington, VA 22209-3901
Phone: (703) 907-7300
E-mail: apa@psych.org
Web: www.psych.org

American Psychiatric Foundation
1000 Wilson Boulevard, Suite 1825
Arlington, VA 22209-3901
Phone: (703) 907-8512
E-mail: apf@psych.org
Web: www.psychfoundation.org

American Psychiatric Nurses Association
1555 Wilson Boulevard, Suite 515
Arlington, VA 22209
Phone: (866) 243-2443
E-mail: inform@apna.org
Web: www.apna.org

American Psychoanalytic Association
309 East 49th Street
New York, NY 10017
Phone: (212) 752-0450
E-mail: info@apsa.org
Web: www.apsa.org

American Psychological Association
750 First Street, N.E.
Washington, DC 20002
Phone: (800) 374-2721 or (202) 336-5500
Web: www.apa.org

American Psychological Society
1010 Vermont Avenue, N.W., 11th Floor
Washington, DC 20005-4918
Phone: (202) 783-2077
Web: www.psychologicalscience.org

American Psychopathological Association
Gary Heiman, Ph.D., Coordinator
E-mail: gah13@columbia.edu
Web: www.appassn.org

American Psychosomatic Society
6728 Old McLean Village Drive
McLean, VA 22101-3906
Phone: (703) 556-9222
E-mail: info@psychosomatic.org
Web: www.psychosomatic.org

American Society of Addiction Medicine
4601 North Park Avenue, Upper Arcade # 101
Chevy Chase, MD 20815-4520
Phone: (301) 656-3920
E-mail: email@asam.org
Web: www.asam.org

American Society for Adolescent Psychiatry
Frances Bell, Executive Director
P.O. Box 570218
Dallas, TX 75357-0218
Phone: (972) 613-0985
E-mail: info@adolpsych.org
Web: www.adolpsych.org

American Society of Clinical Psychopharmacology
P.O. Box 40395
Glen Oaks, NY 11004
Phone: (718) 470-4007
Web: www.ascpp.org

American Society of Psychoanalytic Physicians
13528 Wisteria Drive
Germantown, MD 20874
Phone: (301) 540-3197
E-mail: cfcotter@aspp.net
Web: www.aspp.net

America's Health Insurance Plans
601 Pennsylvania Avenue, N.W., Suite 500, South Building
Washington, DC 20004
Phone: (202) 778-3200
E-mail: ahip@ahip.org
Web: http://www.ahip.org/

Association for Academic Psychiatry
464 Common Street, #147
Belmont, MA 02478
Phone: (617) 393-3935
E-mail: cberney@mah.harvard.edu
Web: www.academicpsychiatry.org

Association for the Advancement of Philosophy and Psychiatry
Department of Psychiatry
UT Southwestern Medical Center
5323 Harry Hines Boulevard
Dallas, TX 75390-9070
Phone: (214) 648-4960
E-mail: Linda.Muncy@UTSouthwestern.edu
Web: www3.utsouthwestern.edu/aapp

Association for Ambulatory Behavioral Healthcare
247 Douglas Avenue
Portsmouth, VA 23707
Phone: (757) 673-3741
E-mail: info@aabh.org
Web: www.aabh.org

Association of Behavioral Healthcare Management
12300 Twinbrook Parkway, Suite 320
Rockville, MD 20852
Phone: (301) 984-6200
E-mail: Communications@thenationalcouncil.org
Web: www.thenationalcouncil.org

Association for Behavioral Health and Wellness
1101 Pennsylvania Avenue, N.W.
Sixth Floor
Washington, DC 20004
Phone: (202) 756-7726
E-mail: info@abhw.org
Web: www.abhw.org

Association for Child Psychoanalysis
7820 Enchanted Hills Blvd. #A-233
Rio Rancho, NM 87144
Phone: (505) 771-0372
E-mail: childanalysis@comcast.net
Web: www.childanalysis.org

Association of Directors of Medical Student Education in Psychiatry
Gary L. Beck, Administrative Consultant
ADMSEP
982183 Nebraska Medical Center
Omaha, NE 68198-2183
Phone: (402) 559-7351
E-mail: gbeck@unmc.edu
Web: www.admsep.org

Association of Gay and Lesbian Psychiatrists
4514 Chester Avenue
Philadelphia, PA 19143-3707
Phone: (215) 222-2800
E-mail: info@aglp.org
Web: www.aglp.org

Canadian Mental Health Association
Phenix Professional Building
595 Montreal Road, Suite 303
Ottawa, Ontario K1K 4L2, Canada
Phone: (613) 745-7750
E-mail: info@cmha.ca
Web: www.cmha.ca

Canadian Psychiatric Association
141 Laurier Avenue West, Suite 701
Ottawa, Ontario K1P 5J3, Canada
Phone: (613) 234-2815
E-mail: cpa@cpa-apc.org
Web: www.cpa-apc.org

College on Problems of Drug Dependence
Martin W. Adler, Ph.D., Executive Officer
Center for Substance Abuse Research
Temple University School of Medicine
3400 North Broad Street
Philadelphia, PA 19140-5104
Phone: (215) 707-3242
E-mail: baldeagl@temple.edu
Web: www.cpdd.org

Depression and Bipolar Support Alliance
730 North Franklin Street, Suite 501
Chicago, IL 60610-7224
Phone: (800) 826-3632
Web: www.dbsalliance.org

Group for the Advancement of Psychiatry
Web: www.groupadpsych.org

Indo-American Psychiatric Association
107 Chesley Drive, Unit 4
Media, PA 19063
Phone: (610) 891-9024 ext. 115
E-mail: shatti1@aol.com
Web: www.myiapa.org

International Association for Group Psychotherapy and
Group Processes
P.O. Box 745
Bukit Merah Central Post Office
Singapore 911539
Republic of Singapore
Phone: 65 6 738 7466 (Singapore)
E-mail: office@iagp.com
Web: www.iagpweb.org

International Federation of Psychoanalytic Societies
Sonia Gojman de Millán, Ph.D., Secretary General
P.O. Box 12788
La Jolla, CA 92039
Phone: (858) 909-0324
E-mail: sgojman@yahoo.com
Web: www.ifp-s.org

International Society for the Study of Trauma and Dissociation
8201 Greensboro Drive, Suite 300
McLean, VA 22102
Phone: (703) 610-9037
E-mail: info@isst-d.org
Web: www.isst-d.org

NAMI: National Alliance on Mental Illness
Colonial Place Three
2107 Wilson Boulevard, Suite 300
Arlington, VA 22201-3042
Phone: (703) 524-7600
Web: www.nami.org

NARSAD: National Alliance for Research on
Schizophrenia and Depression
60 Cutter Mill Road, Suite 404
Great Neck, NY 11021
Phone: (800) 829-8289
E-mail: info@narsad.org
Web: www.narsad.org

National Association of Psychiatric Health Systems
701 13th Street NW, Suite 950
Washington, DC 20005-3903
Phone: (202) 393-6700
E-mail: naphs@naphs.org
Web: www.naphs.org

National Association of State Mental Health Program Directors
Robert W. Glover, Ph.D., Executive Director
66 Canal Center Plaza, Suite 302
Alexandria, VA 22314
Phone: (703) 739-9333
Web: www.nasmhpd.org

National Council on Alcoholism and Drug Dependence
244 East 58th Street, 4th Floor
New York, NY 10022
Phone: (212) 269-7797
E-mail: national@ncadd.org
Web: www.ncadd.org

National Foundation for Depressive Illness
iFred
2017-D Renard Ct.
Annapolis, MD 21401
Phone: (410) 268-0044
E-mail: info@ifred.org
Web: www.depression.org

National Institute on Alcohol Abuse and Alcoholism (NIAAA)
5635 Fishers Lane, MSC 9304
Bethesda, MD 20892-9304
Phone: (301) 443-3860
E-mail: tkli@mail.nih.gov
Web: www.niaaa.nih.gov

National Institute on Drug Abuse (NIDA)
6001 Executive Boulevard, Suite 5213
Bethesda, MD 20892-9561
Phone: (301) 443-1124
E-mail: information@nida.nih.gov
Web: www.nida.nih.gov

National Institute of Mental Health
Science Writing, Press, and Dissemination Branch
6001 Executive Boulevard
Room 8184, MSC 9663
Bethesda, MD 20892-9663
Phone: (866) 615-6464
E-mail: nimhinfo@nih.gov
Web: www.nimh.nih.gov

National Mental Health Association
2000 N. Beauregard Street, 6th Floor
Alexandria, VA 22311
Phone: (800) 969-6642
Web: www.nmha.org

Royal Australian and New Zealand College of Psychiatrists
309 La Trobe Street
Melbourne, Victoria 3000, Australia
Phone: 613 9640 0646
E-mail: ranzcp@ranzcp.org
Web: www.ranzcp.org

Royal College of Psychiatrists
17 Belgrave Square
London, England SW1X 8PG
Phone: 020 7235 2351
E-mail: rcpsych@rcpsych.ac.uk
Web: www.rcpsych.ac.uk

Society of Behavioral Medicine
55 East Wells St., Suite 1100
Milwaukee, WI 53202-3823
Phone: (414) 918-3156
E-mail: info@sbm.org
Web: www.sbm.org

Society of Biological Psychiatry
Maggie Peterson, MBA, Executive Director
c/o Mayo Clinic Jacksonville
Research–Birdsall 310
4500 San Pablo Road
Jacksonville, FL 32224
Phone: (904) 953-2842
E-mail: maggie@mayo.edu
Web: www.sobp.org

Society for Developmental and Behavioral Pediatrics
6728 Old McLean Village Drive
McLean, VA 22101
Phone: (703) 556-9222
E-mail: info@sdbp.org
Web: www.sdbp.org

Society for Neuroscience
1121 14th Street, Suite 1010
Washington, DC 20005
Phone: (202) 962-4000
Web: www.sfn.org

Substance Abuse and Mental Health Services Administration
(SAMHSA)
1 Choke Cherry Road
Rockville, MD 20857
E-mail: info@samhsa.gov
Web: www.samhsa.gov

World Federation for Mental Health
6564 Loisdale Court, Suite 301
Springfield, VA 22150-1812
Phone: (703) 313-8680
E-mail: info@wfmh.com
Web: www.wfmh.org

World Psychiatric Association
WPA Secretariat
Psychiatric Hospital
2, ch. du Petit-Bel-Air
1225 Chêne-Bourg
Switzerland
Phone: 41 22 305 57 30
E-mail: wpasecretariat@wpanet.org
Web: www.wpanet.org

Appendix 10

American Psychiatric Association Assembly Area Councils by Region

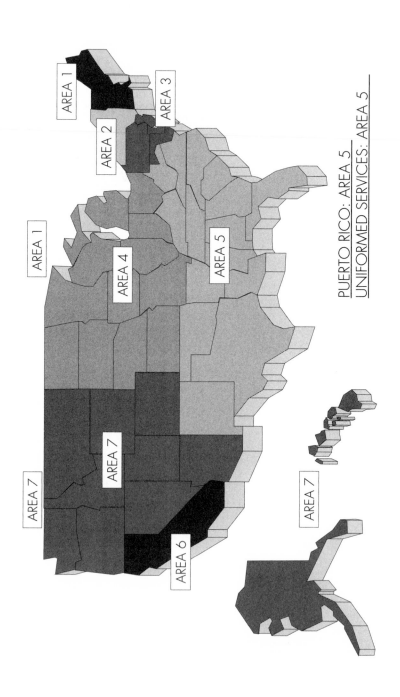

PUERTO RICO: AREA 5
UNIFORMED SERVICES: AREA 5

Appendix 11

Comparison of American Psychiatric Association Area and District Branch Membership, 2002–2007

COMPARISON OF AREA AND DISTRICT BRANCH (DB) MEMBERSHIP, 2002–2007

Area	DB	DB name	Total member count						1-year % change 1/06–1/07	5-year % change 1/02–1/07	Total member count 10/07
			1/02	1/03	1/04	1/05	1/06	1/07			
1	7	Connecticut Psychiatric Society	784	772	792	749	769	769	0.0%	−1.9%	800
1	62	Maine Psychiatric Association	193	199	208	205	201	196	−2.5%	1.6%	203
1	32	Massachusetts Psychiatric Society	1,711	1,691	1,706	1,608	1,588	1,608	1.3%	−6.0%	1,684
1	68	New Hampshire Psychiatric Society	171	162	157	148	151	143	−5.3%	−16.4%	147
1	37	Ontario District Branch	519	510	513	496	535	670	25.2%	29.1%	703
1	39	Quebec and Eastern Canada District Branch	408	384	388	378	377	397	5.3%	−2.7%	411
1	41	Rhode Island Psychiatric Society	251	258	249	242	240	251	4.6%	0.0%	270

COMPARISON OF AREA AND DISTRICT BRANCH (DB) MEMBERSHIP, 2002–2007

Area	DB	DB name	Total member count						1-year % change 1/06–1/07	5-year % change 1/02–1/07	Total member count 10/07
			1/02	1/03	1/04	1/05	1/06	1/07			
1	66	Vermont Psychiatric Association	129	122	127	122	121	129	6.6%	0.0%	133
		Total Area 1	4,166	4,098	4,140	3,948	3,982	4,163	4.5%	−0.1%	4,351
2	2	Bronx District Branch	177	172	171	188	185	171	−7.6%	−3.4%	187
2	3	Brooklyn Psychiatric Society	270	294	303	300	314	305	−2.9%	13.0%	323
2	56	Central New York District Branch	156	158	161	165	160	163	1.9%	4.5%	172
2	5	Genesee Valley Psychiatric Association	203	206	201	190	203	193	−4.9%	−4.9%	207
2	25	Greater Long Island Psychiatric Society	492	499	497	531	556	554	−0.4%	12.6%	597
2	24	Mid-Hudson Psychiatric Society	85	84	85	95	93	97	4.3%	14.1%	95

COMPARISON OF AREA AND DISTRICT BRANCH (DB) MEMBERSHIP, 2002–2007

Area	DB	DB name	Total member count						1-year % change 1/06–1/07	5-year % change 1/02–1/07	Total member count 10/07
			1/02	1/03	1/04	1/05	1/06	1/07			
2	27	New York County District Branch	1,962	1,914	1,942	1,921	1,951	1,915	-1.8%	-2.4%	2,108
2	28	New York State Capital District Branch	184	182	180	176	164	171	4.3%	-7.1%	176
2	59	Northern New York District Branch	43	43	42	44	47	45	-4.3%	4.7%	51
2	40	Queens County District Branch	203	201	216	220	244	234	-4.1%	15.3%	253
2	49	Psychiatric Society of Westchester County	515	507	509	513	505	509	0.8%	-1.2%	532
2	51	Western New York Psychiatric Society	156	154	156	159	161	159	-1.2%	1.9%	173
2	55	West Hudson Psychiatric Society	140	138	137	133	143	133	-7.0%	-5.0%	137
		Total Area 2	4,586	4,552	4,600	4,635	4,726	4,649	-1.6%	1.4%	5,011

COMPARISON OF AREA AND DISTRICT BRANCH (DB) MEMBERSHIP, 2002–2007

Area	DB	DB name	Total member count						1-year % change 1/06–1/07	5-year % change 1/02–1/07	Total member count 10/07
			1/02	1/03	1/04	1/05	1/06	1/07			
3	8	Psychiatric Society of Delaware	89	87	86	91	96	100	4.2%	12.4%	113
3	20	Maryland Psychiatric Society	722	732	732	718	720	745	3.5%	3.2%	772
3	26	New Jersey Psychiatric Association	796	799	840	879	899	939	4.4%	18.0%	996
3	38	Pennsylvania Psychiatric Society	1,697	1,702	1,756	1,693	1,664	1,671	0.4%	–1.5%	1,792
3	48	Washington Psychiatric Society	935	941	970	937	952	924	–2.9%	–1.2%	970
		Total Area 3	4,239	4,261	4,384	4,318	4,331	4,379	1.1%	3.3%	4,643
4	13	Illinois Psychiatric Society	1,231	1,212	1,173	1,121	1,135	1,127	–0.7%	–8.4%	1,170
4	14	Indiana Psychiatric Society	402	412	408	379	386	360	–6.7%	–10.4%	370

COMPARISON OF AREA AND DISTRICT BRANCH (DB) MEMBERSHIP, 2002–2007

Area	DB	DB name	Total member count						1-year % change 1/06–1/07	5-year % change 1/02–1/07	Total member count 10/07
			1/02	1/03	1/04	1/05	1/06	1/07			
4	16	Iowa Psychiatric Society	228	231	238	232	240	213	−11.3%	−6.6%	221
4	17	Kansas Psychiatric Society	265	243	224	225	216	191	−11.6%	−27.9%	201
4	21	Michigan Psychiatric Society	896	856	827	836	810	776	−4.2%	−13.4%	852
4	22	Minnesota Psychiatric Society	457	454	469	445	434	448	3.2%	−2.0%	462
4	9	Eastern Missouri Psychiatric Society	331	313	311	332	323	326	0.9%	−1.5%	327
4	69	Central Missouri Psychiatric Society	80	75	77	77	81	86	6.2%	7.5%	89
4	50	Western Missouri Psychiatric Society	118	114	116	119	113	121	7.1%	2.5%	135
4	34	Nebraska Psychiatric Society	163	161	156	135	139	147	5.8%	−9.8%	161

COMPARISON OF AREA AND DISTRICT BRANCH (DB) MEMBERSHIP, 2002–2007

Area	DB	DB name	Total member count						1-year % change 1/06–1/07	5-year % change 1/02–1/07	Total member count 10/07
			1/02	1/03	1/04	1/05	1/06	1/07			
4	63	North Dakota Psychiatric Society	79	77	71	66	67	66	−1.5%	−16.5%	70
4	35	Ohio Psychiatric Association	1,055	1,038	1,047	1,026	1,024	982	−4.1%	−6.9%	1,031
4	72	South Dakota Psychiatric Association	61	61	59	59	62	60	−3.2%	−1.6%	66
4	52	Wisconsin Psychiatric Association	469	456	461	429	434	425	−2.1%	−9.4%	451
		Total Area 4	5,835	5,703	5,637	5,481	5,464	5,328	−2.5%	−8.7%	5,606
5	60	Alabama Psychiatric Society	270	265	277	266	268	271	1.1%	0.4%	288
5	1	Arkansas Psychiatric Society	183	181	171	157	160	164	2.5%	−10.4%	164
5	10	Florida Psychiatric Society	1,070	1,058	1,093	1,056	1,073	1,117	4.1%	4.4%	1,151

COMPARISON OF AREA AND DISTRICT BRANCH (DB) MEMBERSHIP, 2002–2007

Area	DB	DB name	Total member count						1-year % change 1/06–1/07	5-year % change 1/02–1/07	Total member count 10/07
			1/02	1/03	1/04	1/05	1/06	1/07			
5	11	Georgia Psychiatric Physicians Association	634	641	664	646	647	631	-2.5%	-0.5%	710
5	18	Kentucky Psychiatric Association	336	346	344	340	334	340	1.8%	1.2%	357
5	19	Louisiana Psychiatric Medical Association	462	464	450	392	420	403	-4.0%	-12.8%	408
5	23	Mississippi Psychiatric Association	171	174	196	192	190	182	-4.2%	6.4%	194
5	29	North Carolina Psychiatric Association	809	804	822	812	819	849	3.7%	4.9%	904
5	36	Oklahoma Psychiatric Association	244	238	233	236	252	251	-0.4%	2.9%	261
5	70	Puerto Rico Psychiatric Society	198	181	170	149	144	137	-4.9%	-30.8%	150

COMPARISON OF AREA AND DISTRICT BRANCH (DB) MEMBERSHIP, 2002–2007

Area	DB	DB name	Total member count						1-year % change 1/06–1/07	5-year % change 1/02–1/07	Total member count 10/07
			1/02	1/03	1/04	1/05	1/06	1/07			
5	42	South Carolina Psychiatric Association	348	351	366	348	354	356	0.6%	2.3%	388
5	45	Tennessee Psychiatric Association	403	375	362	338	350	360	2.9%	-10.7%	379
5	46	Texas Society of Psychiatric Physicians	1,463	1,394	1,382	1,280	1,264	1,262	-0.2%	-13.7%	1,300
5	77	Society of Uniformed Services Psychiatrists	205	211	215	212	228	242	6.1%	18.0%	280
5	47	Psychiatric Society of Virginia	573	572	568	564	578	567	-1.9%	-1.0%	619
5	54	West Virginia Psychiatric Association	176	178	170	170	162	149	-8.0%	-15.3%	189
		Total Area 5	7,545	7,433	7,483	7,158	7,243	7,281	0.5%	-3.5%	7,742

COMPARISON OF AREA AND DISTRICT BRANCH (DB) MEMBERSHIP, 2002–2007

Area	DB	DB name	Total member count						1-year % change 1/06–1/07	5-year % change 1/02–1/07	Total member count 10/07
			1/02	1/03	1/04	1/05	1/06	1/07			
6	4	Central California Psychiatric Society	314	312	330	325	335	363	8.4%	15.6%	385
6	30	Northern California Psychiatric Society	1,179	1,182	1,162	1,144	1,132	1,150	1.6%	–2.5%	1,236
6	76	Orange County Psychiatric Society	238	238	243	238	240	243	1.3%	2.1%	268
6	64	San Diego Psychiatric Society	339	343	337	339	345	366	6.1%	8.0%	397
6	43	Southern California Psychiatric Society	1,233	1,230	1,241	1,200	1,209	1,224	1.2%	–0.7%	1,274
		Total Area 6	3,303	3,305	3,313	3,246	3,261	3,346	2.6%	1.3%	3,560
7	71	Alaska District Branch	60	60	61	56	56	61	8.9%	1.7%	62
7	57	Arizona Psychiatric Society	388	383	372	373	376	393	4.5%	1.3%	417

COMPARISON OF AREA AND DISTRICT BRANCH (DB) MEMBERSHIP, 2002–2007

Area	DB	DB name	Total member count							1-year % change 1/06–1/07	5-year % change 1/02–1/07	Total member count 10/07
			1/02	1/03	1/04	1/05	1/06	1/07				
7	6	Colorado Psychiatric Society	506	531	541	507	494	495	0.2%	-2.2%	525
7	12	Hawaii Psychiatric Medical Association	197	197	198	161	162	168	3.7%	-14.7%	181
7	15	Idaho Psychiatric Association	60	57	59	63	62	66	6.5%	10.0%	69
7	73	Montana Psychiatric Association	54	57	63	60	60	56	-6.7%	3.7%	57
7	74	Nevada Psychiatric Association	90	100	108	111	115	126	9.6%	40.0%	133
7	67	Psychiatric Medical Association of New Mexico	146	143	153	161	170	187	10.0%	28.1%	192
7	58	Oregon Psychiatric Association	354	347	351	345	361	383	6.1%	8.2%	403

COMPARISON OF AREA AND DISTRICT BRANCH (DB) MEMBERSHIP, 2002–2007

Area	DB	DB name	Total member count						1-year % change 1/06–1/07	5-year % change 1/02–1/07	Total member count 10/07
			1/02	1/03	1/04	1/05	1/06	1/07			
7	61	Utah Psychiatric Association	131	137	132	142	148	146	-1.4%	11.5%	167
7	33	Washington State Psychiatric Association	505	516	523	522	537	528	-1.7%	4.6%	561
7	53	Western Canada District Branch	287	298	332	315	322	356	10.6%	24.0%	395
7	75	Wyoming Psychiatric Society	28	27	25	25	24	22	-8.3%	-21.4%	24
		Total Area 7	2,806	2,853	2,918	2,841	2,887	2,987	3.5%	6.5%	3,186
		Total District Branch Membership (Areas 1–7)	32,480	32,205	32,475	31,627	31,894	32,133	0.7%	-1.1%	34,099
		Honorary Fellows	32	61	58	59	58	54	-6.9%	68.8%	53
		Medical Student Members	1,805	930	989	1,344	1,980	2,256	13.9%	25.0%	1,768

Appendix 11: APA Area and District Branch Membership 363

COMPARISON OF AREA AND DISTRICT BRANCH (DB) MEMBERSHIP, 2002–2007

Area	DB	DB name	Total member count						1-year % change 1/06–1/07	5-year % change 1/02–1/07	Total member count 10/07
			1/02	1/03	1/04	1/05	1/06	1/07			
		International Members/Fellows	1,173	1,014	1,162	1,313	1,275	1,426	11.8%	21.6%	1,845
		General Members-at-Large (DF, Lifes, etc)	723	597	675	743	609	569	−6.6%	−21.3%	583
		Total At-Large Membership	3,733	2,602	2,884	3,459	3,922	4,305	9.8%	15.3%	4,249
		Total APA Membership (DB and At-Large Members)	36,213	34,807	35,359	35,086	35,816	36,438	1.7%	0.6%	38,348

Appendix 12

DSM Task Forces and Working Groups

DSM-III

Task Force on Nomenclature and Statistics

Robert L. Spitzer, M.D. (Chair)
Nancy Andreasen, M.D., Ph.D.
Robert L. Arnstein, M.D.
Dennis Cantwell, M.D.
Paula J. Clayton, M.D.
Jean Endicott, Ph.D. (Consultant)
Willam A. Frosch, M.D.
Rachel Gittelman, Ph.D. (Consultant)
Donald W. Goodwin, M.D.
Donald F. Klein, M.D.
Morton Kramer, Sc.D. (Consultant)
Z.J. Lipowski, M.D.
Michael L. Mavroidis, M.D.
Theodore Millon, Ph.D. (Consultant)
Henry Pinsker, M.D.
George Saslow, Ph.D.
Michael Sheehy, M.D.
Robert Woodruff, M.D.
Lyman C. Wynne, M.D., Ph.D.

DSM-III-R
Work Group to Revise DSM-III

Robert L. Spitzer, M.D. (Chair)
Jane B.W. Williams, D.S.W (Text Editor)
Dennis Cantwell, M.D.
Allen J. Frances, M.D.
Kenneth S. Kendler, M.D.
Gerald L. Klerman, M.D.
David Kupfer, M.D.
Roger Peele, M.D.
Judith L. Rapoport, M.D.
Darrel A. Regier, M.D., M.P.H.
Bruce Rounsaville, M.D.
George Vaillant, M.D.
Lyman C. Wynne, M.D., Ph.D.
Harold A. Pincus, M.D. (Staff Liaison)
Steven S. Sharfstein, M.D. (Staff Liaison)

DSM-IV
Task Force on DSM-IV

Allen Frances, M.D. (Chairperson)
Harold A. Pincus, M.D. (Vice-Chairperson)
Michael B. First, M.D. (Editor, Text and Criteria)
Nancy C. Andreasen, M.D.. Ph.D.
Magda Campbell, M.D.
Dennis P. Cantwell, M.D.
Ellen Frank, Ph.D.
Judith H. Gold, M.D.
John Gunderson, M.D.
Robert E. Hales, M.D.
Kenneth S. Kendler, M.D.
David J. Kupfer, M.D.
Michael R. Liebowitz, M.D.
Juan E. Mezzich, M.D., Ph.D.
Peter E. Nathan, Ph.D.
Roger Peele, M.D.
Darrel A. Regier, M.D., M.P.H.
A. John Rush, M.D.
Chester W. Schmidt, M.D.

Marc A. Schuckit, M.D.
David Shaffer, M.D.
Robert L. Spitzer, M.D. (Special Adviser)
Gary J. Tucker, M.D.
B. Timothy Walsh, M.D.
Thomas A. Widiger, Ph.D. (Research Coordinator)
Janet B.W. Williams, D.S.W.
John C. Urbaitis, M.D. (Assembly Liaison)
James J. Hudziak, M.D. (Resident Fellow)
Junius Gonzales, M.D. (Resident Fellow)
Ruth Ross, M.A. (Science Editor)
Nancy E. Vetorello, M.U.P. (Administrative Coordinator)
Wendy Wakefield Davis, Ed.M. (Editorial Coordinator)
Cindy D. Jones (Administrative Assistant)
Nancy Sydnor-Greenberg, M.A. (Administrative Consultant)
Miriam Kline, M.S. (Focused Field Trial Coordinator)
James W. Thompson, M.D., M.P.H. (Videotape Field Trial Coordinator)

Anxiety Disorders Work Group

Michael R. Liebowitz, M.D. (Chairperson)
David H. Barlow, Ph.D. (Vice-Chairperson)
James C. Ballenger, M.D.
Jonathan Davidson, M.D.
Edna Foa, Ph.D.
Abby Fyer, M.D.

Delirium, Dementia, and Amnestic and Other Cognitive Disorders Work Group

Gary J. Tucker, M.D. (Chairperson)
Michael Popkin, M.D. (Vice-Chairperson)
Eric Douglas Caine, M.D.
Marshall Folstein, M.D.
Gary Lloyd Gottlieb, M.D.
Igor Grant, M.D.
Benjamin Liptzin, M.D.

Disorders Usually First Diagnosed During Infancy, Childhood, or Adolescence Work Group

David Shaffer, M.D. (Co-Chairperson)
Magda Campbell, M.D. (Co-Chairperson)
Susan J. Bradley, M.D.

Dennis P. Cantwell, M.D.
Gabrielle A. Carlson, M.D.
Donald Jay Cohen, M.D.
Barry Garfinkel, M.D.
Rachel Klein, Ph.D.
Benjamin Lahey, Ph.D.
Rolf Loeber, Ph.D.
Jeffrey Newcorn, M.D.
Rhea Paul, Ph.D.
Judith H. L. Rapoport, M.D.
Sir Michael Rutter, M.D.
Fred Volkmar, M.D.
John S. Werry, M.D.

Eating Disorders Work Group

B. Timothy Walsh, M.D. (Chairperson)
Paul Garfinkel, M.D.
Katherine A. Halmi, M.D.
James Mitchell, M.D.
G. Terence Wilson, Ph.D.

Mood Disorders Work Group

A. John Rush, M.D. (Chairperson)
Martin B. Keller, M.D. (Vice-Chairperson)
Mark S. Bauer, M.D.
David Dunner, M.D.
Ellen Frank, Ph.D.
Donald F. Klein, M.D.

Multiaxial Issues Work Group

Janet B. W. Williams, D.S.W. (Chairperson)
Howard H. Goldman, M.D., Ph.D. (Vice-Chairperson)
Alan M. Gruenberg, M.D.
Juan Enrique Mezzich, M.D., Ph.D.
Roger Peele, M.D.
Stephen Setterberg, M.D.
Andrew Edward Skodol II, M.D.

Personality Disorders Work Group

John Gunderson, M.D. (Chairperson)
Robert M.A. Hirschfeld, M.D. (Vice-Chairperson)

Roger Blashfield, Ph.D.
Susan Jean Fiester, M.D.
Theodore Millon, Ph.D.
Bruce Pfohl, M.D.
Tracie Shea, Ph.D.
Larry Siever, M.D.
Thomas A. Widiger, Ph.D.

Premenstrual Dysphoric Disorder Work Group

Judith H. Gold, M.D. (Chairperson)
Jean Endicott, Ph.D.
Barbara Parry, M.D.
Sally Severino, M.D.
Nada Logan Stotland, M.D.
Ellen Frank, Ph.D. (Consultant)

Psychiatric Systems Interface Disorders (Adjustment, Dissociative, Factitious, Impulse-Control, and Somatoform Disorders and Psychological Factors Affecting Medical Conditions) Work Group

Robert E. Hales, M.D. (Chairperson)
C. Robert Cloninger, M.D. (Vice-Chairperson)
Jonathan F. Borus, M.D.
Jack Denning Burke, Jr., M.D., M.P.H.
Joe P. Fagan, M.D.
Steven A. King, M.D.
Ronald L. Martin, M.D.
Katharine Anne Phillips, M.D.
David Spiegel, M.D.
Alan Stoudemire, M.D.
James J. Strain, M.D.
Michael G. Wise, M.D.

Schizophrenia and Other Psychotic Disorders Work Group

Nancy Coover Andreasen, M.D., Ph.D. (Chairperson)
John M. Kane, M.D. (Vice-Chairperson)
Samuel Keith, M.D.
Kenneth S. Kendler, M.D.
Thomas McGlashan, M.D.

Sexual Disorders Work Group

Chester W. Schmidt, M.D. (Chairperson)
Raul Schiavi, M.D.
Leslie Schover, Ph.D.
Taylor Seagraves, M.D.
Thomas Nathan Wise, M.D.

Sleep Disorders Work Group

David J. Kupfer, M.D. (Chairperson)
Charles F. Reynolds III, M.D. (Vice-Chairperson)
Daniel Buysse, M.D.
Roger Peele, M.D.
Quentin Regestein, M.D.
Michael Sateia, M.D.
Michael Thorpy, M.D.

Substance-Related Disorders Work Group

Marc Alan Schuckit, M.D. (Chairperson)
John E. Helzer, M.D. (Vice-Chairperson)
Linda B. Cottler, Ph.D.
Thomas Crowley, M.D.
Peter E. Nathan, Ph.D.
George E. Woody, M.D.

Committee on Psychiatric Diagnosis and Assessment

Layton McCurdy, M.D. (Chairperson) (1987–1994)
Kenneth Z. Altshuler, M.D. (1987–1992)
Thomas F. Anders, M.D. (1988–1994)
Susan Jane Blumenthal, M.D. (1990–1993)
Leah Joan Dickstein, M.D. (1988–1991)
Lewis J. Judd, M.D. (1988–1994)
Gerald L. Klerman, M.D. (1988–1991)
Stuart C. Yudofsky, M.D. (1992–1994)
Jack D. Blaine, M.D. (Consultant) (1987–1992)
Jerry M. Lewis, M.D. (Consultant) (1988–1994)
Daniel J. Luchins, M.D. (Consultant) (1987–1991)
Katharine Anne Phillips, M.D. (Consultant) (1992–1994)
Cynthia Pearl Rose, M.D. (Consultant) (1990–1994)
Louis Alan Moench, M.D. (Assembly Liaison) (1991–1994)
Steven K. Dobscha, M.D. (Resident Fellow) (1990–1992)
Mark Zimmerman, M.D. (Resident Fellow) (1992–1994)

Joint Committee of the Board of Trustees and Assembly of District Branches on Issues Related to DSM-IV

Ronald A. Shellow, M.D. (Chairperson)
Harvey Bluestone, M.D.
Leah Joan Dickstein, M.D.
Arthur John Farley, M.D.
Carol Ann Bernstein, M.D.

WORK GROUPS FOR THE DSM-IV TEXT REVISION

Michael B. First, M.D. (Co-Chairperson and Editor)
Harold Alan Pincus, M.D. (Co-Chairperson)
Laurie E. McQueen, M.S.S.W. (DSM Project Manager)
Yoshie Satake, B.A. (DSM Program Coordinator)

Anxiety Disorders Text Revision Work Group

Murray B. Stein, M.D. (Chairperson)
Jonathan Abramowitz, Ph.D.
Gordon Asmundson, Ph.D.
Jean C. Beckham, Ph.D.
Timothy Brown, Ph.D., Psy.D.
Michelle Craske, Ph.D.
Edna Foa, Ph.D.
Thomas Mellman, M.D.
Ron Norton, Ph.D.
Franklin Schneier, M.D.
Richard Zinbarg, Ph.D.

Delirium, Dementia, and Amnestic and Other Cognitive Disorders and Mental Disorders Due to a General Medical Condition Text Revision Work Group

Eric Douglas Caine, M.D.
Jesse Fann, M.D., M.P.H.
Jeffrey M. Lyness, M.D.
Anton P. Porsteinsson, M.D.

Disorders Usually First Diagnosed During Infancy, Childhood, or Adolescence Text Revision Work Group

David Shaffer, M.D. (Chairperson)
Donald J. Cohen, M.D.
Stephen Hinshaw, Ph.D.
Rachel G. Klein, Ph.D.
Ami Klin, Ph.D.
Daniel Pine, M.D.
Mark A. Riddle, M.D.
Fred R. Volkmar, M.D.
Charles Zeanah, M.D.

Eating Disorders Text Revision Work Group

Katharine L. Loeb, Ph.D.
B. Timothy Walsh, M.D.

Medication-Induced Movement Disorders Text Revision Work Group

Gerard Addonizio, M.D.
Lenard Adler, M.D.
Burton Angrist, M.D.
Daniel Casey, M.D.
Alan Gelenberg, M.D.
James Jefferson, M.D.
Dilip Jeste, M.D.
Peter Weiden, M.D.

Mood Disorders Text Revision Work Group

Mark S. Bauer, M.D.
Patricia Suppes, M.D., Ph.D.
Michael E. Thase, M.D.

Multiaxial Text Revision Work Group

Alan M. Gruenberg, M.D.

Personality Disorders Text Revision Work Group

Bruce Pfohl, M.D.
Thomas A. Widiger, Ph.D.

Premenstrual Dysphoric Disorder Text Revision Work Group

Sally Severino, M.D.

Psychiatric System Interface Disorders (Adjustment, Dissociative, Factitious, Impulse-Control, and Somatoform Disorders and Psychological Factors Affecting Medical Conditions) Text Revision Work Group

Mitchell Cohen, M.D.
Marc Feldman, M.D.
Eric Hollander, M.D.
Steven A. King, M.D.
James Levenson, M.D.
Ronald L. Martin, M.D. (deceased)
Jeffrey Newcorn, M.D.
Russell Noyes, Jr., M.D.
Katharine Anne Phillips. M.D.
Eyal Shemesh, M.D.
David Spiegel, M.D.
James J. Strain, M.D.
Sean H. Yutzy, M.D.

Schizophrenia and Other Psychotic Disorders Text Revision Work Group

Michael Flaum, M.D. (Co-Chairperson)
Xavier Amador, Ph.D. (Co-Chairperson)

Sexual and Gender Identity Disorders Text Revision Work Group

Chester W. Schmidt, M.D.
R. Taylor Segraves, M.D.
Thomas Nathan Wise, M.D.
Kenneth J. Zucker, Ph.D.

Sleep Disorders Text Revision Work Group

Daniel Buysse, M.D.
Peter Nowell, M.D.

Substance-Related Disorders Text Revision Work Group

Marc Alan Schuckit, M.D.

American Psychiatric Association Committee on Psychiatric Diagnosis and Assessment

David J. Kupfer, M.D. (Chair)
James Leckman, M.D. (Member)
Katharine Anne Phillips, M.D. (Member)
A. John Rush, M.D. (Member)
Daniel Winstead, M.D. (Member)
Bonnie Zima, M.D., Ph.D. (Member)
Barbara Kennedy, M.D., Ph.D. (Consultant)
Janet B. W. Williams, D.S.W. (Consultant)
Louis Alan Moench, M.D. (Assembly Liaison)
Jack Barchas, M.D. (Corresponding Member)
Herbert W. Harris, M.D., Ph.D. (Corresponding Member)
Charles Kaelber, M.D. (Corresponding Member)
Jorge A. Costa e Silva, M.D. (Corresponding Member)
T. Bedirhan Ustun, M.D. (Corresponding Member)
Yeshuschandra Dhaibar, M.D. (APA/Glaxo-Wellcome Fellow)

Appendix 13

American Psychiatric Association Medical Directors

Daniel Blain, M.D.	1948–1958
Matthew Ross, M.D.	1958–1962
Walter E. Barton, M.D.	1963–1974
Melvin Sabshin, M.D.	1974–1997
Steven M. Mirin, M.D.	1997–2002
James H. Scully Jr., M.D.	2003–present

Appendix 14

American Psychiatric Association Association Governance System

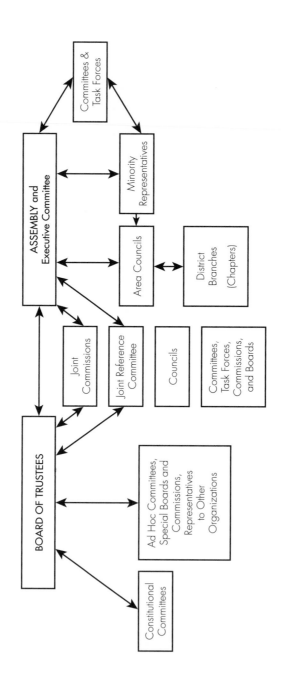

Index

381